Contents

Introduction

This book provides comprehensive listings of the nutrient value of a wide variety of foods. Foods that are not readily available have been excluded, and the remaining foods are listed in the form in which they are usually eaten: beans and grains, for example, are described in cooked form; salad vegetables, raw. The presumed average serving size is 100 grams (slightly more than 3 ounces) for most items, so, with few exceptions (which are clear from their listings), that is the quantity for which the nutrient value has been provided. In this way, readers can look up the quantity of sodium, for example, in a scoop of cottage cheese, and be fairly certain that the list accurately reflects the amount of sodium in the cottage cheese on the plate in front of them.

There are separate listings for carbohydrates, cholesterol, fats, fiber, minerals, protein, sodium, and vitamins.

Each list is organized in such a way that a quick glance at the top of the list will reveal the foods containing the highest quantities of each nutrient. The lists are arranged in descending order; that is, the foods with the largest amount of the nutrient are listed first, and those with less follow. At the bottom of the list are the foods with the least amount. Those who want a high-protein meal would look at the top of the protein list for ideas, while others looking to sharply decrease their cholesterol intake should select foods at the bottom of the cholesterol list in their diet.

To find the listings for particular foods, check the index, where all the foods listed are extensively cross-referenced.

Some 20 to 70 percent of all Americans—no one knows the exact figure, but it is probably on the increase—are allergic to one or more foods. Wheat, corn, citrus fruits, dairy products, beef, and apples are among the most common allergens, but anyone can be allergic to any food. These lists will suggest al-

GARY NULL'S
NUTRITION
SOURCEBOOK
FOR THE '80S

GARY NULL'S
NUTRITION
SOURCEBOOK
FOR THE '80S

Gary Null

Collier Books

Macmillan Publishing Company

New York

Collier Macmillan Publishers

London

Macmillan Publishing Company
866 Third Avenue, New York, N.Y. 10022
Collier Macmillan Canada, Inc.

Library of Congress Cataloging in Publication Data
Null, Gary.
  Gary Null's Nutrition sourcebook for the '80s.
  Includes index.
    1. Food—Composition—Tables. 2. Nutrition—Tables.
I. Title. II. Title: Nutrition sourcebook for the '80s.
[TX551.N74 1983b]   641.1'0212   83-1919
ISBN 0-02-059500-X (pbk.)

First Collier Books Edition 1983

10 9 8 7 6 5 4 3 2 1
Printed in the United States of America

Gary Null's Nutrition Sourcebook for the '80s is also published in a hardcover edition by Macmillan Publishing Company.

ternative ways of obtaining the most important nutrients, so that those who must eliminate particular allergens can do so comfortably and conveniently. Someone allergic to fish and seafood (including cod and other fish liver oils) as well as carrots can find dozens of other less well-known, excellent sources of vitamin A. Someone who has hesitated to eliminate oranges from his or her diet for fear of vitamin C deficiency, yet finds that eating oranges causes symptoms ranging from stuffy nose and watery eyes to skin rashes, will learn that there are more than thirty foods richer in vitamin C than an orange.

Most of the foods available in any supermarket are overly processed, refined, and packaged. They contain too much sodium, sugar, refined or modified food starch, or saturated fat to support good health, and they provide little nutritional value for the dollars spent on them. By indicating the nutrient density of a wide variety of readily available foods, as well as their caloric content, these lists will prove invaluable to every shopper who wants to know whether his food dollars are buying good nutrition. After all, the most basic, important reason for eating is to supply the body with the nutrients it needs for good health and energy. Why spend hard-earned money on foods that do the opposite?

For all these reasons, this in-depth compendium of lists can serve as a companion to every other nutrition book. It stands alone as the most comprehensive nutrient listing guide available.

This book has been written to serve the needs of the eighty million or so people who, on any given day, find themselves on some food-restricting diet. Perhaps twenty-five million of these are suffering from chronic, stable hypertension, and must carefully monitor the amount of sodium they consume. Others, also concerned about their cardiovascular health, or watching their weight for other reasons, are seeking alternatives to the typical American diet, high in cholesterol, high in saturated fats, and high in animal protein, and need to know where they can find the right lipids in the right quantities for optimal health.

Much has been written about high-protein, low-carbohydrate diets. But large numbers of people are now reexamining the word carbohydrate, and eliminating refined, processed starches and sugars from their diets while increasing the amount of natural, whole, fiber- and protein-rich complex carbohydrates they consume. Protein, too, is beginning to be better understood. People who once believed that they could not obtain enough protein for growth and good health without eating roast beef or steak will be able to find here listings of the many foods higher in protein than beef.

Most people have no idea which vitamins and minerals are available naturally from fruits, vegetables, and other foods, but they are concerned that they may be obtaining disproportionate amounts of particular nutrients if they obtain them from supplements rather than from their food. Our aim is to let them know which foods provide the richest sources of each nutrient.

By listing foods according to the major nutrients they contain, we hope not only to enable people to vary and enrich their diets, but also to give them a sense of the wide variety of nutritious foods available, and of the nutrient density of each particular food: that is, of the amount of nutrients supplied by each calorie consumed.

Protein

$$\textcircled{1}$$

When we think of protein, most people envision meat — a thick, rare steak, perhaps a hamburger, or a platter of fried chicken. We associate it, too, with athletic endeavor: Many believe that protein is the most important food for athletes to achieve optimal strength, endurance, and stamina.

In fact, we have been grossly misled on the notion of what our body's protein needs are and how they should be met. Meat is only one of several possible dietary sources of protein. It is the most important source in the average American diet — and unfortunately it is also the most expensive. Our image of protein as the one most important nutrient — the very word is derived from the Greek *protos*, meaning first — has led us to eat so much meat that we often consume more than twice the protein we need each day. On the average, Americans eat nearly 100 grams of protein every day — when all most of us actually need is around 45 to 50 grams a day. Even athletes are better off increasing their carbohydrate rather than their protein consumption if they want to increase their endurance and stamina rather than hinder their performance. One recent study showed that vegetarians have better endurance than meat eaters.

Eggs, dairy products, grain, legumes, nuts, and seeds are all excellent sources of protein that can supplement meat or replace it in the diet. The list we have compiled of protein foods shows the number of grams of usable protein per 3 ounce serving for each food, and is arranged in order, beginning with those foods highest in protein and continuing through those lowest.

How Much Protein Do You Need?

Generally speaking, adults require .9 grams of protein per kilogram of body weight. (A kilogram is 2.2 pounds.) Thus, a 60-kilogram (132-pound) woman probably requires 54 grams of protein a day. During spurts of growth, as in infancy, early childhood, and puberty, that proportion is increased. Others with higher protein needs include pregnant and lactating mothers, for obvious reasons; hypoglycemics; convalescents from surgery and certain types of infection, shock, or fever; and those under any kind of stress.

There are certain conditions, such as kidney disease, which require lower protein intake for a period of time. Whatever your protein requirements, whatever your age, life-style, or special medical problems, this list is designed to be helpful to you in tailoring your diet to your protein needs. You can use it to calculate how much protein you actually consume, and how to increase or decrease your protein intake using either animal or plant sources, or both.

Why We Need Protein

Proteins are the building blocks of life. They are the basic material of which all our cells, tissues, and organs are constructed. In fact, only water represents a larger percentage of our total body weight than protein. Proteins are constantly being replaced, twenty-four hours a day, throughout our entire life. The optimal intake of high-quality proteins allows the body to grow and maintain healthy bones, skin, teeth, muscles, and nerves; it keeps the blood count correct; and it allows the metabolism in general to function at the highest level. Hemoglobin, the part of the red blood cells that provides oxygen to the cells, is made of protein. The protein molecules called enzymes are the catalysts of metabolism: they must be present for hundreds of necessary reactions to occur. For example, they enable energy to be stored and released in each cell; and they allow protein, fats, carbohydrates, and cholesterol to be synthesized by the liver. Protein is responsible for keeping our blood slightly alkaline, and is the raw material out of which the antibodies that shield us from infection are constructed. Hormones, too, the regulators of our metabolism, contain some protein. The building blocks of protein itself, the amino acids, are necessary for certain vitamins and minerals to be utilized: the amino acid tryptophan, for example, initiates the production of the B-vitamin, niacin. Proteins help transport fats through the bloodstream, by combining with them to form lipoproteins. In fact, the only fluids in your body that do not normally contain protein are perspiration, urine, and bile. In short, proteins are needed for growth, for maintenance of body tissues, and for virtually all metabolic functions. It is possible to live without consuming protein — but not for very long.

Complete Protein: The Eight Essential Amino Acids

The hundreds of proteins your body synthesizes are all made up of chains of only twenty-three smaller, basic protein substances, the amino acids. Of these, the body can synthesize fifteen — leaving eight that must be present in your food. These eight are called the essential amino acids.

A protein deficiency can occur when we do not consume enough protein for our body's needs, or when the proteins we do consume lack one or more of these eight essential amino acids.

The eight essential amino acids are threonine, valine, tryptophan, lysine, methionine, histidine, phenylalanine, and isoleucine. Foods which contain all eight of these essential amino acids are called complete protein foods. Eggs, meat, fowl, fish, and dairy products contain complete protein.

For protein to be absorbed and used by the body, all eight essential amino acids must be present in a certain proportion — approximately the same proportion in which they occur in eggs, nature's complete food package for chicken embryos. Partially complete proteins may contain all eight, but not in the correct proportions. Thus foods high in partially complete protein, such as brewer's yeast (also called nutritional yeast), wheat germ, the soy food tofu, peanuts, and certain micro-sea algae, should be eaten in combination with other protein foods which can supplement their limiting amino acids. For example, sprinkle brewer's yeast on your cereal or blend it with milk, combine tofu with algae in salads, add wheat germ to lentil-burgers, and spread your peanut butter on whole wheat bread to increase the usability of the protein in these excellent sources.

Food Combining for Complete Proteins from Non-Animal Sources

The partially complete and incomplete proteins found in grains, beans, nuts, seeds, and tubers, when combined properly, can form complete proteins on a par nutritionally with those in meat, fish, poultry, eggs, milk, yogurt, or cheese. The right combinations are as easy to learn as following a pancake recipe. You don't have to remember that grains, nuts, and seeds are short in isoleucine and lysine, which are contained by dairy products, brewer's yeast, and legumes; or that legumes are short in tryptophan and the sulfur-containing amino acids present in the grains, because the right combinations have been discovered over and over again by the world's people, and are as familiar to us as cereal and milk for breakfast. Grains and legumes complement each other: think of Mexico's corn tortillas with refried beans; Cuba and Puerto Rico's rice and beans; Japanese stir-fried rice with bean sprouts; Boston baked beans with whole-grain black bread; or our universally familiar peanut butter sandwich (best on stone-ground whole wheat bread).

Seeds and legumes also work well together: a favorite Middle Eastern dish is *hummus bi tahini*, that is, mashed chick-peas mixed with sesame paste, often served with pita bread. "Ambrosia" mixes — combinations of roasted legumes, such as peanuts or soybeans, with nuts and seeds of various kinds — mixes of almonds, brazil or cashew nuts with sunflower or pumpkin seeds — don't have to be sweetened with dried fruits or salted with soy sauce to be nutritious and tasty.

Vegetable sources can also be complemented with small amounts of animal protein to greatly increase the usability of the vegetable protein. A little bit of Parmesan cheese sprinkled over the Italian spaghetti makes all the difference, not just in taste, but in the protein available from the spaghetti. Similarly, so do the eggs and milk in that pancake recipe; the milk on your morning cereal; a whole wheat bread and cheese sandwich;

the cheddar melted over your macaroni or bean casserole; the milk mixed into your mashed potatoes; the nibbles of tofu found in Chinese dishes served with rice; and the tiny slices of fish rolled in seaweed and rice of Japanese fare.

Too Little Protein

To summarize, a complete protein, with its full complement of essential amino acids, whether from animal or combined vegetable sources, is capable both of maintaining body tissues and of allowing for optimal growth. Partially complete proteins, such as those found in grains alone, will maintain life, but are deficient in certain amino acids necessary for growth, and must be supplemented with foods containing the limiting amino acids. For example, wheat is a partially complete protein. It can maintain life, and millions of poor people have subsisted on bread or cereal alone for long periods of time. However, wheat alone cannot promote adequate growth, and even adults who restrict their protein to one or two food groups or types of foods — what we call a mono-diet — run the very real risk of lowering their body's immune response: remember, proteins are necessary for antibodies to combat infection. The poor quality of their hair and skin reflects their dietary deficiencies. Indeed, their whole body functions much like a car running on four cylinders rather than six.

Incomplete proteins do poorly at building new tissue or replacing worn-out cells and tissues, and cannot support life: protein deficiency diseases such as kwashiorkor and marasmus have been found in populations attempting to subsist on such incomplete sources as millet (Africa); corn and beans (South America); rice and some legumes (Asia).

Digestion, Utilization, and Absorption

Food is digested in two steps, mechanical and chemical. Mechanical digestion begins in the mouth, when your teeth grind and chop the protein into tiny pieces. The charts below assume that the foods listed are to be properly digested. To aid in complete digestion of protein foods, you should chew each bite until it is fully masticated. This will reduce the stress upon the stomach, allow for better breakdown of the protein into amino acids, and assure a better absorption rate.

Chemical digestion of protein begins in the stomach, where powerful hydrochloric acid begins to break down the proteins into their constituent amino acids. As a person ages, the ability to digest, absorb, utilize, and eliminate protein foods decreases. People over forty become vulnerable to a decrease in secretion of hydrochloric acid. As a result, food takes longer to empty from the stomach, frequently remaining there for six to eight hours, resulting in a heavy, laden feeling. Further digestion of protein takes place in the small intestines, where the enzymes pepsin, trypsin, and chymotrypsin complete the breakdown of proteins into amino acids as they move along the digestive tract. Peristaltic action, the movement of the muscles that propel the food forward, may also slow down with age, so there is greater likelihood of causing chronic constipation. The resultant pressure and strain during evacuation can cause varicose veins and hemorrhoids. Furthermore, a hot, dark, moist medium like the intestine is ideal for the proliferation of bacteria, some of which cause disease. The longer protein foods remain in the intestine, the greater the potential for infections of the intestinal tract such as diverticulosis; for cancer of the colon and rectum; and for toxic reaction. The selection of protein foods are, high in fiber can help prevent these problems by stimulating peristalsis and speeding digestion.

Preparing Protein Foods for Good Digestion

Protein digestion is also improved by correct cooking practices. Moderate heating of most protein foods increases their digestibility. This is especially true for beans, grains, and meat. Beans and other legumes contain several toxins (such as trypsin inhibitors) which can inhibit digestion, but which become harmless when they are cooked or sprouted. Legumes should never be eaten raw: several of them contain even stronger toxins that must be neutralized by heat. Both grains and some legumes contain phytic acid in their outer husks. In the intestines, these can form phytates which bind zinc, calcium, and other minerals and can cause deficiencies. Thus, grains should be sprouted, baked with yeast (unleavened breads contain more phytates than leavened), or cooked thoroughly, and vegetarians should supplement their diet with zinc and calcium or foods containing them. Zinc is present in seafood, peas, corn, egg yolk, carrots, and yeast.

It is also very important to cook meat slowly but thoroughly, because of the microorganisms it contains. Pork, especially, harbors a parasite that can cause trichinosis if the meat is not thoroughly cooked. However, other meats should be broiled or roasted. Excessive heating of any protein, whether of animal or plant origin, may cause what are known as cross-linkages (the same mechanisms that cause your hair to stay curled after a permanent wave). Cross-linkages make it difficult for your protein-digesting enzymes to break down into simple amino acids so it can be absorbed. Therefore, it is best to stay away from deep-fried or overdone protein foods. Milk and milk products are especially sensitive to heat, and should not be heated above the boiling point. If you have trouble digesting milk, you might try yogurt, buttermilk, or other cultured milk products. These contain live, healthy microorganisms that "predigest" lactose, the sugar in milk that many people cannot tolerate, changing it to easily absorbed lactic acid.

On the average, about 90 to 93 percent of the amino acids in the foods you eat are absorbed after digestion commences. However, the absorption rate is slower for plant than for animal sources, so vegetarians may need to increase the actual quantity of protein they consume, even if they combine proteins sufficiently.

Protein Utilization

For your cells to synthesize the proteins they need, all the amino acids necessary must be present simultaneously in sufficient amounts. This is known as the "all or none" law. It means that if any one amino acid is not present, the protein cannot be constructed. Since protein cannot be stored (except, perhaps, by lactating mothers), it is necessary to eat complete protein at each meal, or if you are eating non-animal products, to mix your protein sources to form complete protein. To provide your body with only some of the amino acids it needs is to be like the baker who buys 100 pounds of flour, 100 pounds of shortening, but only 1 ounce of yeast. How many cakes can he bake? Applying the "all or none" law — only one or two — after that he would run out of yeast. And what would he do with all that flour and shortening? In your body, unused amino acids might be excret-

ed or broken down and oxidized for energy or other metabolic
needs.

Too Much Protein

It is estimated that nearly eighty million Americans in any
given year are following some dietary program to lose weight.
Regrettably, many will be going on one version or another of
the high-protein, low-carbohydrate diet, with the misconception
that protein is low in calories. In point of fact, the protein
foods, such as beef or pork, recommended on most of these diets are very high in calories. One gram of protein yields four
calories on utilization. However, most meats are also high in fat
— which yields nine calories per gram. Filet mignon, for example, is nearly 40 to 50 percent fat; a single portion can contain
between four and five hundred calories. However, if you fill up
on a fatty protein food, such as pork, lamb, beef, or even chick-
en or fish, that requires four to six hours for digestion, even
though you consume a large number of calories at one sitting,
you will not crave additional food for several hours. This is the
nutritional sleight of hand that makes those diets work for
some people. Some researchers believe that it is chronic snack-
ing on high-calorie, refined, and sugared foods that contributes
most to overweight and obesity. However, to control obesity, exercise is even more important than limiting calorie intake, since
exercise increases your metabolic efficiency.

In the short run, your body can cope with an excess of protein by burning it for energy. This may be inefficient, since protein takes more energy than carbohydrates or fat to metabolize,
but it is not harmful. However, over the long run, too much
protein *can* hurt. Deaminization of protein releases ammonium.
The ammonium is turned into urea and excreted through the
kidneys. Along with an excess of sodium (meats are naturally
saltier than vegetables), this stepped-up excretion process taxes
the kidneys. Too much protein can also lead to edema and dehydration, as people on high-protein diets require essentially more
water per day than others.

Furthermore, animal foods are much higher in saturated
fats and cholesterol than vegetable protein foods. Especially
when combined with the refined carbohydrates of the typical
American diet, these have been implicated in increasing our risk

of heart disease and arteriosclerosis.

Thus, generally speaking, it is wiser and more advantageous to rely on exercise, on modifying behavior so that living patterns become more disciplined, and on consumption of a higher proportion of complex carbohydrates and vegetable protein sources, with fruits and juices for snacks, rather than to resort to high-protein diets.

Find Reliable Sources

Studies have shown that a low-calorie intake increases life span and diminishes the likelihood of cancer and other diseases of degeneration. However, animal protein has other drawbacks besides its fat content. The animals raised for meat in the United States are given hundreds of chemicals in their food and by injection: hormones, antibiotics, tranquilizers, even arsenic, enzymes, and dyes in the case of poultry. In addition, environmental pollutants such as pesticides and herbicides, found in their feed, are concentrated in their flesh. Further, our rivers and lakes are polluted with mercury and other industrial wastes which fish retain. (Small fish at least are not concentrating many pollutants from other fish's bodies.) Shellfish live by pumping gallons of water through their system, and tend to concentrate viruses and other microorganisms.

When they are sold, both vertebrate fish and shellfish may be dipped in antibiotic solutions to prevent the growth of bacteria. Antibiotics become less effective the more they are used, as microorganisms learn to adapt to their presence. Meat, too, may be packaged with preservatives, nitrites (which can lower blood pressure and hemoglobin efficiency, or combine with amines to form carcinogenic nitrosamines), artificial flavorings, and other chemicals. For all these reasons, it is highly recommended to find reliable sources of fresh, organically produced flesh foods.

The unit value for protein is given in grams. Any food having less than 1 gram of protein per 100-gram portion is considered to have a trace protein content and is listed as having .00 for its unit value.

Where the symbol N. A. appears in the calorie column, the information was not available.

All these figures are based on an edible portion equaling 100 grams, or approximately 3 ounces. In the case of some of the listed foods, one would not consume 100 grams in one serving. Calculations should be adjusted accordingly.

Protein

FOOD ITEM	CALS.	UNITS
Gelatin dry	335	85.60
Soybean protein	322	74.90
Dried eggs whole	592	48.90
Soybean flour defatted	326	47.00
Sunflower seed flour partially defatted	339	45.20
Soybean flour low fat	356	43.40
Soybean milk powder	429	41.80
Wheat flour 45% gluten, 55% patent	378	41.40
Soybean flour high fat	380	41.20
Rice cereal with casein	382	40.00
Safflower seed meal partially defatted	355	39.60
Almond meal partially defatted	408	39.50
Brewer's yeast debittered	283	38.80
Torula yeast	277	38.60
Baker's yeast dry	282	36.90
Smoked herring hard	300	36.90
Soybean flour full fat	421	36.70
Skim milk dry, regular	363	35.90
Skim milk dry, instant	359	35.80
Baby cereal high protein, added nutrients	357	35.20
Caviar (sturgeon), pressed	316	34.40
Chipped beef dried, uncooked	203	34.30
Lamb liver broiled	261	32.30
Sirloin steak wedge and round bone, choice grade, roasted	207	32.30
Beef round, choice grade, broiled	189	31.30
Smoked sturgeon	149	31.20
Pinenuts (pignolias)	552	31.10
Beef hind shank, choice grade, simmered	184	30.70
Chicken (fryers), flesh and skin, fried	250	30.60
Pork loin, medium fat class, broiled	270	30.60
Sirloin steak double-bone, loin end, choice grade, broiled	216	30.60

FOOD ITEM	CALS.	UNITS
Beef chuck, arm, choice grade, braised or pot-roasted	193	30.50
Bacon cured, broiled or fried	611	30.40
T-bone steak short loin, choice grade, broiled	223	30.40
Beef Porterhouse, short loin, choice grade, broiled	224	30.20
Turkey all classes, dark meat, roasted	203	30.00
Wheat germ toasted	391	30.00
Beef short plate, choice grade, simmered	222	29.70
Ham medium fat content, roasted	217	29.70
Club steak short loin, choice grade, broiled	244	29.60
Calf liver fried	261	29.50
Chicken roaster, without skin, roasted	183	29.50
Pork loin, medium fat class, roasted	254	29.40
Cod dried, salted	130	29.00
Pork picnic, medium fat class, simmered	212	29.00
Pumpkin and squash seed kernels dried	553	29.00
Tuna canned in oil, drained solids	197	28.80
Lamb leg, choice grade, roasted, separable lean	186	28.70
Veal foreshank, medium fat content, stewed	216	28.70
Beef round, choice grade, broiled	261	28.60
Pork lean cuts, roasted	228	28.60
Cod broiled	170	28.50
Beef rib, choice grade, braised	263	28.40
Pork cured, picnic cut, medium fat class, roasted	211	28.40
Lamb loin, choice grade, broiled, separable lean	188	28.20
Sweetbreads (lamb), braised	175	28.10
Lamb loin, prime grade, broiled, separable lean	197	28.00
Pork lean cuts, medium fat class, roasted	236	28.00
Swordfish broiled	174	28.00
Tuna canned in water, solids and liquid	127	28.00
Turkey liver simmered	174	27.90
Veal chuck, medium fat content, braised	235	27.90
Peanut butter	581	27.80
Pork Boston butt, medium fat class, roasted	243	27.80
Canadian bacon broiled or fried, drained	277	27.60
Swiss cheese (domestic), unprocessed	370	27.50
Hamburger lean, cooked	219	27.40
Chicken (roasters), with skin	242	27.20
Beef chuck, arm, choice grade, braised or pot-roasted	289	27.10
Veal round with rump, medium fat content, broiled	216	27.10
Salmon cooked, broiled, or baked	182	27.00

FOOD ITEM	CALS.	UNITS
Caviar (sturgeon), granular	262	26.90
Lamb rib, prime grade, broiled	224	26.90
Lamb shoulder, choice grade, roasted	205	26.80
Wheat germ raw, commercially milled	363	26.60
Chicken liver simmered	165	26.50
Beef liver fried	229	26.40
Corned beef boneless, lean, canned	185	26.40
Swiss cheese pasteurized, processed	355	26.40
Whole dry milk	502	26.40
Peanuts without skins, raw	568	26.30
Bluefish baked or broiled	159	26.20
Peanuts with skins, roasted	582	26.20
Beef chuck, ribs 1 to 5, neck and arm, choice grade, braised	327	26.00
Peanuts roasted and salted	585	26.00
Peanuts with skins, raw	564	26.00
Peanut butter with small amount of sweetener added	582	25.50
Sturgeon steamed	160	25.40
Corned beef medium fat content, canned, boneless	216	25.30
Pork ham, roasted	187	25.30
Halibut (Atlantic and Pacific), broiled	171	25.20
Beef hindshank, choice grade, simmered	361	25.10
Beef roast, canned	224	25.00
Cheddar cheese unprocessed	398	25.00
Pork composite of lean cuts, medium fat class, broiled	391	24.70
Weakfish broiled	208	24.60
Shrimp canned, drained solids	116	24.20
Tuna canned in oil, solids and liquids	288	24.20
Sunflower seed kernels dried	560	24.00
Calf tongue braised	160	23.90
Lamb leg, prime grade, roasted	319	23.90
Chicken (broiler), broiled	136	23.80
Salami dry	450	23.80
Butternuts	629	23.70
Corned beef fat canned	263	23.50
American cheese pasteurized, processed	370	23.20
Scallops (bay and sea), steamed	112	23.20
Smoked haddock	103	23.20
Veal flank, medium fat content, stewed	390	23.20
Cornflakes	378	23.00

FOOD ITEM	CALS.	UNITS
Corned beef medium fat content	372	22.90
Brick cheese	370	22.20
Herring kippered	211	22.20
Roe (cod and shad), baked or broiled	126	22.00
Mackerel (Atlantic), broiled	236	21.80
Chicken canned, boned	198	21.70
Smoked salmon	176	21.60
Bass (striped), fried	196	21.50
Beef tongue medium fat content, braised	244	21.50
Blue cheese or Roquefort cheese	369	21.50
Limburger cheese	345	21.20
Mackerel (Pacific), canned, solids and liquid	180	21.10
Turkey meat only, canned	202	20.90
Whitefish smoked	155	20.90
Pork spareribs braised, medium fat class	440	20.80
Salmon (Coho), canned, solids and liquid	153	20.80
Shrimp paste or lobster paste canned	180	20.80
Smoked halibut	224	20.80
Lamb shoulder, prime grade, roasted	374	20.70
Club steak choice grade, broiled	454	20.60
Giblets simmered	233	20.60
Sardines (Atlantic), canned in oil, solids and liquid	311	20.60
Trout (rainbow or steelhead), canned	209	20.60
Black walnuts	628	20.50
Pickled herring (Bismarck)	223	20.40
Soybean milk powder, sweetened	452	20.40
Peanut spread	601	20.30
Salmon (sockeye), canned, solids and liquid	171	20.30
Vegetables with wheat protein and nuts, canned	212	20.30
Cocoa powder low fat	187	20.20
Rice cereal with wheat gluten	386	20.00
Herring canned, solids and liquid	208	19.90
Porterhouse steak choice grade, broiled	465	19.70
Haddock fried	165	19.60
Salmon (chinook), canned, solids and liquid	210	19.60
Smoked herring (bloaters)	196	19.60
Lamb chops prime grade, broiled	420	19.50
Beef (baby food), commercial	118	19.30
Mackerel (Atlantic), canned, solids and liquid	183	19.30
Pistachio nuts	594	19.30

FOOD ITEM	CALS.	UNITS
Anchovies	176	19.20
Cocoa (Dutch process), low to medium fat content	215	19.20
Cocoa powder low to medium fat content	220	19.20
Beef tripe commercial	62	19.10
Boiled ham (luncheon meat)	234	19.00
Herring salted or brined	218	19.00
Ocean perch (Atlantic)	227	19.00
Ocean perch (Atlantic), breaded, frozen fried	319	18.90
Sardines (Pacific), canned in brine or mustard, solids and liquid	196	18.80
Shredded oats (cereal)	279	18.80
Lobster (northern), canned or cooked	95	18.70
Menhaden (Atlantic), canned, solids and liquid	84	18.70
Sardines (Pacific), canned in tomato sauce, solids and liquid	197	18.70
Almonds roasted and salted	627	18.60
Sesame seeds dry, whole	563	18.60
Shad baked	170	18.60
Smelt (Atlantic, jack, and bay), raw	98	18.60
Smoked eel	330	18.60
Tongue potted or deviled	290	18.60
Lobster Newburg	194	18.50
Mackerel salted	305	18.50
Smelt (Atlantic, jack, and bay), canned, solids and liquid	200	18.40
Ham canned	193	18.30
Pork sausage canned, drained solids	381	18.30
Mussels (Pacific), canned, drained solids	114	18.20
Sesame seeds dry, hulled	582	18.20
Pork sausage links or bulk	476	18.10
Scallops frozen, breaded, fried	194	18.00
Camembert cheese	299	17.50
Peanut bars	515	17.50
Potted luncheon meats	248	17.50
Salami cooked	311	17.50
Swordfish canned, solids and liquid	102	17.50
Crab canned	101	17.40
Cocoa (Dutch process), high to medium fat content	261	17.30
Cocoa powder high to medium fat content	265	17.30
Crab steamed	93	17.30
Beef tongue smoked	N.A.	17.20
Cashew nuts	561	17.20

FOOD ITEM	CALS.	UNITS
Cottage cheese uncreamed	86	17.00
Ham country style, medium fat class	389	16.90
Shad creole	152	16.90
Cocoa (Dutch process), high fat content	295	16.80
Cocoa powder high fat content	299	16.80
Brown and serve sausage	422	16.50
Oatmeal (baby food), commercial	375	16.50
Peanuts (chocolate-coated)	561	16.40
Pork and gravy canned	256	16.40
Ham croquette	251	16.30
Rye flour dark	327	16.30
Bass (black sea), stuffed, baked	259	16.20
Liverwurst	307	16.20
Shrimp canned, solids and liquid	80	16.20
Vegetables with wheat and soy protein, canned	104	16.10
Abalone canned	80	16.00
Wheat bran crude, commercially milled	213	16.00
Meatloaf	200	15.90
Clams canned, drained solids	98	15.80
Herring canned in tomato sauce, solids and liquid	176	15.80
Polish-style sausage	304	15.70
Pork and beef chopped together	336	15.60
Strained veal (baby food), commercial	91	15.50
Strained pork (baby food), commercial	118	15.40
Chicken fricassee homemade	161	15.30
Cereal (baby food), commercial	368	15.20
Peanut and cheese crackers	491	15.20
Whitefish (lake), stuffed, baked	215	15.20
Country-style sausage	345	15.10
Puffed wheat (cereal)	363	15.00
Flaked oats (cereal)	397	14.90
Cheese fondue homemade	265	14.80
Liverwurst smoked	319	14.80
Oats (cereal), maple flavored	383	14.80
Walnuts	651	14.80
Malted milk dry	410	14.70
Oats and wheat (cereal)	364	14.70
Strained beef (baby food), commercial	99	14.70
Crab imperial	147	14.60
Strained lamb (baby food), commercial	107	14.60

FOOD ITEM	CALS.	UNITS
Tuna salad	170	14.60
Frankfurters made with cereal, raw	248	14.40
Brazil nuts	654	14.30
Frankfurters made with nonfat dry milk and cereal	248	14.20
Fish loaf cooked	124	14.10
Knockwurst	278	14.10
Milk chocolate with peanuts	543	14.10
Strained liver (baby food), commercial	97	14.10
Vienna sausage canned	240	14.00
Cream substitutes	509	13.90
Creamed pollock	128	13.90
Deviled ham canned	351	13.90
Eggs fried	216	13.80
Pork sausage canned, solids and liquid	415	13.80
Chicken (baby food), commercial	127	13.70
Minced ham	228	13.70
Strained liver and bacon (baby food), commercial	123	13.70
Cottage cheese creamed	106	13.60
Strained beef heart (baby food), commercial	93	13.50
Barley cereal (baby food), commercial	348	13.40
Bologna made with nonfat dry milk	N.A.	13.40
Frankfurters canned	221	13.40
Bologna all meat	277	13.30
Rice bran	276	13.30
Whole wheat flour	333	13.30
Chow mein noodles canned	489	13.20
Hickory nuts	673	13.20
Frankfurters all meat, raw	296	13.10
Green peppers stuffed with beef and bread cereal crumbs	170	13.00
Pinenuts	635	13.00
Rye wafers whole grain	344	13.00
Bread stuffing mix	371	12.90
Eggs hard-boiled	163	12.90
Popcorn plain	386	12.70
Bran sugar and malt extract added	240	12.60
Filberts (hazelnuts)	634	12.60
Chicken chow mein without noodles, homemade	102	12.40
Pastina (spinach)	368	12.40
Almonds (chocolate-covered)	569	12.30

FOOD ITEM	CALS.	UNITS
Shrimp breaded, frozen	139	12.30
Baker's yeast compressed	86	12.10
Rye whole grain	334	12.10
Pizza homemade	236	12.00
Carrot pastina	371	11.90
Puffed oats (cereal)	397	11.90
Beef tripe pickled	435	11.80
Bread flour	365	11.80
Buckwheat flour whole grain	335	11.70
Vegetables with peanuts and soya, canned	303	11.70
Clam fritters	311	11.40
Rye flour medium	350	11.40
Chicken a la king homemade	191	11.20
Eggs scrambled	173	11.20
Clams hard, meat only	80	11.10
Teething biscuits (baby food)	378	11.10
Soybeans dry, cooked	130	11.00
Bran sugar and defatted wheat germ added	238	10.80
Whole wheat bread toasted	287	10.80
Zwieback	423	10.70
French or Vienna bread toasted	338	10.60
Oysters (Pacific and Western), raw	91	10.60
Rye bread (American), toasted	338	10.60
Miso (fermented soybean product)	171	10.50
Wheat flour all purpose	364	10.50
White bread 5% - 6% nonfat dry milk, toasted	320	10.50
Whole wheat bread commercial	243	10.50
Bulgur	357	10.40
Chop suey with meat, homemade	120	10.40
Cracked wheat bread toasted	313	10.40
Turkey potpie homemade	237	10.40
Chili con carne without beans, canned	200	10.30
Bran flakes cereal	303	10.20
Wheat flakes (cereal)	354	10.20
Beef potpie homemade	246	10.10
Chicken potpie homemade	235	10.10
Lobster salad	110	10.10
Strained egg yolks (baby food), commercial	210	10.10
White bread made with 1% - 2% nonfat dry milk, toasted	314	10.10
Ice cream cones	377	10.00

FOOD ITEM	CALS.	UNITS
Strained egg yolks with ham or bacon (baby food), commercial	208	10.00
Whole wheat rolls	257	10.00
Cheese souffle homemade	218	9.90
Shredded wheat (cereal)	354	9.90
Hard rolls enriched, commercial	312	9.80
Popcorn with oil and salt	456	9.80
Pretzels	390	9.80
Barley pearled	348	9.60
Pizza frozen	245	9.50
Gelatin dessert powder	371	9.40
Hot chocolate mix	392	9.40
Pork luncheon meat	498	9.40
Rye flour light	357	9.40
Chicken and noodles homemade	153	9.30
Flour self rising	352	9.30
Milk chocolate with almonds	532	9.30
Waffles homemade	279	9.30
Cornmeal whole ground, unbolted	355	9.20
Pecans	687	9.20
Soda crackers	439	9.20
French or Vienna bread commercial	290	9.10
Italian bread enriched or unenriched, commercial	276	9.10
Pumpernickel bread commercial	246	9.10
Rye bread (American), commercial	243	9.10
Shredded wheat (cereal), sweetened	366	9.10
Cornmeal bolted	362	9.00
Rolls from mix, made with water	299	9.00
Saltine crackers	433	9.00
Soybeans canned, drained solids	103	9.00
White bread made with 5% - 6% nonfat dry milk	275	9.00
Cowpeas boiled	130	8.90
Bread salt-rising, toasted	297	8.80
Wheat and malted barley flakes (cereal)	392	8.80
Brown-and-serve buns browned	328	8.70
Bulgur made from club wheat	359	8.70
Corn bread (Johnny cake), homemade	267	8.70
Corn grits degermed	362	8.70
Cracked wheat bread commercial	263	8.70
Onions dried	350	8.70

FOOD ITEM	CALS.	UNITS
White bread made with 1% - 2% nonfat dry milk, toasted	269	8.70
Clams soft, meat and liquid	54	8.60
Bacon canned	685	8.50
Cornmeal whole ground, self-rising	347	8.50
Cream substitutes dry	508	8.50
Oysters canned, solids and liquid	76	8.50
Sweet rolls commercial	316	8.50
Whole wheat crackers	403	8.40
Bran flakes with raisins (cereal)	287	8.30
Barley pearled, light	349	8.20
Cream chipped beef	154	8.20
Lima beans dry, boiled and drained	138	8.20
Rolls homemade	339	8.20
Condensed milk canned, sweetened	32	8.10
Cowpeas cooked	130	8.10
Puffed corn (cereal)	399	8.10
Cream cheese	374	8.00
Graham crackers plain	384	8.00
Meatloaf TV dinner with tomato sauce, mashed potatoes, and peas	131	8.00
Potato flour	351	8.00
Raisin bread toasted	316	8.00
Split peas cooked	115	8.00
Bittersweet chocolate	477	7.90
Clams canned, solids and liquid	52	7.90
Cornflakes	386	7.90
Cornmeal degermed	364	7.90
Rye bread salt-rising	267	7.90
Corn flour	368	7.80
Corn fritters	377	7.80
Ladyfinger cookies	360	7.80
Macadamia nuts	691	7.80
Muffins homemade, plain	294	7.80
Pizza with sausage, homemade	234	7.80
Red beans dry, boiled and drained	118	7.80
Sugar-coated almonds	456	7.80
Tofu (soybean curd)	72	7.80
Bran muffins homemade	261	7.70
Cornmeal degermed, self-rising, with soft white flour	348	7.70
Fudge (chocolate-coated) with caramel and peanuts	433	7.70

FOOD ITEM	CALS.	UNITS
Milk chocolate plain	520	7.70
Frankfurters and beans canned	144	7.60
Lima beans boiled and drained	111	7.60
Sponge cake homemade	297	7.60
Chili con carne with beans, canned	133	7.50
Cornmeal degermed, self-rising	348	7.50
Spaghetti with meatballs in tomato sauce, homemade	134	7.50
Baby lima beans frozen, boiled and drained	118	7.40
Baking-powder biscuits homemade	369	7.40
Beef with vegetables (baby food)	87	7.40
Cake or pastry flour	364	7.40
Chicken with vegetables (baby food), commercial	100	7.40
Corn, rice, and wheat flakes (cereal)	389	7.40
Cornbread (southern style), homemade	207	7.40
Danish pastry commercial	422	7.40
White rice parboiled	369	7.40
Blueberry muffins homemade	281	7.30
Coconut meat dried, unsweetened	662	7.20
Corn muffins homemade	288	7.20
Pancakes from mix, made with eggs and milk	225	7.20
Piecrust mix	522	7.20
Biscuits homemade, from self-rising flour	372	7.10
Biscuits from mix, made with milk	325	7.10
Cookies (chocolate), commercial	445	7.10
Pancakes homemade, from enriched or unenriched flour	231	7.10
Veal with vegetables (baby food), commercial	63	7.10
Waffles frozen	253	7.10
Evaporated milk canned, unsweetened	137	7.00
Lemon chiffon pie commercial	313	7.00
Shredded corn (cereal)	389	7.00
Split pea soup canned, condensed	118	7.00
Muffins from mix, made with eggs and milk	200	6.90
Raisin rolls homemade	275	6.90
Buckwheat pancakes from mix, made with eggs and milk	200	6.80
Pie chocolate chiffon, commercial	328	6.80
Chestnuts dried	377	6.70
Cornbread homemade	195	6.70
Graham crackers honey coated	411	6.70

FOOD ITEM	CALS.	UNITS
Puffed oats (cereal), sugar coated	396	6.70
Turkey with vegetables (baby food), commercial	86	6.70
Animal crackers commercial	429	6.60
Carrots dried	341	6.60
Pineapple chiffon pie commercial	288	6.60
Rice cereal (baby food), commercial	371	6.60
Brownies with nuts, homemade	485	6.50
Cream puffs commercial	233	6.50
Stuffing dry	358	6.50
Beef and vegetable stew homemade	89	6.40
Buckwheat flour light	347	6.40
Cottage pudding without sauce	344	6.40
Molasses cookies commercial	422	6.40
Potato sticks	544	6.40
Pound cake commercial	411	6.40
Coffee cake from mix	322	6.30
Doughnuts yeast leavened	414	6.30
Beans with pork in sweet sauce, canned	150	6.20
Bulgur canned	168	6.20
Coconut bar commercial	494	6.20
Eclairs with custard filling and chocolate frosting, commercial	239	6.20
Garlic cloves raw	137	6.20
Oatmeal cookies with raisins, commercial	451	6.20
Puffed corn (cereal), cocoa flavored	390	6.20
Soybean sprouts raw	46	6.20
Beans with pork in tomato sauce, canned	122	6.10
Butter cookies thin, commercial	457	6.10
Chestnut flour	362	6.10
Cornbread from mix	233	6.10
Custard pie commercial	218	6.10
Oysters frozen, solids and liquid	N.A.	6.10
Pancakes from mix, made with milk	202	6.10
Piecrust	500	6.10
Popcorn sugar coated	383	6.10
Coconut custard pie commercial	235	6.00
Light fruitcake homemade	389	6.00
Malt extract dried	367	6.00
Puffed rice (cereal)	399	6.00
Puffed wheat (cereal)	376	6.00
Sugar cookies thick, homemade	444	6.00

FOOD ITEM	CALS.	UNITS
Brown mustard prepared	91	5.90
Charlotte russe with ladyfingers and whipped cream filling	286	5.90
Rice flakes (cereal)	390	5.90
Beef and vegetable stew canned	79	5.80
Turkey potpie commercial	197	5.80
Angel food cake from mix	259	5.70
Peanut brittle	421	5.70
Pound cake homemade	473	5.70
Red beans canned, solids and liquid	90	5.70
Bread pudding with raisins, commercial	187	5.60
Puffed corn (cereal), fruit flavored	395	5.60
Soy sauce	68	5.60
Baked custard	115	5.50
Boston brown bread commercial	211	5.50
Ginger snaps commercial	420	5.50
Chocolate chip cookies homemade from enriched flour	516	5.40
Lima beans canned, drained solids	96	5.40
Peas	71	5.40
Raisins (chocolate-coated)	425	5.40
Vanilla wafers commercial	462	5.40
Cottage pudding with chocolate sauce	318	5.30
Macaroons	475	5.30
Potato chips	568	5.30
Potatoes au gratin	145	5.30
Soybean sprouts boiled and drained	38	5.30
Shredded rice (cereal)	392	5.20
Assorted cookies commercial	480	5.10
Chocolate syrup (fudge)	330	5.10
Cottage pudding with fruit sauce	292	5.10
Cowpeas dry, cooked	76	5.10
Graham crackers (chocolate-covered)	475	5.10
Pecan pie commercial	418	5.10
Boston cream pie	302	5.00
Dried apricots uncooked	260	5.00
Macaroni enriched or unenriched, cooked until firm	148	5.00
Tapioca cream pudding	134	5.00
Brownies with nuts and chocolate icing, commercial	419	4.90
Chocolate fudge (chocolate-coated), with nuts	452	4.90
Oyster stew prepared with milk, homemade	86	4.90
Sugar wafers commercial	485	4.90

FOOD ITEM	CALS.	UNITS
Blue cheese salad dressing	504	4.80
Chocolate cake homemade	366	4.80
Chocolate meringue pie	252	4.80
Cookies (sandwich), commercial	495	4.80
Dark fruitcake homemade	379	4.80
Dried peaches	340	4.80
Ice milk	152	4.80
Waffles from mix, made with water	305	4.80
Malted milk	104	4.70
Yellow mustard prepared	75	4.70
Doughnuts cake type	391	4.60
White cake homemade	375	4.60
Banana custard pie commercial	221	4.50
Caramel cake homemade	385	4.50
Caramels (plain or chocolate) with nuts	428	4.50
Carob flour	180	4.50
Chocolate cake with chocolate frosting, homemade	369	4.50
Corn pone	204	4.50
Ice cream fat content 10%	193	4.50
Puffed rice (cereal), cocoa flavored	401	4.50
Sweet potato pie commercial	213	4.50
Yellow cake homemade	363	4.50
Banana powder	340	4.40
Butterscotch pie commercial	267	4.40
Chocolate sweet	528	4.40
Chop suey with meat, canned	62	4.40
Coconut cream	334	4.40
Cornflakes sugar coated	386	4.40
Devil's food cake with chocolate frosting, from mix	339	4.40
Marble cake with white frosting	331	4.40
Raisin cookies	379	4.40
Stuffing moist	208	4.40
French fried potatoes	274	4.30
Brussels sprouts boiled	36	4.20
Chocolate (semi-sweet)	507	4.20
Milk part skim	59	4.20
Strained peas (baby food), commercial	54	4.20
Succotash frozen, boiled and drained	93	4.20
Vanilla fudge with nuts	424	4.20

FOOD ITEM	CALS.	UNITS
Yellow cake with chocolate frosting, homemade	365	4.20
Egg noodles enriched, cooked	125	4.10
Honey spice cake with caramel frosting, from mix	352	4.10
Yellow cake with chocolate frosting, from mix	337	4.10
Caramels (plain or chocolate)	399	4.00
Caramels Chocolate-coated	416	4.00
Cocoa powder	347	4.00
Corn pudding	104	4.00
Marshmallow cookies commercial	409	4.00
Nougats and caramels (chocolate-coated)	416	4.00
Oyster stew frozen, prepared with milk	84	4.00
Pineapple custard pie commercial	220	4.00
Puffed corn (cereal), sweetened	379	4.00
Pumpkin pie commercial	211	4.00
Split peas with ham or bacon (baby food), commercial	80	4.00
White sauce thick	198	4.00
Yellow cake with caramel frosting, homemade	362	4.00
Chocolate fudge with nuts, homemade	426	3.90
Fig bars commercial	358	3.90
Macaroni and cheese canned	95	3.90
White cake with chocolate frosting, from mix	351	3.90
Chocolate cake with white frosting, homemade	369	3.80
Chocolate fudge (chocolate-coated)	430	3.80
Cocoa	97	3.80
Creamed shrimp soup frozen, made with milk	99	3.80
Gingerbread homemade	317	3.80
Green pea soup with ham, frozen	57	3.80
Lichees dried	277	3.80
Mung bean sprouts raw	35	3.80
Vanilla creams (chocolate-coated), commercial	435	3.80
Caramel cake with caramel frosting, homemade	379	3.70
Lemon meringue pie commercial	255	3.70
New England clam chowder frozen, made with milk	86	3.70
Buttermilk cultured	36	3.60
Coconut meat dried, sweetened	548	3.60
Collard greens boiled	33	3.60
French fried potatoes frozen	220	3.60
Parsley raw	44	3.60
Rice pudding with raisins, commercial	146	3.60
Skim milk	36	3.60

FOOD ITEM	CALS.	UNITS
Coconut meat fresh	346	3.50
Figs candied	299	3.50
Spaghetti with cheese in tomato sauce, homemade	104	3.50
Vanilla pudding homemade	111	3.50
Whole milk	65	3.50
Chicken vegetable soup canned, condensed	62	3.40
Chocolate malt cake with white frosting, from mix	346	3.40
Chocolate milk whole	85	3.40
Chocolate pudding from mix	124	3.40
Chocolate rennet custard from mix	102	3.40
Macaroni enriched or unenriched, cooked until tender	111	3.40
Soybean milk fluid	33	3.40
Tomato paste canned	82	3.40
Yogurt made from partially skimmed milk	50	3.40
Hot chocolate homemade	95	3.30
Milk (chocolate), made with skim	76	3.30
Oatmeal with wheat germ and soy grits, (cereal)	62	3.30
Prunes	344	3.30
White cake with white frosting, homemade	375	3.30
Bean soup with pork	67	3.20
Chocolate frosting	376	3.20
Coconut milk	252	3.20
Corn sweet, boiled	83	3.20
Creamed potato soup frozen, made with milk	76	3.20
Goat's milk	67	3.20
Half-and-half cream	134	3.20
Mixed vegetables (carrots, corn, peas, green snap beans, and lima beans), frozen, boiled and drained	64	3.20
Mung bean sprouts boiled and drained	28	3.20
Peas and carrots boiled	53	3.20
Spinach raw	26	3.20
Broccoli boiled	26	3.10
Chocolate pudding homemade	148	3.10
Dried pears	268	3.10
Gingerbread cake from mix	276	3.10
Hash-browned potatoes	229	3.10
Vegetables and liver with cereal (baby food), commercial	47	3.10
Blue cheese dressing low calorie, commercial	76	3.00
Cream of chicken soup made with milk, commercial	73	3.00
Light cream	211	3.00

FOOD ITEM	CALS.	UNITS
Potatoes scalloped, without cheese	104	3.00
Spinach boiled and drained	23	3.00
Yogurt made from whole milk	62	3.00
Chestnuts fresh	194	2.90
Egg yolk and bacon (baby food), commercial	82	2.90
Peas cooked	43	2.90
Artichokes (globe or French), boiled and drained	44	2.80
Asparagus soup made with milk, commercial	60	2.80
Beef noodle dinner (baby food), commercial	48	2.80
Chicken noodle soup canned, condensed	53	2.80
Coconut (chocolate-coated)	438	2.80
Cream of mushroom soup made with milk, commercial	88	2.80
Fennel leaves, raw	28	2.80
Vegetables and ham with cereal (baby food), commercial	64	2.80
Chocolate fudge	400	2.70
Dandelion greens raw	45	2.70
Mushrooms raw	28	2.70
Vegetables and beef with cereal (baby food), commercial	56	2.70
Baked potatoes	93	2.60
Bamboo shoots raw	27	2.60
Blackberry pie commercial	243	2.60
Celery soup made with milk	69	2.60
Chicken chow mein without noodles, canned	38	2.60
Chicken gumbo canned, condensed	46	2.60
Chicken with rice soup canned, condensed	39	2.60
Cowpeas pods, boiled	34	2.60
Cress raw	32	2.60
Dandelion greens boiled and drained	33	2.60
Elderberries raw	72	2.60
Macaroni, tomatoes, meat, and cereal (baby food), commercial	67	2.60
Oat and wheat cereal cooked	65	2.60
Oat flakes (cereal), maple flavored, cooked	69	2.60
Raisin pie commercial	270	2.60
Tomato soup canned, condensed, prepared with milk	69	2.60
Brown rice	119	2.50
Light whipping cream	300	2.50
Mince pie commercial	271	2.50
Peach pie commercial	255	2.50
Raisins	289	2.50

FOOD ITEM	CALS.	UNITS
Rhubarb pie commercial	253	2.50
Shallots bulbs, raw	72	2.50
Tomato chili sauce bottled	104	2.50
Blueberry pie commercial	242	2.40
Vegetables, liver and bacon with cereal (baby food), commercial	57	2.40
Cauliflower boiled and drained	22	2.30
Chocolate syrup (thin)	245	2.30
Custard (baby food), commercial	100	2.30
Green pea soup canned, condensed	53	2.30
Jerusalem artichokes raw, freshly harvested	7	2.30
Oyster stew frozen, prepared with water	51	2.30
Pokeberry shoots boiled	20	2.30
Spinach (baby food), creamed, commercial	43	2.30
Apple pie commercial	256	2.20
Asparagus spears, boiled and drained	20	2.20
Caramels (chocolate-flavored)	396	2.20
Dates (domestic), dry	274	2.20
Greek olives	338	2.20
Heavy whipping cream	352	2.20
Leeks	52	2.20
Mustard greens boiled and drained	23	2.20
Onion soup canned, condensed	27	2.20
Pineapple pie commercial	253	2.20
Spaghetti with cheese and tomato sauce, canned	76	2.20
Swamp cabbage boiled and drained	21	2.20
Turnip greens leaves and stems, boiled and drained	20	2.20
Vegetables and lamb with cereal (baby food), commercial	58	2.20
Watercress leaves and stems, raw	19	2.20
Avocado	167	2.10
Beef bouillon	13	2.10
Chicken noodle dinner (baby food), commercial	49	2.10
Corn canned	82	2.10
Mashed potatoes milk added	65	2.10
Mashed potatoes made with milk and table fat	94	2.10
Potatoes with skin, boiled	76	2.10
Potatoes without skin, boiled	67	2.10
Red cabbage raw	31	2.10
Sweet potatoes with skin, baked	141	2.10
Vegetable beef soup canned, prepared with equal volume of water	32	2.10

FOOD ITEM	CALS.	UNITS
Vegetables and chicken with cereal (baby food), commercial	52	2.10
Vegetables and turkey with cereal (baby food), commercial	44	2.10
Yams tuber, raw	101	2.10
Cream of shrimp soup frozen, prepared with water	66	2.00
Hash-browned potatoes frozen, cooked	224	2.00
Marshmallows	319	2.00
Minestrone soup	43	2.00
Okra boiled and drained	29	2.00
Potatoes instant, prepared with milk and fat	96	2.00
Tomato catsup bottled	106	2.00
Wheat and malted barley (hot cereal)	65	2.00
White rice	109	2.00
Coconut frosting	364	1.90
Cream of mushroom soup canned, condensed	111	1.90
Ground cherries raw	53	1.90
Mushrooms canned	17	1.90
Potatoes flaked, prepared with water, milk, and fat	93	1.90
Strawberry pie commercial	198	1.90
Tomato soup (baby food), commercial	54	1.90
Welsh onions	34	1.90
Celeriac root, raw	40	1.80
Chard boiled and drained	18	1.80
Chicory greens raw	20	1.80
Chives raw	28	1.80
Cress boiled	22	1.80
New England clam chowder frozen, made with water	54	1.80
Spanish rice homemade	87	1.80
Sugar apples	94	1.80
Turkey noodle soup	33	1.80
Whole wheat cereal cooked	45	1.80
Winter squash	63	1.80
Apple custard	101	1.70
Beet greens	18	1.70
Currants	54	1.70
Escarole raw	20	1.70
Fondant (chocolate-coated)	410	1.70
Kohlrabi boiled	24	1.70
Mustard spinach boiled and drained	16	1.70
New Zealand spinach boiled and drained	13	1.70
Sweet potatoes boiled with skin	114	1.70

FOOD ITEM	CALS.	UNITS
Tomato puree canned, regular or low sodium	39	1.70
Vegetables and bacon with cereal (baby food), commercial	68	1.70
Apple brown betty	151	1.60
Beef noodle soup	28	1.60
Dried apricots sulfured, cooked, sugar added	122	1.60
Green beans boiled and drained	25	1.60
Mixed vegetables (baby food), commercial	37	1.60
Russian salad dressing commercial, regular	494	1.60
Barbecue sauce	91	1.50
Gelatin dessert	59	1.50
Green onions (bunching variety), young, raw	36	1.50
Onions raw	38	1.50
Parsnips boiled and drained	66	1.50
Beans (baby food), commercial	22	1.40
Beets (baby food), commercial	37	1.40
Blue cheese salad dressing low calorie	19	1.40
Boiled white frosting	316	1.40
Cabbage (spoon), boiled and drained	14	1.40
Celery soup canned, condensed	72	1.40
Chicken consomme	9	1.40
Creamed potato soup frozen	44	1.40
Dried apples sulfered, cooked, sugar added	112	1.40
Ginger root fresh	49	1.40
Green olives pickled, canned or bottled	116	1.40
Red peppers	31	1.40
Tartar sauce regular	531	1.40
Water chestnuts raw	79	1.40
Yambean tuber, raw	55	1.40
Cabbage raw	24	1.30
Cherries (sweet), raw	70	1.30
Coleslaw made with mayonnaise	144	1.30
Dried apricots cooked, without sugar added	85	1.30
Farina enriched, regular, cooked	42	1.30
Frosting (caramel)	360	1.30
Grapes (American), raw	69	1.30
Horseradish prepared	38	1.30
Lettuce (cos and romaine)	18	1.30
Pears candied	303	1.30
Sweet potatoes candied	168	1.30
Tomatoes red, boiled	26	1.30

FOOD ITEM	CALS.	UNITS
Blackberries	58	1.20
Boysenberries frozen	48	1.20
Casaba melon	27	1.20
Chinese cabbage raw	14	1.20
Corn grits cooked	51	1.20
Cream of chicken soup prepared with water	39	1.20
Figs raw	80	1.20
Fruit pudding (baby food), commercial	96	1.20
Green peppers (sweet), raw	22	1.20
Prunes stewed	180	1.20
Red raspberries raw	57	1.20
Bananas	91	1.10
Beets boiled	32	1.10
Black olives	129	1.10
Carrots raw	42	1.10
Coleslaw made with French dressing	129	1.10
Cornmeal degermed, cooked	50	1.10
Lemons	27	1.10
Mayonnaise	718	1.10
Milk human	77	1.10
Plantain	119	1.10
Potatoes canned, solids and liquid	44	1.10
Tomatoes ripe, raw	22	1.10
Vegetables with beef broth	32	1.10
Apricots raw	51	1.00
Asparagus soup canned, condensed	39	1.00
Belgian endive	15	1.00
Cream of mushroom soup canned, condensed	56	1.00
Dried apples uncooked	275	1.00
Eggplant boiled and drained	19	1.00
Guavas (strawberry), whole, raw	65	1.00
Loganberries raw	62	1.00
Longans raw	61	1.00
Oranges raw	49	1.00
Pumpkin canned	33	1.00
Radishes raw	17	1.00
Sauerkraut canned, solids and liquid	18	1.00
Sweet potatoes (baby food), commercial	67	1.00
Apple butter	186	.00
Apple juice canned or bottled	47	.00

FOOD ITEM	CALS.	UNITS
Apple sauce	41	.00
Apple tapioca commercial	117	.00
Apricot nectar canned	57	.00
Baking powder	129	.00
Beer	42	.00
Beets	34	.00
Blackberries	40	.00
Blackberry juice	37	.00
Blueberries	62	.00
Boysenberries	36	.00
Butterscotch candy	367	.00
Cantaloupe	30	.00
Carrots (baby food), commercial	29	.00
Carrots boiled and drained	31	.00
Celery (green and yellow varieties), raw	17	.00
Chayote raw	28	.00
Cherries (sweet), canned in water, with or without artificial sweetener, fruit and liquid	48	.00
Chili pepper canned, pods and liquid	25	.00
Coffee instant	1	.00
Cornstarch	362	.00
Cranberries	46	.00
Cucumbers	14	.00
Figs canned in water, with or without artificial sweetener, fruit and liquid	48	.00
Fondant	N.A.	.00
Fruit salad	35	.00
Fruit-flavored ices	78	.00
Gooseberries raw	39	.00
Grape juice canned or bottled	66	.00
Grapefruit raw	41	.00
Grapefruit juice	39	.00
Grapes (European), raw	67	.00
Grapes canned	51	.00
Guavas whole, raw	62	.00
Gum drops	347	.00
Hard candy	386	.00
Honey	304	.00
Honeydew melon	33	.00
Jelly beans	367	.00

FOOD ITEM	CALS.	UNITS
Kumquats	65	.00
Lard	902	.00
Lemon candied	314	.00
Lemon juice	25	.00
Lemon peel candied	316	.00
Lemonade	44	.00
Lettuce (iceberg), raw	13	.00
Lichees raw	64	.00
Lime juice canned or bottled, unsweetened	26	.00
Limeade frozen concentrate	41	.00
Limes raw	28	.00
Loquats raw	48	.00
Mangoes raw	66	.00
Margarine	720	.00
Nectarines raw	64	.00
Oils	884	.00
Orange juice	45	.00
Oranges	49	.00
Papayas raw	39	.00
Peach nectar canned	48	.00
Peaches raw	38	.00
Pear nectar canned	52	.00
Pears raw	61	.00
Persimmons	77	.00
Pickles	10	.00
Pimientos	27	.00
Pineapple	52	.00
Pineapple juice	55	.00
Plums	66	.00
Pomegranate pulp	63	.00
Prickly pears	42	.00
Quinces raw	57	.00
Radishes (Oriental, including daikon and Chinese), raw	19	.00
Raspberries (red), canned	35	.00
Rhubarb raw	16	.00
Rose apples raw	56	.00
Rutabagas boiled and drained	35	.00
Sauerkraut juice canned	10	.00
Sherbet orange	134	.00

FOOD ITEM	CALS.	UNITS
Squash (summer), boiled and drained	14	.00
Strawberries raw	37	.00
Sugar (cane), granulated	385	.00
Sweet potatoes canned in liquid, solids and liquid, unsweetened	46	.00
Syrup cane and maple (blend)	252	.00
Tangerine juice	43	.00
Tangerines	46	.00
Tartar sauce low calorie	224	.00
Tomato juice canned, condensed	20	.00
Tomato soup canned, condensed	36	.00
Tomato vegetable soup with noodles from mix	27	.00
Turnips boiled and drained	23	.00
Vegetable juice cocktail canned	17	.00
Vinegar cider	14	.00
Watermelon raw	26	.00
White frosting	397	.00
Wine	85	.00

Carbohydrates

Carbohydrates have generally gotten bad press, and are only recently being rehabilitated. Highly sugared, refined carbohydrates like candy, soft drinks, pastries, sugared cereals, and refined bread and pasta have been lumped together with fresh fruits and nutritious starchy vegetables and whole grains and tubers. As a result, when we think of carbohydrates, we tend to think "calories—fattening." Hypoglycemics, diabetics, and the overweight or obese have been instructed by their doctors to stay away from all carbohydrate foods, considered too high in calories, and the concept that "carbohydrate intolerance" is a widespread problem has been promulgated by advocates of high-protein, low-carbohydrate diets.

Most people still do not understand the distinction between the two forms of carbohydrates, the refined starches and sugars that have given carbohydrates their bad name, and the complex carbohydrates whose health benefits are finally beginning to be appreciated. Because carbohydrates are so important in our diet, it is essential to understand what they are, their sources in nature, their nutritional benefits, and the amount we require.

What Carbohydrates Are

Carbohydrates are one of the most abundant compounds in living things. They include nondigestible cellulose, the fibrous material that gives plants their shape (which is discussed in the Fiber section), and starches and sugars, two of the storable fuels that supply living things with immediate energy for all the body's needs. Supplying energy is the primary purpose of foods. Each gram of carbohydrate supplies the body with four calories of energy when it is oxidized in our cells. In this country, half of our caloric intake — half of our energy — comes from carbohydrate foods. Many carbohydrate-rich foods also contain substantial units of amino acids, the building blocks of protein. In fact, for over half of the world's people, carbohydrate foods are the major source of protein as well as energy.

We need carbohydrates in our diet. They are our most important source of energy for all our activities, for sustaining our metabolism; and the foods in which they are found — fruits, cereals, seeds and nuts, vegetables, and tubers — are important sources of vitamins, minerals, and other nutrients as well.

Classification of Carbohydrates

Carbohydrate foods are classified as either complex or refined. Complex carbohydrates are the whole starches, sugars, and fibers of the above-mentioned food sources, as they are found in nature, having undergone minimal or no processing.

The starches and sugars of all carbohydrates supply energy. But complex carbohydrates also offer fiber for good digestive functioning, B- and C-complex and other vitamins, and protein, the building material of which our bodies are constructed. Our bodies are best adapted to consume carbohydrates in their complex form, since refinement is an extremely recent innovation in our long history of evolution. When carbohydrates are refined, they are stripped of both their outer shell (the bran layer which contains most of the fiber) and their oil and B-vitamin-rich germ.

For example, refined flour contains no wheat germ; refined cane sugar is chemically pure sucrose crystals. Thus, refined flour or sugar is no more than a skeleton of the complex carbohydrate that exists in nature. Refined carbohydrates may also be bleached, milled, baked (like bread), puffed (like some cereals), or otherwise processed (like sugar). In short, complex carbohydrates are close to their natural state. Refined carbohydrates are highly processed foods, depleted of nutrients and fiber, and containing little more than pure starch or sugar — energy sources on which no animal can subsist.

Unfortunately, it is the refined carbohydrates that predominate in the American diet. Our breakfast cereals are generally made from wheat, corn, oats, or rice. But (with the exception of real oatmeal and a few hot wheat cereals) these are rarely served in their natural form. They are dried, refined, bleached, steamed, puffed, flaked, or sugared; occasionally a small percentage of the recommended daily allowance of certain minerals and (usually synthetic) vitamins is re-added, so the cereals can be labeled "enriched"; but most of the nutrients available from such breakfasts comes from the milk that people add rather than from the cereal itself. Our breads (even "rye" and "whole wheat") are usually produced from refined flour and are loaded with chemical additives. Similarly, the potato chips we munch are a far cry from the vitamin- and fiber-rich whole potatoes from which they are manufactured. Most of the white rice that graces our plates may look pretty but lacks the fiber, protein, vitamins, and minerals found in whole, brown rice. Because refined carbohydrates contain no fiber, overreliance on them as a source of energy can lead to poor intestinal health and a myriad of digestive disorders. In addition, overconsumption of refined sugar is linked to hypoglycemia, diabetes, and other blood-sugar disorders.

Complex Carbohydrates

If you want to increase the amount of complex carbohydrates in your diet, there is a wide assortment from which to choose. There are many varieties of basic whole grains easily available, and you may wish to try those with which you are unfamiliar. Grains include whole wheat (to which, unfortunately, many people are allergic because they have consumed so much refined flour in breads, cakes, pastas, and packaged, processed foods), rye, triticale (a cross between rye and wheat that you may be able to tolerate if you are allergic to wheat), corn, barley, brown rice, oats, millet, and buckwheat. These can be served whole, as cereals or side dishes, or mixed in soups and casseroles, ground into whole flour and baked into bread, or rolled into whole-grain pastas. Legumes are also more varied than most people realize. Some of the most common varieties include soybeans and soy products such as tofu, tempeh, and miso, mung beans, lentils, aduki beans, split peas, black-eyed peas, kidney beans, navy beans, red beans, pink beans, pinto beans, black beans, turtle beans, fava beans, chick-peas (garbanzos), and peanuts. Seeds such as sunflower and sesame seeds are high in protein as well as carbohydrates; alfalfa, chia and flax seeds (those grown organically as food, not for fabric, to avoid pesticides) are highly nutritious when sprouted. Most nuts are mainly fat, but almonds, cashews, pistachios, and pine nuts are high in carbohydrates as well. Grains, legumes, and seeds are high in protein as well as carbohydrates.

The entire vegetable family contains carbohydrates. Those lowest in calories, such as celery, broccoli, and mushrooms, contain mostly water and fiber; the starchier, root vegetables like carrots, beets, potatoes, and yams, tend to be higher in unrefined starches and sugars as well as fiber.

Fruits are an excellent source of natural sugar, minerals, vitamins, and fiber. You should choose from among a selection of apples, pears, peaches, nectarines, plums, grapes, or citrus fruits. Although the sugar content of these fruits is fairly high, it is diluted with water and released relatively slowly into your system as you chew and digest the cellulose-encased cells of the pulp. That way your body doesn't get the sudden jolt it does from refined, pure sugar. Bananas and other tropical fruits should be eaten in moderation by those sensitive to sugar, since their sugar content is higher. Similarly, dried figs, prunes, raisins, dates, apricots, pears, or apples contain three times the sugar dose of fresh fruit: like refined sugar, they are highly concentrated carbohydrates, which should only be eaten occasionally, and of which hypoglycemics and diabetics especially must beware.

There is little need to fear the caloric consequences of eating too much fruit. An apple may contain the equivalent of three teaspoons of sugar, but it is much harder to down three whole apples than nine teaspoons of sugar. Some people consume that much sugar in one cup of coffee, one mug of cocoa, or one doughnut — none of which contains the beneficial vitamins, minerals, and enzymes of the apple.

Kinds of Sugar

Fructose, the form of sugar predominant in fruits and honey, has been much praised recently as superior to sucrose (cane sugar) or glucose (corn sugar). Dr. John Yudkin, Professor Emeritus of the University of London and an eminent authority on sugar, is among those who have refuted these claims. Dr. Yudkin points out that, like other forms of refined sugar, refined fructose tends to raise blood triglyceride and cholesterol levels — two factors implicated in cardiovascular disease. The only advantage of fructose is that it is sweeter than sucrose (the sucrose molecule is half fructose and half glucose) or glucose. This is why honey, which contains mostly fructose, is sweeter than table sugar and much sweeter than corn syrup.

"Glucose"; "corn syrup"; "dextrose"; "corn sugar" — all those are names for the same inexpensive, refined sweetener, used in large quantities in packaged foods. You may find more than one of them deceptively listed on the label of refined-carbohydrate foods, along with sugar, honey, sucrose, maltose, or lactose. If more than one of these is listed, the chances are that refined sugar is the main ingredient of the product, even if it is not listed first on the label. Though it is not very sweet, pure glucose has the same effect on your metabolism as other refined sugars.

Digestion, Storage, and Utilization of Starches and Sugars

Starches, like sugars, are one form in which plants store the energy they absorb from the sun. They are similar to sugar in chemical composition, containing carbon, hydrogen, and oxygen. However, they are based on much longer carbon chains than sugars. This is why they can be broken down into sugars.

Digestion of carbohydrate foods is usually swift and simple. It begins in the mouth, with the conversion of some starch to sugar: the enzyme amylase, from the salivary gland, breaks the long-carbohydrate-chain starch into the double sugar maltose. This breakdown continues in the intestine. (Very little carbohydrate digestion takes place in the stomach, except for acidification and a slight amount of hydrolysis.) All carbohydrates are absorbed into the bloodstream as the simple sugars glucose or fructose.

How to Facilitate Digestion of Carbohydrate Foods

Cooked starches are easier to digest than uncooked, since heat ruptures the cell walls of plants and allows the mouth and intestine's enzymes to convert the starch to sugar more easily. Normally, carbohydrates are digested quickly: the carbohydrates in fruit or fruit juice may be digested in as little as forty minutes; starchy foods, such as beans or grains, may take up to one and one-half hours. Cooked and eaten properly, the digestion time of a carbohydrate meal may be only eighty to ninety minutes. The more fiber you consume with your meals, the faster the digestion process will be, since fiber absorbs water and stimulates the peristaltic action of the digestive tract, which pushes food along. Proteins and fats take much longer to digest, and if sweet or starchy foods are eaten at the same time as meat and fish, they can remain in the stomach for the entire time the protein foods take to digest. This can cause gas and indigestion, since the sugar from the carbohydrates may begin to ferment in the warm environment of the digestive tract. For this reason, it's a good idea, if you eat meat, fish, or fowl, to serve your meal with only a salad and vegetables, and to save carbohydrate foods for other meals.

If you begin your meal with a beverage, this can dilute briefly the acid in your stomach and slow digestion. Cold beverages can suspend the digestion temporarily, since the acids and enzymes of your digestive system usually operate at body temperature.

The typical American dinner, consisting of meat, potatoes, vegetables, and perhaps a salad, with dessert afterward, mixes up all four digestive processes at once, weakening them all. The acid from the meat's protein neutralizes the amylase in your mouth, and starch digestion is limited. When a sugary dessert is added, the simple sugars start fermenting and the result may be a hyperacid reaction in the stomach. If you then take an antacid, this plays havoc with the digestive process; such habits can eventually lead to chronic indigestion and stress on the gastrointestinal tract.

It is preferable to eat complex carbohydrates at one meal, protein foods at another, and fruits as snacks in between meals. Protein meals take a long time to digest, and can leave you with no less energy for several hours after eating them, since much of your energy is absorbed in digesting the protein, and blood must be channeled from other parts of the body to the digestive organs. If you eat some fruit ten to fifteen minutes before such a meal, you can prevent your blood-glucose levels from declining during the time you are digesting your meal. Someone who eats complete protein at every meal may spend the whole day with part of his or her energy involved in digestion. If, on the other hand, you eat a few small meals including complex carbohydrates, your energy levels are likely to be higher and more constant throughout the day, and your intestines will not be taxed to do their job.

How Much Carbohydrate Do You Need? From Which Foods Should You Obtain It?

In the United States, we consume, on the average, about 50 percent of our calories from carbohydrates. Unfortunately, most people obtain most of their carbohydrates in refined form. The breads most people still eat are 55 percent carbohydrate, since the refined flour from which they are made is 75 percent carbohydrate. Our refined cereals are 80 percent carbohydrate; our spaghetti and pastas are 75 percent carbohydrate. Jam, candies, and some pastries may be 90 percent refined carbohydrate. If we ate more vegetables and fewer starchy refined flour products, we would not be losing the enzymes that are refined out of our flours and packaged desserts.

In contrast to these refined products, fresh fruit is only 15 percent carbohydrate; dry legumes — even before being doubled or tripled in size by the addition of water in cooking — are just 60 percent carbohydrate; and uncooked whole grains, before the absorption of water, are 70 percent carbohydrate. It would be better to try to eliminate candies, cookies, sodas, refined pastas, refined breads and cereals, and sugary beverages (including so-called fruit drinks which consist mostly of sugar water) from our diets and replace them with complex carbohydrates.

The ideal diet obtains 75 to 80 percent of its calories from the complex carbohydrates; 12 to 15 percent from complete protein sources such as animal sources; and 10 to 12 percent from the fats found in the animal sources such as butter and fish, or in nuts, seeds, and oils. This would mean getting fewer of our calories from fats, fewer from complete protein foods, and allowing complex carbohydrates to be the mainstay of our diet. This was the recommendation of the Senate Select Committee on Nutrition that met during the Carter administration.

We have not placed as much emphasis on carbohydrates as we should have. When you consider that breads are about 55 percent carbohydrates, cereals about 80 percent, flour products 75 percent, and spaghetti and pastas around 75 percent, while on the other hand, candy and sugar products are about 90 percent, they are, unfortunately, the foods from which we derive the greatest percentage of our carbohydrate intake. A higher percentage of our carbohydrates should come from vegetables, fruits, and legumes. Green, leafy vegetables average 8 percent carbohydrate or less; starchy vegetables such as potatoes or corn, 20 percent or less; fresh fruit, 15 percent average, legumes (dry) around 60 percent; and grains (dry) about 70 percent. Try to eliminate sugars, beverages, candies, cookies, pasta, crackers, cereals, and breads as much as possible.

Like plants, your body stores much of its energy in the form of simple sugars and starches. Everyone is aware that one of our backup energy reserves is the fat in our adipose tissues; but the form of stored energy immediately available and most easily converted to energy is carbohydrate. The sugar we absorb from our food may be converted into energy, starch, or fat by the body. At any given time, we usually have available about a thirteen-hour supply of glycogen (starch) and glucose (sugar). About 225 grams of glycogen will be stored in our cardiac and skeletal muscles; about 100 grams in the liver. In addition, our blood levels of glucose are supposed to remain stable, with about 15 grams of this simple sugar circulating at all times. Each gram of glycogen or glucose, when oxidized by the cells, provides four calories of energy for all the body's needs.

As we mentioned earlier, supplying energy is the number one purpose of eating foods. This is one reason why high-protein diets can be dangerous: protein is mainly a building material. Although it can be oxidized as fuel, this is an inefficient way to provide energy to our systems: it requires extra energy, and it results in a waste product called urea which must be disposed of through the kidneys. Over the long term, eating too much protein and burning protein as fuel overstresses and weakens the kidneys. In contrast, carbohydrates yield immediately available energy; if they are oversupplied, the body builds up its glycogen reserves or converts the extra to fat.

We should have three to four servings a day of fruits and vegetables, and one to three servings daily of whole grains or legumes, preferably combined with each other for protein complementarity. (See Protein section.)

Preparing Complex Carbohydrate Foods

Grains should be rinsed before use, and the larger legumes soaked overnight before cooking. (Cooking time can be shortened by pressure cooking.)

People who eat meat and wish to switch to a more complex carbohydrate-oriented, vegetarian diet often worry that they will be bored, aesthetically, by a diet that seems more limited in variety. However, with the large number of vegetarian cookbooks now available featuring foods from all nationalities, no one need worry about lack of variety or aesthetic appeal. Those who must restrict their sodium intake may still have a wide variety of herbs and spices from which to choose for seasoning these foods. A few of the liveliest are leeks, dill, oregano, cumin, curry, and chili peppers. Vegetables may be mixed with legumes for stews and casseroles as well as soups; seasoned grains, such as millet (perhaps combined with soy granules or lentils for protein enhancement), are delicious stuffed into peppers, tomatoes, or hollowed-out zucchini.

Some people complain that they have trouble digesting beans, and that flatulence is a problem for them. When these products ferment in the large intestines, gas is produced. To prevent it, it is important to soak the beans for at least fifteen hours before cooking them — even the smaller beans such as lentils and split peas — and then to cook them slowly to avoid altering the protein, but thoroughly so that their fiber is completely softened.

Most people find bean sprouts easier to digest than cooked dried beans. Sprouting increases the nutrient content as well as digestibility of beans (or of grains and seeds). Alfalfa and mung beans are two of the most popular. Alfalfa sprouts are a nutrition powerhouse, containing five times the amount of vitamin C of alfalfa seeds. Two ounces of sprouts a day will supply you with vitamins and enzymes you might not otherwise obtain from your diet, as well as chlorophyll, which is considered an intestine and blood cleanser. Always steam bean sprouts briefly before serving them, since raw beans contain digestion inhibitors and other natural toxins that are neutralized by heat.

The Myth of Carbohydrate Intolerance

There are some people who are allergic to one or more grains, legumes, seeds, or nuts; however, most people who have been considered "carbohydrate intolerant" can actually benefit from complex as opposed to refined carbohydrates. Hypoglycemics, for whom a high-protein diet is often recommended, can usually do well on a complex carbohydrates diet when they maintain a moderate daily exercise program. Many hypoglycemics are more energetic, healthier, and less toxin-ridden on such a complex carbohydrate/exercise regimen than they are on the traditional high-protein diet. Even diabetics are being reeducated today to include carbohydrates in their diet.

The unit value for carbohydrates is given in grams. Any food having less than 1 gram of carbohydrates per 100-gram serving is considered to have a trace carbohydrate content and is listed as having a .00 unit value.

Where the symbol N. A. appears in the calorie column, the information was not available.

All figures are based on an edible portion equaling 100 grams, or approximately 3 ounces. In the case of some of the listed foods, one would not consume 100 grams in one serving. Calculations should be made accordingly.

Carbohydrates

FOOD ITEM	CALS.	UNITS
Sugar (beet or cane), granulated	385	99.50
Sugar (beet or cane), powdered	385	99.50
Brown sugar	373	96.40
Chewing gum	317	95.20
Butterscotch	397	94.80
Cornflakes sugar coated	386	91.30
Maple sugar	348	90.00
Puffed rice (cereal)	399	89.50
Cocoa powder	347	89.40
Corn flakes	386	85.30
Honey	304	82.30
Puffed wheat (cereal), with malt and sugar added	366	81.70
Raisin cookies commercial	379	80.80
Carob flour	180	80.70
40% bran flakes (cereal)	303	80.60
Wheat flakes (cereal)	354	80.50
Animal crackers commercial	429	79.90
Shredded wheat (cereal)	354	79.90
Gingersnaps commercial	420	79.80
Buckwheat flour dark	333	79.50
Pastry flour (wheat)	364	79.40
Chestnuts dried	377	78.60
Puffed wheat (cereal)	363	78.50
Barley light	349	78.10
Teething biscuits (baby food)	378	78.00
Ice cream cones	377	77.90
Rye flour light	357	77.90
Malt dry	368	77.40
Raisins uncooked	289	77.40
Whole wheat flour	364	76.90
Corn flour	368	76.80
Popcorn plain	386	76.70
Caramels plain or chocolate	399	76.60
Rye wafers whole grain	344	76.30
All-purpose flour (wheat), unenriched	364	76.10
Fig bars commercial	358	75.40
Puffed oats (cereal)	397	75.20
Corn syrup (light or dark)	290	75.00

FOOD ITEM	CALS.	UNITS
Rye flour medium	350	74.80
Bread flour from enriched wheat	365	74.70
Wheat flour from straight, hard wheat	365	74.50
Zwieback	423	74.30
Cornmeal whole	355	73.70
Bread crumbs commercial	392	73.40
Rye whole grain	334	73.40
Millet whole grain	327	72.90
Buckwheat flour light	347	72.00
Dried apples uncooked	275	71.80
Saltine crackers	433	71.50
Whole wheat flour from hard wheat	333	71.00
Cocoa powder with nonfat dry milk	359	70.80
Malted milk powder	410	70.80
Dried lichees	277	70.70
Soda crackers	439	70.60
Dried figs	274	69.10
Chocolate fudge with nuts, commercial	426	69.00
Dried peaches uncooked	262	68.30
Whole wheat crackers	403	68.20
Rye flour dark	327	68.10
Cane syrup	263	68.00
Sorghum syrup	257	68.00
Dried prunes uncooked	255	67.40
Dried pears	268	67.30
Dried apricots uncooked	260	66.50
Dried apricots uncooked	260	66.50
Oatmeal (baby food), commercial	375	66.00
Beef noodle soup from mix	387	65.30
Shortbread cookies commercial	498	65.10
Light molasses	252	65.00
Maple syrup	252	65.00
Raisin bread toasted	316	64.60
French bread enriched or unenriched, toasted	338	64.40
Lima bean flour	343	63.00
Chocolate syrup (thin)	245	62.70
Wheat bran crude, commercially milled	213	61.90
Cheese crackers commercial	479	60.40
Angel food cake homemade	269	60.20
Chocolate chip cookies homemade from enriched flour	516	60.10

FOOD ITEM	CALS.	UNITS
Molasses medium	232	60.00
Chili peppers (hot), dry, pods	321	59.80
Popcorn cooked in oil	456	59.10
White bread made with 3% - 4% nonfat dry milk, toasted	314	58.80
White bread made with 1% - 2% nonfat dry milk, toasted	314	58.70
Whole wheat bread made with water	287	58.70
White bread made with 5% - 6% nonfat dry milk, toasted	320	58.40
Devil's food cake from mix	339	58.30
Bread (salt rising), toasted, commercial	297	58.00
Chow mein noodles canned	489	58.00
Salt sticks (Vienna bread)	304	58.00
Chocolate (sweet)	528	57.90
Chocolate (semisweet)	507	57.00
Milk chocolate plain	520	56.90
Whole wheat bread made with 2% nonfat milk, toasted	289	56.70
Italian bread	276	56.40
Rolls homemade	339	56.10
French bread enriched or unenriched	290	55.40
Blackstrap molasses	213	55.00
Rice with casein	382	54.80
Rolls from mix	299	54.50
Condensed milk sweetened	321	54.30
Raisin bread commercial	262	53.60
Pumpernickel bread commercial	246	53.10
Biscuits made with whole milk, commercial	325	52.30
Skim milk dry, regular	363	52.30
Cracked wheat bread commercial	263	52.10
Rye bread (American), commercial	243	52.10
Corn muffins made with eggs and water, commercial	297	51.90
Skim milk instant, dry	359	51.60
Doughnuts cake type	391	51.40
Milk chocolate with almonds	532	51.30
Pecan pie commercial	418	51.30
Gingerbread commercial	317	51.10
Brownies with nuts, homemade	485	50.90
Potato chips	568	50.80
Rice bran	276	50.80
White bread made with 3% - 4% nonfat dry milk	270	50.50
White bread made with 1% - 2% nonfat dry milk	269	50.40
White bread made with 5% - 6% nonfat dry milk	275	50.20

FOOD ITEM	CALS.	UNITS
Corn muffins made with eggs and milk, commercial	324	50.00
Boston cream pie homemade	302	49.90
Whole wheat bread made with water, commercial	241	49.30
Cocoa powder high fat content	299	48.30
Whole wheat bread made with nonfat dry milk, commercial	243	47.70
Peanut bars	515	47.20
Pound cake homemade	473	47.00
Apple butter	186	46.80
Bittersweet chocolate	505	46.80
Wheat germ raw, commercially milled	363	46.70
Biscuits homemade	369	45.80
Boston brown bread commercial	211	45.60
Danish pastry commercial	422	45.60
Cranberry sauce sweetened, homemade	178	45.50
Cocoa powder high fat content, processed with alkali	295	45.40
Cranberry orange relish	178	45.40
Piecrust from mix, prepared with water	464	44.00
Lemon chiffon pie commercial	313	43.80
Piecrust	500	43.80
Bran muffins homemade	261	43.10
Raisin pie commercial	270	43.00
Corn muffins homemade with whole ground cornmeal	288	42.50
Muffins plain, homemade	294	42.30
Chestnuts fresh	194	42.10
Waffles frozen, commercial	253	42.00
Blueberry muffins homemade	281	41.90
Waffles from mix, made with water	305	40.20
Apple pie frozen, baked	254	40.00
Corn fritters commercial	368	39.70
Almonds (chocolate-coated)	569	39.60
Peanuts (chocolate-coated)	561	39.10
Pineapple chiffon pie commercial	288	39.10
Baker's yeast dry, commercial	282	38.90
Brewer's yeast debittered	283	38.40
Cherry pie commercial	261	38.40
Butterscotch pie commercial	267	38.30
Peach pie commercial	255	38.20
Rhubarb pie commercial	253	38.20
Whole milk dry	502	38.20

FOOD ITEM	CALS.	UNITS
Apple pie commercial	256	38.10
Pineapple pie commercial	253	38.10
Soybean flour defatted	326	38.10
Doughnuts yeast leavened,	414	37.70
Lemon meringue pie commercial	255	37.70
Sunflower seed flour partially defatted	339	37.70
Waffles homemade	279	37.50
Lemon juice concentrate	116	37.40
Torula yeast	277	37.00
Soybean flour low fat	356	36.60
Safflower seed meal partially defatted	355	36.50
Pizza commercial	245	36.30
Corn pone from white, whole-ground cornmeal	204	36.20
Waffles from mix, made with eggs and milk	275	36.20
French fried potatoes	274	36.00
Rhubarb cooked, sugar added	141	36.00
Bulgur canned, from hard red winter wheat	168	35.00
Blueberry pie commercial	242	34.90
Cornbread homemade from degermed cornmeal	224	34.70
Grapefruit juice frozen	145	34.60
Blackberry pie commercial	243	34.40
Sweet potatoes candied	168	34.20
Pancakes homemade from enriched or unenriched flour	231	34.10
Charlotte russe with ladyfingers and whipped cream filling	286	33.50
Chocolate meringue pie commercial	252	33.50
Persimmons native, raw	127	33.50
Soybean flour high fat	380	33.30
Cottonseed flour	356	33.00
Bulgur canned, from hard red winter wheat, seasoned	182	32.80
Potatoes fried	268	32.60
Sweet potatoes with skin, baked	141	32.50
Pancakes from mix, made from milk and eggs	225	32.40
Pineapple custard pie commercial	220	32.10
Pears cooked	126	31.70
Peanut flour defatted	371	31.50
Prunes cooked	119	31.40
Clam fritters	311	30.90
Strawberry pie commercial	198	30.90
Garlic cloves raw	137	30.80
Orange sherbet	134	30.80

FOOD ITEM	CALS.	UNITS
Banana custard pie commercial	221	30.70
Soybean flour full fat	421	30.40
Macaroni enriched or unenriched, cooked until firm	148	30.10
Pizza with sausage, homemade	234	29.60
Apple tapioca commercial	117	29.40
Maraschino cherries bottled, fruit and liquid	116	29.40
Cashew nuts	561	29.30
Cornbread homemade from whole-ground meal	207	29.10
Hash browned potatoes	229	29.10
Almond meal partially defatted	408	28.90
Bitter chocolate	505	28.90
Bread pudding with raisins, commercial	187	28.40
Soybean milk powder	429	28.00
Rice pudding with raisins, commercial	146	26.70
Popovers homemade	224	25.80
Chocolate pudding homemade	148	25.70
Brown rice cooked	119	25.50
Tomato catsup bottled	106	25.40
Coconut custard pie commercial	235	24.90
Tomato chili sauce bottled	104	24.80
Raspberries frozen, sweetened	98	24.60
Pumpkin pie commercial	211	24.50
Pudding (chocolate), instant made with milk, without cooking	125	24.40
White rice cooked	119	24.20
Sweet potato pie	213	23.70
Strawberries whole, frozen, sweetened	92	23.50
Egg noodles enriched, cooked	125	23.30
Eclairs with custard filling and chocolate frosting, commercial	239	23.20
Coconut dried, unsweentened	662	23.00
Spaghetti enriched, cooked until tender	111	23.00
Pudding (custard dessert), made with milk, commercial	131	22.60
Sweet potatoes dehydrated	95	22.60
Ice milk	152	22.40
Bananas raw	85	22.20
Pineapple frozen, sweetened	85	22.20
Apricots cooked, without added sugar, fruit and liquid	85	21.60
Dried apricots cooked, no sugar added	85	21.60
Sesame seeds dry, whole	563	21.60
Dried peaches cooked, no sugar added	82	21.40
Red beans dry, boiled and drained	118	21.40

FOOD ITEM	CALS.	UNITS
Baked potatoes with skin	93	21.10
Corn on the cob	91	21.00
Ice cream fat content 10%	193	20.80
Split peas cooked	115	20.80
Peanuts with skins, roasted	582	20.60
Cream puffs commercial	233	20.50
Pinenuts (pignolias)	635	20.50
Figs raw	80	20.30
Macaroni and cheese baked, homemade	215	20.10
Sunflower seed kernels dried	560	19.90
Horseradish raw	87	19.70
Almonds dried	598	19.50
Pistachio nuts raw	594	19.00
Prune juice bottled	77	19.00
Water chestnuts raw	79	19.00
Tomato paste canned	82	18.60
Turkey potpie baked, homemade	237	18.50
Red peppers (hot), pods	93	18.10
Pickles fresh	73	17.90
Crabapples raw	68	17.80
Plums (damson)	66	17.80
French salad dressing commercial, regular	410	17.50
Cherries (sweet), raw	70	17.40
Grapes (European), raw	67	17.30
Kumquats raw	65	17.10
Potatoes with skin, boiled	76	17.10
Tapioca cream pudding	134	17.10
Mangoes raw	66	16.80
Shallots bulbs, raw	72	16.80
Filberts (hazelnuts)	634	16.70
Jerusalem artichokes raw, freshly harvested	7	16.70
Pomegranates pulp, raw	63	16.70
Spanish rice homemade	87	16.60
Macadamia nuts	691	15.90
Vanilla pudding homemade	111	15.90
Black raspberries raw	73	15.70
Thousand Island salad dressing commercial, regular	502	15.40
Winter squash baked	63	15.40
Blueberries raw	62	15.30
Quinces raw	57	15.30

FOOD ITEM	CALS.	UNITS
Pumpkin seeds raw	553	15.00
Parsnips cooked	66	14.90
Black walnuts	628	14.80
Spaghetti with cheese in tomato sauce, homemade	104	14.80
Apples freshly harvested, with skin, raw	58	14.50
Acorn squash baked	55	14.00
Pineapple raw	52	13.70
Pineapple juice canned, unsweetened	55	13.50
Mixed vegetables frozen, boiled and drained	64	13.40
Potato salad with mayonnaise, homemade	145	13.40
Grape juice frozen concentrate, sweetened	53	13.30
Apricots raw	51	12.80
Dried safflower seeds	615	12.40
Orange raw	49	12.20
Sodas fruit flavors (10% to 13% sugar)	46	12.00
Apple juice canned or bottled	47	11.90
Hubbard squash baked	50	11.70
Pinenuts raw	552	11.60
Bass (black sea)	259	11.40
Lemonade frozen	44	11.40
Colas	90	11.00
Corn grits cooked	51	11.00
Limeade frozen concentrate	41	11.00
White sauce thick	198	11.00
Brazil nuts	654	10.90
Applesauce canned, unsweetened	41	10.80
Cranberries raw	46	10.80
Grapefruit raw	41	10.80
Soybeans dry, cooked	130	10.80
Grapefruit juice and orange juice blend, frozen, unsweetened	44	10.50
Root beer soda	41	10.50
Butternut squash boiled	41	10.40
Russian salad dressing commercial, regular	494	10.40
Orange juice frozen concentrate, unsweetened	45	10.30
Tangerine juice fresh	43	10.10
Cheese fondue homemade	265	10.00
French fried shrimp	225	10.00
Papayas raw	39	10.00
Artichokes (globe or French), boiled and drained	44	9.90

FOOD ITEM	CALS.	UNITS
Beets raw	43	9.90
Carrots raw	42	9.70
Peaches raw	38	9.70
Ginger root	49	9.50
Soy sauce	68	9.50
Greek olives	338	8.70
Onions raw	38	8.70
Parsley raw	44	8.50
Green pea soup from mix	50	8.40
Strawberries raw	37	8.40
Brussels sprouts raw	45	8.30
Scallions raw	36	8.20
Honeydew melon	33	7.70
Okra raw	36	7.60
Cantaloupe raw	30	7.50
Collards raw	45	7.50
Beets cooked	32	7.20
Carrots boiled and drained	31	7.10
Green beans raw	32	7.10
Kohlrabi raw	29	6.60
Onions cooked	29	6.50
Brussels sprouts cooked	36	6.40
Dandelion greens cooked	33	6.40
Watermelon raw	26	6.40
Broccoli raw	32	5.90
Cider vinegar	14	5.90
Chives raw	28	5.80
Pimentos canned	27	5.80
Cabbage raw	24	5.40
Green beans boiled and drained	25	5.40
Kale frozen, boiled and drained	31	5.40
Beef liver	229	5.30
Kohlrabi cooked	24	5.30
Soybean sprouts raw	46	5.30
Bamboo shoots raw	27	5.20
Yogurt made from partially skimmed milk	50	5.20
Skim milk	36	5.10
Tomato vegetable soup with noodles from mix	27	5.10
Asparagus raw	26	5.00
Turnips boiled and drained	23	4.90

FOOD ITEM	CALS.	UNITS
Whole milk	66	4.90
Yogurt made from whole milk	62	4.90
Green peppers (sweet), raw	22	4.80
Chard (Swiss), raw	25	4.60
Goat's milk	67	4.60
Broccoli cooked	26	4.50
Mushrooms raw	28	4.40
Cabbage shredded, boiled and drained	20	4.30
Spinach raw	26	4.30
Radishes (Oriental, including daikon and Chinese), raw	19	4.20
Eggplant boiled and drained	19	4.10
Bologna	277	3.70
Soybean sprouts boiled and drained	38	3.70
Asparagus spears, boiled and drained	20	3.60
Radishes raw	17	3.60
Spinach boiled and drained	23	3.60
Turnip greens leaves and stems, boiled and drained	20	3.60
Zucchini raw	17	3.60
Romaine lettuce	18	3.50
Tuna salad	170	3.50
Chicken liver simmered	165	3.10
Heavy whipping cream	352	3.10
Summer squash cooked	14	3.10
Parmesan cheese	393	2.90
Cottage cheese	86	2.70
Black olives ripe	129	2.60
Zucchini cooked	12	2.50
Tofu (soybean curd)	72	2.40
Abalone canned	80	2.30
Cheddar cheese unprocessed	398	2.10
Cream cheese	374	2.10
Blue cheese	368	2.00
Clams soft, meat and liquid	54	2.00
Frankfurters	304	1.60
Swiss cheese pasteurized, processed	355	1.60
Salami cooked	311	1.40
Green olives pickled, canned or bottled	116	1.30
Eggs hard-boiled	163	.90
Tomatoes ripe, raw	22	.50
Anchovies	176	.30

FOOD ITEM	CALS.	UNITS
Cauliflower raw	27	.20
Alcoholic beverages (gin, rum, vodka, and whiskey)	231	.00
Beef all cuts	327	.00
Bluefish baked or broiled	159	.00
Boiled ham	234	.00
Cod broiled	170	.00
Coffee instant	1	.00
Corned beef medium fat content, cooked	372	.00
Country-style sausage	345	.00
Crab steamed	93	.00
Deviled ham canned	351	.00
Eggs whole, fresh	163	.00
Finnan haddie (smoked haddock)	103	.00
Fish flour from whole fish	336	.00
Flounder baked	202	.00
Frankfurters made with cereal	248	.00
Frankfurters canned	221	.00
Haddock fried	165	.00
Halibut (Atlantic and Pacific), broiled	171	.00
Herring (Atlantic), canned	208	.00
Lamb leg, prime grade, roasted	319	.00
Lard	902	.00
Lobster canned or cooked	95	.00
Mackerel broiled	236	.00
Oils salad or cooking	884	.00
Polish-style sausage	336	.00
Pompano	N.A.	.00
Pork medium fat class, roasted	373	.00
Pork sausage cooked	476	.00
Potted meats (beef, chicken, and turkey)	248	.00
Salmon (Atlantic), canned, solids and liquids	203	.00
Salt	0	.00
Shrimp canned, solids and liquid	80	.00
Smelt (Atlantic, jack, and bay), canned, solids and liquid	200	.00
Sturgeon steamed	160	.00
Sweetbreads (calf), braised	168	.00
Swordfish broiled	174	.00
Tongue medium fat content	62	.00
Tripe commercial	100	.00
Trout (rainbow or steelhead), canned	209	.00

CARBOHYDRATES 55

FOOD ITEM	CALS.	UNITS
Tuna canned in water, solids and liquid	127	.00
Turkey all classes, dark meat, roasted	203	.00
Veal chuck, medium fat content, braised	235	.00
Vienna sausage canned	240	.00
Weakfish broiled	208	.00
White fish smoked	155	.00

Fat

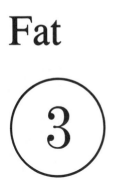

When we think of fat, what is the first thing that comes to mind? A creamy, velvety, delicious bowl of ice cream? Cream cheese with lox, a juicy steak? Perhaps bacon, fried crisp? People are hooked on fat, that is, the substance that provides foods such as butter, eggs, meats, nuts, and oils with their smooth consistency. Americans receive nearly 45 percent of their total caloric intake from fats.

For decades we indulged in highly saturated fatty foods. We felt no fear — only occasional guilt depending on our weight. We now know that we had deceived ourselves; that our overindulgence in highly fatty foods contributed not only to overweight, but also in no small part to the degeneration of our heart and blood vessels. The resulting conditions such as atherosclerosis, a fatty plaque buildup inside the arteries, reduce the blood flow through the arteries (and increase blood pressure). The American Heart Association in April 1982 declared that we should reduce the amount of saturated fat and cholesterol in our diet to help prevent heart disease.

Let's examine fat to see how we can monitor our intake of that substance using the list that follows to know which foods have high, moderate, or low fat content so that we can intelligently choose our foods to consume only a healthy level.

We should not avoid fat completely. Reducing the fat in

your diet doesn't mean eliminating it. People have a tendency to overreact, much as they did with the cholesterol scare, completely abandoning highly nutritious foods such as eggs, which contain cholesterol, out of the fear that the eggs would give them a heart attack or some other degenerative disease. So, too, with fat. Now that we have been able to show a correlation between degenerative disease and excess saturated fat in the diet, what then is the proper amount and why do we need fat at all?

Benefits of Fat

Fat is one of the primary nutrients to the body. We need it in small amounts because it allows us to use the fat-soluble vitamins A, D, E, and K which are essential for the health of our immune system. Fat helps prevent viral infections, protects our heart, blood vessels, and internal organs, slows down the aging process, and keeps the skin healthy. In fact, people who severely deprive themselves of fat can suffer the reverse of all the above conditions. Most important, fats, like carbohydrates, are a usable essential source of energy. Fats serve as a backup — a reserve supply of energy deposited in various locations throughout the body called adipose tissue.

There have been periods of time throughout history, especially during prolonged wars and famine, when nutritional survival was correlated to the amount of "stored energy" fat in the body. Because the body could burn its stored fat for energy, protein was spared from being oxidized as an energy source.

Fat is a concentrated source of energy. It yields 9 calories per gram upon oxidation, whereas protein and carbohydrates yield 4 calories. Therefore a little bit of fat goes a long way in allowing you to carry on normal body functions.

Fat is also essential in padding the body. Nearly 40 to 45 percent of your internal abdominal cavity is filled with fat; it cushions the kidneys, preventing them from being bruised or damaged from the constant shaking and jarring of walking or the more rigorous strains of jogging, biking, and other athletic activity. You need some fat around your internal organs to prevent bruising, hemorrhage, or rupture. Fat acts as a great shock absorber, but you don't want too much, because it then not only surrounds the organs but penetrates them. It laces itself through the organs and through the muscle tissue. With too much intramuscular fat your risks of disease (heart disease, diabetes, etc.) increase.

Your body fat also acts as an insulator. In colder climates such as found in Alaska, Sweden, Finland, Siberia, Norway, Iceland, Greenland, and other Arctic areas, the population may seem, by our standards, overweight. However, it may be necessary to be slightly fatter for added insulation to help prevent excessive heat loss. Of course, the opposite is true in tropical climates. You would not want any excess fat there because the body needs to perspire to cool itself. The fat would have the same effect as wearing thermal underwear. It could raise the blood pressure. It could create excess strain on the heart and cardiovascular system in cooling the body, adding to the risk of stroke or heart attack.

Fats are essential in the utilization of nutrients and the production of hormones. In fact, much of your body's chemistry revolves around the proper utilization of fat. Therefore, fat, in the proper quality and quantity is healthy.

Saturated vs. Unsaturated Fats

Saturated fats are basically found in animal food sources such as meat and dairy products, which constitute half of the USDA's dietary recommendations for the "basic four food groups." "Saturated fat" means that the carbon atom chain that composes the fat is saturated with hydrogen atoms. Generally speaking, fat is saturated if it is solid at room temperature. Examples include butter; the fatty part of chicken, fish, veal, lamb, pork, and beef — the actual marbled fat that you can see; lard; and coconut oil. The unsaturated fats are primarily found in grains, legumes, seeds, nuts, and the oils derived from them, including corn oil, safflower, sunflower, and soy oil, which are liquid at room temperature. These are the oils that should represent the majority of our fat intake, the unsaturated fats. Essential fatty acids are provided by the unsaturated fats. These are linoleic acid, linolenic acid, and oleic acid. They have several vital functions: controlling high blood pressure; precursor of prostaglandins; regulator of cell permeability. The body is capable of manufacturing those fatty acids not considered "essential" if your diet is not providing them.

How Much Fat to Consume

No one, including nutritionists or medical authorities, can agree on how much fat is necessary in the diet. Some state that it should be 25 percent of our total caloric intake, others say 30 percent, and still others say as little 10 percent.

Your consumption of calories from fat should be limited to 15 percent and 25 percent of these calories should be saturated. The other three-fourths should come from the unsaturated fats found in cooking and salad oils or, more beneficially, from those naturally occurring in vegetables, grains, legumes, nuts, and seeds. In their natural state, if they are unbleached, unadulterated, and have not been clarified or chemically altered to destroy their nutritive benefits, oils not only provide you with fat that the body can utilize, but also supply vitamin E, which has antioxidant properties. From a properly balanced diet, you will obtain more than enough fats without the need to supplement more.

Hydrogenation

You may wonder what's the importance of "hydrogenated" fats. Once a vegetable oil has been hydrogenated (a process carried out in the presence of a metal catalyst such as nickel) and becomes solid it is no longer a polyunsaturated fat. It is now a saturated fat. The problem or confusion lies in that it was originally made from a polyunsaturated oil but now it is no longer polyunsaturated. So be wary of those food labels declaring the product to be made from polyunsaturates — including salad oils, margarine, and egg and cream substitutes. That part of the statement is true. What they may fail to mention is that now you are eating a saturated fat.

Although the consumption of unsaturated fats is essential for meeting our requirements for fatty acids, they are very easily oxidized and highly reactive. The overconsumption of unsaturated fats may result in premature aging, liver damage, blood disease, and possibly breast cancer.

Fats for Dieters

One of the reasons doctors prescribe high-fat, high-protein, low-carbohydrate diets is because of the satiety or "staying power" of that fat and protein in a meal. If you eat a complex carbohydrate in the form of a grain or vegetable, it is digested and goes through your system in a matter of thirty to eighty minutes. You benefit from the energy and you're not taxing your digestive system. But it also means there's a tendency to get hungry sooner. Do you remember the last time you had a Chinese meal of vegetables and an hour later were hungry again? But we have a tendency to gain weight because of our preoccupation with in-between meal snacks. Those snacks are usually in the form of high-sugar, refined carbohydrate foods like jelly rolls, candy bars, and soft drinks. These can put 200 to 400 calories per snack back into our system, adding to our total caloric load, and we gain weight. But a fatty or high-protein food eaten at mealtime will require four to six hours of digestion just to empty out the stomach. As long as we have that much food in our stomach, our appetite is repressed so we do not feel hungry. Therefore we can bypass the midmorning snack, midafternoon snack, and late evening snack and eliminate 400 to 900 calories. In a period of a week you would be able to knock off a pound just by modifying the diet to reduce snacks and the protein and fat content. This is not necessarily ideal or healthy but it does explain why we don't feel hungry on a high-protein, high-fat diet.

Fat's Danger

But there are certain things about fats that could be harmful in this process. Many people like deep-fried foods: french fries, onion rings, fried fish, potato chips, doughnuts, and other foods. These are prepared with fatty oils heated to high temperatures, which alter the chemical structure of the fat, creating free fatty acids, which can produce an irritating effect upon the stomach and sensitive mucous lining of the intestine. If you frequently eat fried foods, you can set into motion the ultimate dysfunction of your intestine. Colitis, spastic colon, or some other form of irritable intestine condition may be the result.

Heated fats also slow down the digestive time. The longer fat is cooked, the more difficult it is for the enzymes in the stomach and the intestine to break down the fat. Liquid fats are easier to digest. Oils go through the system much more rapidly than saturated fat.

As people age they lose the capacity to digest both protein and fats. There is a lessening of the secretion of hydrochloric acid and certain enzymes necessary for hydrolyzing fat. Gall bladder problems can inhibit fat digestion, since the gall bladder stores and secretes bile, which helps break down fats.

The amount of fat in the intestine determines at what speed food will go through the intestine, because bile and fat both have the capacity to affect peristaltic action. Hence, people who eat too much fat have a tendency to be constipated. (The lack of fiber in meat, our major source of saturated fat, also contributes to this problem.) Chronic constipation increases the likelihood of developing diseases of the intestine, including colon-rectal cancer.

When you have a lot of fat in your stomach after a meal, you will find yourself lacking in energy. This is due to the fact that your energy is relegated to facilitating the proper digestion, utilization, absorption, and elimination of your food. The blood and oxygen cannot be drawn to your brain to energize you.

Older people should eliminate saturated fat as much as possible, because they are simply unable to digest it as well as they did when they were younger and it will cause them intestinal distress.

Upwards of 95 percent of the fat consumed is digested and utilized by the system. It is perfectly fine to have a certain amount of body fat as reserve, but in the absence of regular, daily exercise the muscles begin to atrophy and fat infiltration into the muscle occurs. Fat then takes the place of unused, atrophied muscles. We lose our strength, endurance and stamina, and we become more susceptible to bodily injury, accident, and disease. In order to be truly healthy we must restrict not only the amount of saturated fat in the diet but also the amount of fat that ends up as part of our muscular and body structure. Even models who are very thin can have fat-infiltrated muscles if they fail to exercise for fear of developing their muscles. No matter what your age, you should try to develop, with the guidance of a qualified health professional, a daily exercise program for total body fitness, to burn up muscle fat and to strengthen existing muscles. Good appearance is not merely a matter of being the right weight. A football player could weigh 200 pounds and have a very low percentage of total body fat, but if a year after retiring from football he still weighed 200 pounds but his muscles had atrophied and fat had taken their place, then he would be not only overweight but overfat.

There are now centers throughout the U.S. where you can check to see what your ideal body fat and muscle content is. Muscle is more dense and heavier than fat, so don't be surprised if with the proper diet and exercise regimen you actually gain a little weight. That is not a disadvantage as long as the weight is muscle and not fat.

The unit value for fat is given in grams. Any food having less than 1 gram of fat per 100-gram portion is considered to have a trace fat content and is listed as having .00 for its unit value.

Where the symbol N. A. appears in the calorie column, the information was not available.

All figures are based on an edible portion equaling 100 grams, or approximately 3 ounces. In the case of some of the listed foods, one would not consume 100 grams in one serving. Calculations should be adjusted accordingly.

Fat

FOOD ITEM	CALS.	UNITS
Lard	902	100.00
Butter oil dehydrated	876	99.50
Butter	716	81.00
Margarine	720	81.00
Mayonnaise	718	79.90
Beef fat cooked	729	78.10
Lamb fat cooked	709	75.60
Macadamia nuts	691	71.60
Bacon cured, canned	685	71.50
Pecans	687	71.20
French salad dressing homemade	632	70.10
Hickory nuts	673	68.70
Brazil nuts	654	66.90
Coconut meat dried, unsweetened	662	64.90
Walnuts	651	64.00

FOOD ITEM	CALS.	UNITS
Filberts (hazelnuts)	634	62.40
Butternuts	629	61.20
Pinenuts	635	60.50
Italian salad dressing commercial, regular	552	60.00
Safflower seed kernels	615	59.50
Black walnuts	628	59.30
Tartar sauce regular	531	57.80
Almonds roasted and salted	627	57.20
Almonds dried	598	54.20
Pistachio nuts	594	53.70
Sesame seeds dry, hulled	582	53.40
Bitter or baking chocolate	505	53.00
Blue cheese or Roquefort salad dressing commercial, regular	504	52.30
Bacon cured, broiled or fried, drained	611	52.00
Russian salad dressing commercial, regular	494	50.80
Peanut butter fat and sweetener added	589	50.60
Thousand Island salad dressing commercial, regular	502	50.20
Peanuts roasted and salted	585	49.80
Peanut butter small amount of fat and sweetener added	582	49.50
Sesame seeds whole, dried	563	49.10
Peanuts with skins, roasted	582	48.70
Peanuts without skins, raw	568	48.40
Peanuts with skins, raw	564	47.50
Dried sunflower seed kernels	560	47.30
Dried pumpkin and squash seed kernels	553	46.70
Lamb rib, prime grade, broiled	492	46.50
Capicola (sausage meat)	499	45.80
Cashew nuts	561	45.70
Beef hip, choice grade, broiled	487	44.90
Beef ribs 11 to 12, choice grade, roasted	481	44.70
Country style ham long cured dry, fat class	460	44.00
Chocolate-coated almonds	569	43.70
Beef T-bone, choice grade, broiled	473	43.20
Pork spareribs fat class, braised	467	42.50
Beef Porterhouse, choice grade, broiled	465	42.20
Peanuts chocolate-coated	561	41.30
Beef club steak, choice grade, broiled	454	40.60
Potato chips	568	39.80

FOOD ITEM	CALS.	UNITS
Beef Porterhouse steak, good grade, broiled	446	39.70
Bittersweet chocolate	477	39.70
Beef loin, ribs 6 to 12, choice grade, roasted	440	39.40
Beef T-bone steak, good grade, broiled	442	39.20
Coconut meat shredded, sweetened	548	39.10
Beef sirloin steak, good grade, roasted	441	39.00
French salad dressing regular, commercial	410	38.90
Pork spareribs medium fat class, braised	440	38.90
Pork sausage canned, solids and liquids	415	38.40
Salami dry	450	38.10
Beef 6th rib, choice grade, braised	437	38.00
Brown-and-serve sausage	422	37.80
Cream cheese	374	37.70
Heavy whipping cream	352	37.60
Sausage (cervelat), dry, commercial	451	37.60
Lamb loin, prime grade, broiled	420	37.30
Beef chuck, 5th rib, choice grade, braised	427	36.70
Potato sticks	544	36.40
Beef loin end or sirloin, ribs 11 to 12, good grade, roasted	417	36.30
Pork picnic, fat class, simmered	420	36.20
Greek olives	338	35.80
Chocolate (semi-sweet)	507	35.70
Lamb chops rib, choice grade, broiled	407	35.60
Coconut meat fresh	346	35.30
Chocolate (sweet)	528	35.10
Country-style ham long cured, dry, medium fat class	389	35.10
Pork spareribs thin fat class, broiled	410	35.10
Ham dry, long cured, medium fat class	380	35.00
Ham medium fat class, roasted	389	35.00
Beef sirloin steak, double-bone, choice grade, broiled	408	34.70
Piecrust commercial	500	33.40
Beef club steak, good grade, broiled	398	33.30
Pork Boston butt, fat class, roasted	389	33.20
Pork sausage canned, drained solids	381	32.80
Deviled ham canned	351	32.30
Milk chocolate plain	520	32.30
Cheddar cheese unprocessed	398	32.20
Coconut cream liquid expressed, from grated coconut meat	334	32.20
Beef loin end or sirloin, choice grade, broiled	387	32.00
Peanut bars	515	32.00

FOOD ITEM	CALS.	UNITS
Lamb chops rib, good grade, broiled	378	31.90
Lamb shoulder, prime grade, roasted	374	31.70
Peanuts boiled	376	31.50
Brownies with nuts, homemade	485	31.30
Light whipping cream	300	31.30
Country-style sausage	345	31.10
Egg yolks raw	348	30.60
Ham medium fat class, roasted	374	30.60
Blue cheese or Roquefort cheese	368	30.50
Brick cheese	370	30.50
Pork picnic, medium- fat class, roasted	374	30.50
Corned beef medium fat content, boneless, cooked	372	30.40
Beef chuck, 5th rib, good grade, braised	377	30.30
Chocolate chip cookies homemade from enriched flour	516	30.10
American cheese pasteurized, processed	370	30.00
Beef 6th rib, choice grade, braised	373	29.90
Pound cake homemade	473	29.50
Lamb loin, choice grade, broiled	359	29.40
Piecrust from mix, prepared with water	464	29.10
Beef tongue smoked	N.A.	28.80
Pork Boston butt, medium fat class, roasted	353	28.50
Beef hindshank, choice grade	361	28.10
Limburger cheese	345	28.00
Swiss cheese (domestic), unprocessed	370	28.00
Cream substitute from skim milk	509	27.70
Bologna	304	27.50
Whole milk dry	502	27.50
Liverwurst smoked	319	27.40
Beef rump, choice grade, roasted	347	27.20
Lamb shoulder, choice grade, roasted	338	27.20
Lamb loin, good grade, broiled	341	27.00
Swiss cheese pasteurized, processed	355	26.90
Cream substitute from skim milk, dry	508	26.70
Doughnuts yeast leavened	414	26.70
Parmesan cheese	393	26.00
Polish-style sausage	304	25.80
Ham Boston butt, medium fat class, roasted	330	25.70
Liverwurst	307	25.60
Salami cooked	311	25.60
Mackerel salted	305	25.10

FOOD ITEM	CALS.	UNITS
Cookies plain	496	25.00
Country-style pork long-cured, dry, lean	310	25.00
Ham long cured, thin	310	25.00
Mortadella	315	25.00
Coconut milk	252	24.90
Cured ham canned, spiced or unspiced	294	24.90
Camembert cheese	299	24.70
Pork picnic, thin class, simmered	329	24.70
Beef loin end or sirloin, wedge and round bone, good grade	353	24.50
Coconut bar cookies	494	24.50
Sausage (cervelat), soft	307	24.50
Sardines (Atlantic), canned in oil, solids and liquid	311	24.40
American cheese food pasteurized, processed	323	24.00
Lamb leg, prime grade, roasted	319	24.00
Beef chuck, ribs 1 to 5, choice grade, braised	327	23.90
Peanut cheese crackers commercial	491	23.90
Cocoa powder high fat	299	23.70
Pork Boston butt, thin class, roasted	317	23.70
Chow mein noodles canned	489	23.50
Danish pastry commercial	422	23.50
Graham crackers (chocolate-coated)	475	23.50
Beef rump, good grade, roasted	317	23.40
Knockwurst	278	23.20
Macaroons commercial	475	23.20
Sweetbreads (beef), braised	320	23.20
Cookies (shortbread), commercial	498	23.10
Fudge (chocolate-coated), with caramel and peanuts	459	23.10
Tongue potted or deviled	290	23.00
Pecan pie commercial	418	22.90
Bologna all meat	277	22.80
Cookies (sandwich), commercial	495	22.50
Tartar sauce low calorie, commercial	224	22.40
Bread stuffing from mix	358	21.80
Popcorn popped, oil and salt added	456	21.80
Corn fritters commercial	377	21.50
American cheese spread pasteurized, processed	288	21.40
Cheese crackers commercial	479	21.30
Beef hindshank, good grade, simmered	307	21.20
Lamb shoulder, good grade, roasted	322	21.10

FOOD ITEM	CALS.	UNITS
Chocolate chip cookies commercial	471	21.00
Chocolate fudge (chocolate-coated), with nuts	452	20.80
Bologna made with cereal	262	20.60
Light cream	211	20.60
Tuna canned in oil, solids and liquids	288	20.50
Hamburger regular, ground, broiled	286	20.30
Soybean flour	421	20.30
Soybean milk powder, sweetened	429	20.30
Assorted cookies commercial	480	20.20
Mission olives large	184	20.10
Vienna sausage canned	240	19.80
Sugar wafers	485	19.40
Beef chuck, arm, choice grade, braised	289	19.20
Peanut cookies commercial	473	19.10
Cocoa powder medium fat content	265	19.00
Ocean perch breaded, frozen, fried, reheated	319	18.90
Doughnuts cake type	391	18.60
Lamb leg, choice grade, roasted	279	18.60
Strained egg yolk (baby food), commercial	210	18.40
Almond meal partially defatted	408	18.30
Cheese fondue homemade	265	18.30
Egg yolk with ham or bacon (baby food), commercial	208	18.10
Frankfurters canned	221	18.10
Fudge (chocolate-coated), with caramel and peanuts	433	18.10
Fish cakes frozen, fried, reheated	270	17.90
Butter crackers commercial	458	17.80
Pork and gravy (90% pork), canned	256	17.80
Coconut (chocolate-coated)	438	17.60
Canadian bacon broiled or fried, drained	277	17.50
Baking-powder biscuits homemade	372	17.40
Chocolate fudge with nuts	426	17.40
Caramel cake homemade	385	17.30
Lamb leg good grade, roasted	266	17.30
Devil's food cake homemade	366	17.20
Eggs fried	216	17.20
Cheese souffle homemade	218	17.10
Raisins (chocolate-coated)	425	17.10
Vanilla creams (chocolate-coated)	435	17.10
Butter cookies thin, rich, commercial	457	16.90
French salad dressing low calorie	228	16.90

FOOD ITEM	CALS.	UNITS
Veal rib, medium fat content, roasted	269	16.90
Sugar cookies thick, homemade	444	16.80
Beef tongue medium fat content, braised	344	16.70
Caviar pressed	316	16.70
Light fruitcake homemade	389	16.50
Devil's food cake with chocolate frosting, homemade	369	16.40
Vanilla fudge with nuts	424	16.40
Caramels plain or chocolate, with nuts	428	16.30
Ice cream fat content 16%	222	16.10
Vanilla wafers commercial	462	16.10
Chocolate fudge (chocolate-coated)	430	16.00
White cake homemade	375	16.00
Bass (black sea), baked	259	15.80
Herring smoked, hard	300	15.80
Mackerel (Atlantic), boiled	236	15.80
Cookies (chocolate), commercial	445	15.70
White sauce thick	198	15.60
Beef round, choice grade, broiled	261	15.40
Chicken ribs, fried	298	15.40
Oatmeal cookies with raisins, commercial	451	15.40
Dark fruitcake homemade	379	15.30
Pie (chocolate chiffon), commercial	328	15.30
Herring salted or brined	218	15.20
Ham croquette	251	15.10
Pickled herring (Bismarck)	223	15.10
Caviar (sturgeon)	262	15.00
Clam fritters	311	15.00
Smoked halibut	224	15.00
Caramel cake with caramel frosting, homemade	379	14.80
Chile con carne without beans, canned	200	14.80
Beef chuck, arm, good grade, braised	253	14.60
Charlotte russe	286	14.60
Devil's food cake with white frosting, homemade	369	14.60
Beef potpie homemade	246	14.50
Potatoes fried	268	14.20
Chicken a la king homemade	191	14.00
Coleslaw made with mayonnaise	144	14.00
Salmon (Chinook), canned, solids and liquid	210	14.00
Whitefish (lake), stuffed, baked	215	14.00
Caramel (chocolate-coated)	416	13.90

FOOD ITEM	CALS.	UNITS
Cream puffs with custard pudding, commercial	233	13.90
Frosting (chocolate), homemade	376	13.90
Nougats (chocolate-coated)	416	13.90
Oysters fried	239	13.90
Plain cake with chocolate frosting	368	13.90
Plain cake or cupcake homemade	364	13.90
Manzanilla olives ripe	129	13.80
Olives ripe, extra large	129	13.80
Whole wheat crackers commercial	403	13.80
Chocolate syrup (fudge)	330	13.70
Thousand Island salad dressing commercial, low calorie	180	13.70
Eclairs with custard filling and chocolate frosting, commercial	239	13.60
Herring canned, solids and liquid	208	13.60
Chicken potpie homemade	235	13.50
Smelt (Atlantic, jack, and bay), canned, solids and liquid	200	13.50
Turkey potpie homemade	237	13.50
Trout (rainbow), canned	209	13.40
Veal loin, medium fat content, broiled	234	13.40
Ocean perch fried	227	13.30
Calf liver fried	261	13.20
French fried potatoes	274	13.20
Marshmallow cookies commercial	409	13.20
Meatloaf	200	13.20
Beef roast, canned	224	13.00
Smoked mackerel	219	13.00
Soda crackers	439	13.00
Eggs scrambled	173	12.90
Kippered herring	211	12.90
Omelets	173	12.90
Bread stuffing from mix, made with water, eggs, and table fat	208	12.80
Cocoa low to medium fat content	220	12.70
Green olives pickled, canned or bottled	116	12.70
Mayonnaise salad dressing commercial, low calorie	136	12.70
Yellow cake homemade	363	12.70
Ice cream fat content 12%	207	12.60
Lemon chiffon pie commercial	313	12.60
Coconut custard pie commercial	235	12.50
Frozen custard fat content 12%	162	12.50
Turkey canned	202	12.50
Smoked herring (bloaters)	196	12.40

FOOD ITEM	CALS.	UNITS
Coleslaw homemade, with French dressing	129	12.30
Chocolate fudge	400	12.20
Ham canned	193	12.20
Salmon (Atlantic), canned, solids and liquid	203	12.20
Sardines (Pacific), canned in tomato sauce, solids and liquid	197	12.20
Pineapple chiffon pie commercial	288	12.10
Soybean flour high fat content	380	12.10
Cherry pie frozen, commercial	291	12.00
Coconut custard pie frozen, commercial	249	12.00
Corned beef canned, medium fat content, cooked	216	12.00
Kidneys braised	252	12.00
Saltine crackers commercial	433	12.00
Sardines (Pacific), canned in brine, solids and liquid	196	12.00
Chicken (fryers), with skin, fried	249	11.80
Chicken canned, boned	198	11.70
Half-and-half cream	134	11.70
Poached eggs	163	11.60
Eggs hard-boiled	163	11.50
Hash-browned potatoes frozen, cooked	224	11.50
Mince pie commercial	271	11.50
Wheat germ toasted	391	11.50
Chicken (thighs), fried	237	11.40
Graham crackers honey-coated, commercial	411	11.40
Spoonbread white whole-ground cornmeal, homemade	195	11.40
Cherry pie commercial	261	11.30
Corned beef hash with potatoes, canned	181	11.30
Cottage pudding homemade	344	11.30
Hamburger lean, cooked	219	11.30
Shad baked	201	11.30
Sweet potato pie commercial	213	11.30
Chicken (giblets), fried	252	11.20
Pumpkin pie commercial	211	11.20
Apple pie commercial	256	11.10
Macaroni and cheese baked, homemade	215	11.10
Mackerel canned, solids and liquid	183	11.10
Sardines (Atlantic), canned in oil, drained solids	203	11.10
Vanilla fudge	398	11.10
Blackberry pie commercial	243	11.00
Wheat germ raw, commercially milled	363	10.90
Blueberry pie commercial	242	10.80

FOOD ITEM	CALS.	UNITS
French fried shrimp	225	10.80
Gingerbread homemade from enriched flour	317	10.70
Peach pie commercial	255	10.70
Pineapple pie commercial	253	10.70
Raisin pie commercial	270	10.70
Beef liver fried	229	10.60
Frozen custard fat content 10%	193	10.60
Ice cream fat content 10%	193	10.60
Lobster Newburg	194	10.60
Molasses cookies commercial	422	10.60
Fondant (chocolate-coated)	410	10.50
Herring canned in tomato sauce, solids and liquid	176	10.50
Tuna salad	170	10.50
Peanut brittle	421	10.40
Caramels plain or chocolate	399	10.20
Chicken (fryer), drumstick, fried	235	10.20
Lemon meringue pie commercial	255	10.20
Menhaden (Atlantic), canned, solids and liquid	172	10.20
Corn muffins homemade from enriched, degermed cornmeal	314	10.10
Mackerel Pacific, canned, solids and liquid	180	10.00
Bran muffins homemade	261	9.80
Animal crackers commercial	384	9.40
Boston cream pie commercial	302	9.40
Crackers plain, commercial	384	9.40
Deviled crab	188	9.40
Banana custard pie commercial	221	9.30
Blueberry muffins homemade	281	9.30
Pizza with sausage topping, homemade	234	9.30
Smoked salmon	176	9.30
Peanut flour defatted	371	9.20
Popovers commercial	224	9.20
Potato salad made with hard-boiled eggs and mayonnaise, homemade	145	9.20
Buckwheat pancakes from mix	200	9.10
Red pepper pods dried	340	9.10
Sweet rolls commercial	316	9.10
Fish sticks cooked	176	8.90
Ginger snaps commercial	420	8.90
Cottage pudding with chocolate sauce	318	8.80

FOOD ITEM	CALS.	UNITS
Cottage pudding with fruit sauce	292	8.80
Zwieback	423	8.80
Condensed milk sweetened	321	8.70
Pineapple custard pie commercial	220	8.70
Rolls homemade	339	8.70
Shad creole	152	8.70
Bass oven fried	196	8.50
Cornbread from mix	233	8.40
Cream of asparagus soup canned, condensed	54	8.40
French fried potatoes frozen, heated	220	8.40
Scallops fried	194	8.40
Malted milk powder	410	8.30
Pizza with a cheese topping, homemade	236	8.30
Turkey all classes, dark meat, roasted	203	8.30
Caramels (chocolate-flavored)	396	8.20
Flounder baked	202	8.20
Safflower seed meal partially defatted	355	8.20
Tuna canned in oil, drained solids	197	8.20
Corned beef lean	185	8.00
Cream of mushroom soup canned, condensed	111	8.00
Fish cakes fried	172	8.00
Cocoa powder low fat	187	7.90
Coconut custard pie from mix	203	7.90
Evaporated milk canned, unsweetened	137	7.90
Potatoes au gratin with cheese	145	7.90
Strawberry pie commercial	198	7.90
Brown-and-serve rolls	328	7.80
Corn muffins from mix, made with eggs and water	297	7.80
Ladyfinger cookies commercial	360	7.80
Chicken and noodles	153	7.70
Coconut frosting commercial	364	7.70
Chicken (baby food), commercial	127	7.60
Crab imperial	147	7.60
Natto (fermented soybean product)	167	7.40
Salmon cooked, broiled, or baked	182	7.40
Pancakes from mix	225	7.30
Smoked whitefish (lake)	155	7.30
Soybean milk concentrated, sweetened	126	7.30
Cornbread made from whole-ground meal	207	7.20
Coho salmon canned	153	7.10

FOOD ITEM	CALS.	UNITS
Frankfurters and beans canned	144	7.10
Pizza frozen, baked	245	7.10
Barbecue sauce	91	6.90
Chop suey with meat, homemade	120	6.80
Cream of shrimp soup frozen, made with milk	99	6.70
Frosting (caramel), commercial	360	6.70
Soybean flour	356	6.70
Cottonseed flour	356	6.60
Dried cranberries	368	6.60
White frosting uncooked, commercial	376	6.60
Biscuits canned	277	6.40
Haddock fried	165	6.40
Lobster salad	110	6.40
Oyster stew made with milk, homemade	97	6.40
Brown mustard	91	6.30
Bread pudding with raisins, commercial	187	6.10
Chili con carne with beans, canned	133	6.10
Corn bread made with degermed meal	224	6.00
Swordfish broiled	174	6.00
Blue cheese salad dressing low calorie, commercial	76	5.90
Pink salmon canned	141	5.90
Pork (baby food), commercial	134	5.90
Cream of mushroom soup canned, condensed, prepared with milk	88	5.80
Flaked oats (cereal)	397	5.70
Soybeans dry, cooked	130	5.70
Sponge cake homemade	297	5.70
Fig bars commercial	358	5.60
Vegetables with wheat and soy protein	150	5.60
Custard baked, commercial	115	5.50
Green peppers stuffed with beef and bread crumbs, home-made	170	5.50
Oatmeal (baby food), commercial	375	5.50
Puffed oats (cereal)	397	5.50
Cod broiled	170	5.30
Corn pone made from white whole-ground cornmeal, home-made	204	5.30
Raisin cookies commercial	379	5.30
Bluefish baked or broiled	159	5.20
Johnnycake made with yellow degermed cornmeal	267	5.20

FOOD ITEM	CALS.	UNITS
Salmon (chum), canned, solids and liquid	139	5.20
Ice milk	152	5.10
Lamb (baby food), commercial	121	5.10
Tapioca cream pudding commercial	134	5.10
Cream of shrimp soup frozen, made with water	66	5.00
Hot chocolate homemade	95	5.00
New England clam chowder frozen, made with milk	86	5.00
Popcorn plain	386	5.00
Cereal, egg yolk, and bacon dinner (baby food), commercial	82	4.90
Oyster stew with milk, commercial	84	4.90
Cream of chicken soup canned, condensed	79	4.80
Turkey liver simmered	174	4.80
Chocolate pudding homemade	148	4.70
Corn pudding commercial	104	4.70
Italian salad dressing commercial, low calorie	50	4.70
Spaghetti with meatballs in tomato sauce, homemade	134	4.70
White beans with pork and sweet sauce	150	4.70
Bread crumbs	392	4.60
Chicken with vegetables (baby food), commercial	100	4.60
Hot cocoa homemade	97	4.60
Miso (fermented soybean product)	171	4.60
Wheat bran crude, commercially milled	213	4.60
Pretzels	390	4.50
Rolls from mix	299	4.50
Salmon rice loaf	122	4.50
Malted milk	104	4.40
Yellow mustard prepared	75	4.40
Beef and vegetable stew homemade	89	4.30
French salad dressing commercial, low calorie	96	4.30
Mashed potatoes made with milk and table fat, homemade	94	4.30
Cottage cheese creamed	106	4.20
Cream of celery soup canned, condensed	72	4.20
Cream of chicken soup made with milk	73	4.20
Puffed corn (cereal)	399	4.20
Tofu (soy bean curd)	72	4.20
Chestnuts dried	377	4.10
Spaghetti with meatballs in tomato sauce, canned	103	4.10
Beef (baby food), commercial	118	4.00
Chicken chow mein without noodles, homemade	102	4.00
Cream of mushroom soup canned, condensed	56	4.00

FOOD ITEM	CALS.	UNITS
Goat's milk	67	4.00
Macaroni and cheese canned	95	4.00
Puffed rice (cereal), honey or cocoa added	401	4.00
Cornmeal whole ground, unbolted	355	3.90
Cream of potato soup frozen, prepared with milk	72	3.90
Potatoes scalloped, without cheese	104	3.90
Vanilla pudding homemade	111	3.90
Chocolate rennet custard from mix	102	3.80
Cream of celery soup made with milk	69	3.80
Beef with vegetables (baby food), commercial	87	3.70
Chestnut flour	362	3.70
Fish loaf cooked	124	3.70
High-protein cereal (baby food), commercial	357	3.70
Mashed potatoes made from granules	96	3.60
Whole milk	66	3.60
Whole wheat bread toasted, made with milk	289	3.60
Apple brown betty	151	3.50
French bread toasted, commercial	338	3.50
Popcorn (sugar-coated)	383	3.50
Spaghetti with cheese in tomato sauce, homemade	104	3.50
Cornmeal whole ground, bolted	362	3.40
Oat cereal sugar coated	396	3.40
Raisin bread toasted	316	3.40
Strained liver (baby food), commercial	97	3.40
Sunflower seed flour partially defatted	339	3.40
Yogurt made from whole milk	62	3.40
Mussels (Pacific), canned, drained solids	114	3.30
Sweet potatoes (candied)	168	3.30
Chop suey with meat, canned	62	3.20
Cornmeal whole ground, self-rising	347	3.20
Dulse (seaweed)	0	3.20
Hard rolls enriched, commercial	312	3.20
Mashed potatoes made from flakes	93	3.20
New England clam chowder frozen, made with water	54	3.20
Oyster stew prepared with water, commercial	51	3.20
Turkey with vegetables (baby food), commercial	86	3.20
White bread made with 3% - 4% nonfat dry milk	270	3.20
Rice pudding with raisins, commercial'	146	3.10
Salt sticks (Vienna bread)	304	3.10
Whole wheat bread made with water, toasted	287	3.10

FOOD ITEM	CALS.	UNITS
Bouillon cubes or powder	120	3.00
Bran, sugar, and malt extract (cereal)	240	3.00
French bread enriched or unenriched	290	3.00
Swordfish canned, solids and liquid	102	3.00
Veal (baby food), commercial	107	3.00
Whole wheat bread made with milk, commercial	243	3.00
Baby cereal mixed grains	368	2.90
Cornmeal whole ground, self-rising, with soft white flour added	347	2.90
Millet whole grain	327	2.90
Raisin rolls homemade	275	2.90
Shredded wheat (cereal), sweetened	366	2.90
Vegetables and bacon with cereal (baby food), commercial	68	2.90
Mashed potatoes frozen	93	2.80
Raisin bread commercial	262	2.80
Roe (cod and shad), baked or broiled	126	2.80
Tomato soup canned, condensed, prepared with milk	69	2.80
Whole wheat rolls commercial	257	2.80
Puffed corn (cereal), fruit flavored	395	2.70
Salt rising bread toasted, commercial	297	2.70
Corn flour	368	2.60
Cracked wheat bread toasted, commercial	263	2.60
Green pea soup canned, condensed, prepared with milk	85	2.60
Split pea soup canned, condensed	118	2.60
White beans with pork and tomato sauce	122	2.60
Whole wheat bread made with water, commercial	241	2.60
Buckwheat flour dark	333	2.50
Crab canned	101	2.50
Rockfish oven steamed	107	2.50
Bread (salt rising), commercial	267	2.40
Cream of asparagus soup made with milk	60	2.40
Cream of chicken soup canned, condensed	39	2.40
Ice cream cones	377	2.40
Bean with pork soup made with water	67	2.30
Chocolate milk skim	76	2.30
Red chili peppers raw	93	2.30
Teething biscuits (baby food)	378	2.30
Cracked wheat bread commercial	263	2.20
Cream of potato soup frozen	44	2.20
Mashed potatoes made from granules, prepared with milk	79	2.20
Puffed corn (cereal), chocolate flavored	390	2.20

FOOD ITEM	CALS.	UNITS
Vegetables and ham, with cereal (baby food), commercial	64	2.20
Cream of celery soup prepared with water	36	2.10
Puffed wheat (cereal), sweetened	376	2.10
Shredded oats (cereal)	379	2.10
Split peas with ham or bacon (baby food), commercial	80	2.10
Chicken vegetable soup canned, condensed	62	2.00
Chocolate syrup thin	245	2.00
Cocoa powder	347	2.00
Fondant	364	2.00
Macaroni, tomatoes, meat, and cereal (baby food)	67	2.00
Milk partially skimmed	59	2.00
Shredded wheat (cereal)	354	2.00
Tripe commercial	100	2.00
Whole wheat flour	333	2.00
Crab	93	1.90
Gluten flour	378	1.90
Malt dry	368	1.90
Vegetables, liver and bacon with cereal (baby food), commercial	57	1.90
Bran, sugar, and defatted wheat germ (cereal)	238	1.80
Custard (baby food), commercial	100	1.80
Dried pears	268	1.80
Irish moss (seaweed), raw	N.A.	1.80
Smoked sturgeon	149	1.80
40% bran flakes (cereal)	303	1.80
Cabbage dried	308	1.70
Rye whole grain	334	1.70
Spanish rice homemade	87	1.70
Yogurt made from partially skimmed milk	50	1.70
Baker's yeast dry or active	282	1.60
Chicken noodle soup canned, condensed	53	1.60
Cornflakes with protein concentrate	378	1.60
Dried apples uncooked	275	1.60
Rice (baby food), commercial	371	1.60
Veal with vegetables (baby food), commercial	63	1.60
Vegetables and beef and cereal (baby food), commercial	56	1.60
Wheat flakes (cereal)	354	1.60
Chestnuts fresh	194	1.50
Noodles cooked	125	1.50
Oat cereal with toasted wheat germ and soy grits, cooked	62	1.50

FOOD ITEM	CALS.	UNITS
Puffed wheat (cereal)	363	1.50
Soybean milk fluid	33	1.50
Black raspberries raw	73	1.40
Bran flakes (cereal), with raisins	287	1.40
Carob flour	180	1.40
Lima bean flour	343	1.40
Minestrone soup	43	1.40
Scallops (bay and sea), steamed	112	1.40
Soybean sprouts raw	46	1.40
Vegetables and chicken with cereal (baby food), commercial	52	1.40
Boston brown bread commercial	211	1.30
Carrots dried	341	1.30
Chicken gumbo canned, condensed	46	1.30
Chicken noodle dinner (baby food), commercial	49	1.30
Dried figs	274	1.30
Onions dried	350	1.30
Rye bread (American), toasted	282	1.30
Soy sauce	68	1.30
Tripe pickled	62	1.30
Wheat and malted barley flakes (cereal)	392	1.30
Wheat flour	365	1.30
Barley (baby food), commercial	348	1.20
Buckwheat flour light	347	1.20
Cornmeal degermed, enriched	364	1.20
Green pea soup with ham, frozen	57	1.20
Lichees dried	277	1.20
Orange sherbet	134	1.20
Pumpernickel bread commercial	246	1.20
Rye wafers whole grain	344	1.20
Turkey noodle soup	33	1.20
Vegetable with beef soup frozen	35	1.20
Barley pearled	348	1.10
Beef noodle dinner (baby food), commercial	48	1.10
Beef noodle soup made with water, commercial	28	1.10
Black raspberries canned in water	51	1.10
Blue cheese salad dressing low calorie, commercial	19	1.10
Bread flour	365	1.10
Cornmeal degermed, self-rising	348	1.10
Hard candy	386	1.10
Kelp raw	N.A.	1.10

FOOD ITEM	CALS.	UNITS
Rye bread (Amercian), commercial	243	1.10
Whey dried	349	1.10
Brewer's yeast debittered	283	1.00
Chicken with rice soup canned, condensed	39	1.00
Corn on the cob sweet	91	1.00
Flour self-rising	352	1.00
Ginger root fresh	49	1.00
Grapes (American), raw	69	1.00
Manhattan clam chowder canned, condensed	33	1.00
Oatmeal or rolled oats	55	1.00
Onion soup canned, condensed	27	1.00
Torula yeast	277	1.00
Wheat flour soft, all purpose	364	1.00
Green pea soup canned, condensed	53	.90
Apples freshly harvested, pared, raw	54	.30
Agar (seaweed), raw	N.A.	.00
Angel food cake homemade	269	.00
Apple butter	186	.00
Apple juice canned or bottled	47	.00
Applesauce sweetened	91	.00
Applesauce (baby food), commercial	72	.00
Applesauce and apricots (baby food), commercial	86	.00
Apricot nectar canned	57	.00
Asparagus spears, boiled and drained	20	.00
Baker's yeast compressed	86	.00
Bamboo shoots raw	27	.00
Bananas (baby food), commercial	84	.00
Bananas raw	85	.00
Bananas and pineapple (baby food), commercial	80	.00
Bean sprouts raw	35	.00
Beef noodle soup from mix	28	.00
Beets (baby food), commercial	37	.00
Beets raw	43	.00
Blackberries raw	58	.00
Blueberries raw	62	.00
Boysenberries raw	36	.00
Broccoli raw	32	.00
Brown rice	119	.00
Brussels sprouts boiled and drained	36	.00

FOOD ITEM	CALS.	UNITS
Buttermilk cultured from skim milk	36	.00
Cabbage raw	24	.00
Cabbage (spoon), boiled and drained	14	.00
Cake flour or pastry flour	364	.00
Cantaloupe	30	.00
Carambola	35	.00
Carrots (baby food), commercial	29	.00
Carrots boiled and drained	31	.00
Cauliflower boiled and drained	22	.00
Celeriac root, raw	40	.00
Celery (green and yellow varieties), raw	17	.00
Chard, Swiss boiled and drained	18	.00
Chayote raw	28	.00
Cherries (sweet), fresh	70	.00
Chewing gum	317	.00
Chicken chow mein without noodles, canned	38	.00
Chicken gizzard simmered	148	.00
Chicken noodle soup from mix	22	.00
Chicken with rice soup from mix	20	.00
Chicory (endive), raw	15	.00
Chicory greens raw	20	.00
Chili pepper hot, canned in chili sauce	21	.00
Chili sauce	20	.00
Chinese cabbage raw	14	.00
Chives raw	28	.00
Clams canned, solids and liquid	52	.00
Coconut water	22	.00
Collards boiled and drained	33	.00
Corn	83	.00
Corn grits degermed	51	.00
Corn, wheat, and rice flakes (cereal)	389	.00
Cornflakes plain and sugar coated	386	.00
Cornmeal degermed, cooked	50	.00
Cornstarch	362	.00
Cottage cheese uncreamed	86	.00
Crabapples raw	68	.00
Cranberries raw	46	.00
Cranberry juice cocktail	65	.00
Cranberry orange relish	178	.00
Cranberry sauce	146	.00

FAT 81

FOOD ITEM	CALS.	UNITS
Cream of asparagus soup prepared with water	27	.00
Creamed corn	82	.00
Cress raw	32	.00
Cucumber raw	14	.00
Currants	54	.00
Dandelion greens raw	45	.00
Dates (domestic), natural, dry	274	.00
Dried apples cooked, no sugar added	78	.00
Eggplant boiled and drained	19	.00
Elderberries raw	72	.00
Escarole raw	20	.00
Farina enriched, regular, cooked	42	.00
Fennel leaves, raw	28	.00
Figs raw	80	.00
Finnan haddie (smoked haddock)	103	.00
Fish flakes	111	.00
Fish flour from whole fish	336	.00
French salad dressing low fat, with artificial sweetener	10	.00
Frogs legs raw	73	.00
Fruit cocktail canned in water, with or without artificial sweetener, fruit and liquid	37	.00
Fruit dessert (baby food), commercial	84	.00
Fruit pudding (baby food), commercial	96	.00
Garlic cloves raw	137	.00
Gelatin dry	335	.00
Ginger root (candied)	340	.00
Gooseberries raw	39	.00
Grapefruit raw	41	.00
Green beans (baby food), commercial	22	.00
Green beans raw	32	.00
Green pea soup prepared with water	53	.00
Green pea soup from mix	50	.00
Green peppers (sweet), raw	22	.00
Green tomatoes	24	.00
Ground cherries raw	53	.00
Guavas whole, raw	62	.00
Gum drops	347	.00
Honeydew melon	33	.00
Horseradish prepared	38	.00
Italian bread enriched or unenriched	276	.00

FOOD ITEM	CALS.	UNITS
Jams and preserves	272	.00
Jellies	273	.00
Jelly beans	367	.00
Jerusalem artichokes raw, freshly harvested	7	.00
Kale frozen, boiled and drained	31	.00
Kohlrabi raw	29	.00
Kumquats	65	.00
Laver (seaweed)	N.A.	.00
Leeks	52	.00
Lemon candied	314	.00
Lemon juice	25	.00
Lemon peel candied	316	.00
Lemons	27	.00
Lettuce	14	.00
Lichees raw	64	.00
Lime juice canned or bottled, unsweetened	26	.00
Limes raw	28	.00
Loganberries	62	.00
Longans	61	.00
Macaroni enriched or unenriched, cooked until firm	148	.00
Mangoes raw	66	.00
Maraschino cherries bottled, fruit and liquid	116	.00
Marmalade citrus	257	.00
Marshmallows	319	.00
Mixed vegetables (baby food), commercial	37	.00
Mixed vegetables (carrots, corn, peas, green snap beans, and lima beans), frozen, boiled and drained	64	.00
Mushrooms canned, solids and liquid	17	.00
Mustard greens boiled and drained	23	.00
Mustard spinach (tendergreen), raw	22	.00
New Zealand spinach boiled and drained	13	.00
Oat and wheat cereal cooked	65	.00
Oat flakes (cereal), maple flavored	69	.00
Oat granules (cereal), maple flavored	60	.00
Okra boiled and drained	29	.00
Onion soup from mix	15	.00
Onions raw	38	.00
Orange and apricot drink (40% fruit juice), canned	50	.00
Orange juice	45	.00
Oranges	49	.00

FOOD ITEM	CALS.	UNITS
Papayas raw	39	.00
Parsley raw	44	.00
Parsnips raw	76	.00
Peaches (baby food), commercial	81	.00
Peaches raw	38	.00
Pear nectar	52	.00
Pears (baby food), commercial	66	.00
Pears raw	61	.00
Pears and pineapple (baby food), commercial	69	.00
Peas (baby food), commercial	54	.00
Peas	71	.00
Peas and carrots	53	.00
Persimmons	77	.00
Pickle relish (sweet)	138	.00
Pickles (sweet)	146	.00
Pickles (sour)	10	.00
Pimientos	27	.00
Pineapple	52	.00
Pineapple and orange drink	54	.00
Pineapple juice	55	.00
Plantains	119	.00
Plums	66	.00
Plums with tapioca (baby food), commercial	94	.00
Pomegranates	63	.00
Potato flour	351	.00
Prickly pears	42	.00
Prune juice	77	.00
Prunes	344	.00
Prunes with tapioca (baby food), commercial	86	.00
Puffed corn (cereal), plain and sweetened	390	.00
Puffed rice (cereal), plain and presweetened	390	.00
Pumpkin	33	.00
Purslane leaves	15	.00
Quinces raw	57	.00
Radishes raw	17	.00
Raisins	289	.00
Red beans boiled and drained	118	.00
Red peppers	31	.00
Red raspberries raw	57	.00
Rhubarb raw	16	.00

FOOD ITEM	CALS.	UNITS
Rice flakes (cereal)	390	.00
Rice with casein (cereal)	382	.00
Rutabagas boiled and drained	35	.00
Sapotes (marmalade plums)	125	.00
Sauerkraut canned, solids and liquid	18	.00
Shallots bulbs, raw	72	.00
Shredded corn (cereal), plain	389	.00
Shredded rice (cereal)	392	.00
Shrimp canned, solids and liquids	80	.00
Skim milk	36	.00
Skim milk dry, regular	363	.00
Soybean flour defatted	326	.00
Spaghetti enriched, cooked until firm	148	.00
Spaghetti with cheese in tomato sauce, canned	76	.00
Spinach (baby food), creamed, commercial	43	.00
Spinach raw	26	.00
Split peas cooked	115	.00
Squash (baby food), commercial	25	.00
Strawberries raw	37	.00
Succotash frozen, boiled and drained	93	.00
Sugar apples	94	.00
Summer squash boiled and drained	14	.00
Swamp cabbage boiled and drained	21	.00
Sweet potatoes (baby food), commercial	67	.00
Sweet potatoes baked with skin	141	.00
Tamarinds	239	.00
Tangerine juice	43	.00
Tangerines	46	.00
Tomato catsup bottled	106	.00
Tomato chili sauce bottled	104	.00
Tomato juice canned, concentrate	20	.00
Tomato paste canned	82	.00
Tomato puree canned, regular or low sodium	39	.00
Tomato soup (baby food), commercial	54	.00
Tomato vegetable soup with noodles from mix	27	.00
Tomatoes ripe, raw	22	.00
Tuna canned in water, solids and liquid	127	.00
Turnip greens leaves and stems, raw	28	.00
Turnips boiled and drained	23	.00
Vegetable beef soup canned, condensed	32	.00

FOOD ITEM	CALS.	UNITS
Vegetable juice cocktail canned	17	.00
Vegetable soup (baby food), commercial	37	.00
Vegetable soup with beef broth, canned	32	.00
Vegetables with wheat protein, canned	109	.00
Vegetables and liver with cereal (baby food), commercial	47	.00
Vegetables and turkey with cereal (baby food), commercial	44	.00
Vegetarian vegetable soup canned, condensed	32	.00
Welsh onions	34	.00
Wheat cereal cooked	75	.00
Whey fluid	26	.00
White beans boiled and drained	118	.00
White icing boiled	316	.00
White rice	109	.00
Whole-meal wheat (cereal)	45	.00
Winter squash baked	63	.00
Yellow beans raw	27	.00

Cholesterol

There is no one word that has caused more panic in dietary circles in the past ten years than the word cholesterol. Many people will avoid foods that contain cholesterol. Over the past thirty years, butter consumption has been down; egg consumption has been down; and dairy consumption has been down, while consumption of egg substitutes, bacon substitutes, and cream substitutes was up. In other words, sales of foods that can be chemically imitated without the use of cholesterol are booming. When the word cholesterol is used today, it was usually in a negative context. Frequently, you'll see a gentleman on television — often against a natural background, perhaps a corn field or a vegetable stand — extolling the virtues of some vegetable oil or margarine and promising that what he's selling contains no cholesterol; that it is absolutely 100 percent polyunsaturated; and that consuming this oil or margarine is one way of keeping your dietary cholesterol in check.

In point of fact, these ads do not present nearly the full story of a very misunderstood nutrient.

Cholesterol is, indeed, a nutrient. In fact, dietary cholesterol levels may have little bearing on blood cholesterol. But even if you tried, you could not eliminate all the cholesterol from your diet. Unfortunately, many Americans have tried to do just that: eliminate all foods that contain cholesterol. Many individuals on a low-protein, high-complex carbohydrate diet eliminate a substantial amount of fat from the diet — often too much. When less than 10 percent of the calories in your diet come from fat, there is reason to believe that is too low for proper body function and optimal health of the cells.

Why We Need Cholesterol

Cholesterol is a member of the fat family: it is a waxlike, solid alcohol. We call it a phospholipid, and it belongs to a group of compounds called steroids. It is a natural and essential part of all the cells in your body. You'll find cholesterol in all animal cells, including human, where it provides the framework that helps support each cell.

Cholesterol is a substantial part of the dry weight of the brain. You couldn't have proper nerve function without cholesterol. It allows the impulses to be transmitted throughout the body in uninterrupted, smooth patterns.

In addition, 80 percent of the cholesterol in your body is used by the liver. The liver is the key organ for metabolism of nutrients. It helps metabolize proteins, fats, carbohydrates, vitamins, and minerals. In particular, fat digestion depends on a secretion called bile, manufactured by the liver. The bile salts lower the surface tension of fats, emulsifying and breaking them down in the intestines. Bile also helps stimulate peristalsis, the wavelike movement of the intestine that allows food to pass at a normal rate. Whether the fat you've eaten comes from the butter on your bread, a marbled steak, or a glass of whole milk, it may be hours before it reaches your intestines, depending on what and how much you've eaten — so by then you need that bile. The liver uses cholesterol — upwards of 80 percent of the serum cholesterol circulating in the blood — to produce bile. Thus cholesterol is indispensable to fat digestion, absorption, utilization, and elimination.

Of the remaining cholesterol some is used to synthesize vitamin D and to produce adrenocortical hormones. Your sex hormones are also partially produced through the utilization of cholesterol. Your brain, your nerves, your liver, your intestines, your adrenal glands, your skin, and your sex glands all depend in large or smaller part on the substance called cholesterol for healthy functioning. So you see that a substance we have avoided, feared, and tried to eliminate is, in fact, a very necessary nutrient that is a natural part of our body's chemistry.

How the Cholesterol Scare Began

Why is it then that we fear cholesterol? Have we simply been manipulated by the financial interests of people who benefit from our lack of knowledge? The cholesterol scare all started with the famous Framingham study, a classic epidemiological analysis of risk factors in the American diet contributing to coronary heart disease. The fourteen-year study, completed in 1960, found that the major risk factors affecting middle class, suburban males were cigarette smoking, alcohol consumption, a diet in which most of the protein came from meat, and cholesterol. This study received enormous publicity in scientific circles. The data were interpreted as if they represented the final word on the entire male population of the United States. On that basis, the American Heart Association recommended that the public should be encouraged to avoid the consumption of certain foods, including eggs, that contain cholesterol.

That AHA proclamation was quickly picked up and taken advantage of by the processed food industry. Margarine and artificial cream were promoted with the message, "Look, if you don't want to get a heart attack, if you don't want heart disease, stay away from cholesterol. Here are completely safe, healthy alternatives to it."

But the AHA's warning against dietary cholesterol was premature. As a result, the American public was unjustifiably frightened away from eggs, milk, and cheese, high quality sources of protein, vitamins, and minerals. Subsequent studies have shown that dietary cholesterol does not necessarily increase serum cholesterol levels.

Dr. Roslyn Alfin-Slater of the School of Public Health at UCLA, led a group studying the effects of egg consumption on blood cholesterol over a three-month period. She divided a number of men aged twenty to sixty-six into several groups and had them consume various amounts of eggs in their diet. At various periods they would abstain from eating the eggs. She found that there was virtually no difference in the blood cholesterol levels of the various groups.

Even though eggs contain close to 250 milligrams (mg.) of

cholesterol per egg — a higher amount than almost any other food — this does not mean that we should immediately restrict consumption of eggs or eliminate them from our diet. Eggs have not been shown to be a direct cause of arteriosclerosis, atherosclerosis, or other forms of heart disease, nor necessarily to raise blood cholesterol levels. The majority of the cholesterol in your body is synthesized and produced by your body cells, and is not affected in a major way by the exogenous cholesterol coming from your food. That is really the major flaw in the whole anticholesterol argument.

Another study involved a group of burn victims. They were fed thirty-five eggs a day for nearly a month in a highly concentrated high-protein, high-calorie diet. Their cholesterol levels, below normal before the test because of the substantially altered metabolism of burn victims, were monitored throughout the study. No matter how many eggs they consumed, their cholesterol levels remained within normal limits. No adverse reactions were noted.

All the evidence either to indict or to acquit cholesterol is not in yet. But the commercials that try to manipulate us into buying cholesterol-free foods are motivated by economic interests and are pseudoscientific half-truths.

These ads have convinced many homemakers that instead of risking having their children develop heart disease, they should feed them egg substitutes instead of eggs.

Such parents would be well advised to refer to an article in *Pediatrics* in 1974 reporting a study of three groups of newborn rats placed on three different diets — Egg Beaters, whole eggs, and standard laboratory chow. The group that had consumed the standard Purina rat chow averaged about 70 grams in weight (about 2.5 ounces); those on whole eggs weighed 66.5 grams; but those on the Egg Beaters were 31.6 grams, less than half the weight of the others. The rats were weaned at five weeks; all those fed only Egg Beaters died within three to four weeks. Egg Beaters may taste like eggs — but eggs beat them hands down for nutrition.

Sources of Cholesterol

Animal foods are the primary source of cholesterol in our diet. You'll find cholesterol in eggs, cream, dairy products, organ meats (highest sources — the brain, kidney, liver, and animal fat). If you want to lower the cholesterol content of your food, the list below will show you which foods contain the most. But remember, you will produce cholesterol in your own liver, muscles, skin, and virtually all the cells of your body; the average person synthesizes nearly 1,600 to 1,700 mg. of cholesterol daily, whereas a typical low-cholesterol diet adds only 200 to 500 more mg. a day. If you're on a cholesterol-free diet you probably won't be receiving any cholesterol. But don't go overboard in eliminating cholesterol: the body can sense when it is not receiving an adequate amount from the diet, and may overcompensate and produce more cholesterol than normal. By eliminating cholesterol from the diet you may in fact be stimulating the body's internal chemistry to produce additional amounts over a short period of time.

Normal Cholesterol Levels

How do you know that your cholesterol is normal and what is normal? Cardiologists and others studying the effect of fat on the diet disagree so we don't really have a figure we can say is a normal cholesterol level. However, generally speaking, if your level is between 125 and 250 mg. per 100 milliliters of blood it would be considered in the normal range. The blood serves as the transportation for cholesterol from one part of the body to another and thus the level fluctuates constantly. One day you might have a cholesterol test and it will read high. The same test given the next day without any dietary changes, may read normal. The next it might be low. Why can you have three different readings in three days when your diet and life-style have remained the same? And how scientifically accurate can such tests be for a physician to use in deciding whether you should be on a restrictive diet or medically supervised program? What doctors fail to take into account is that your state of mind — whether you are calm or anxious, whether you are under normal everyday stress or under severe distress — can affect your cholesterol level by as much as 100 points. In fact, if you went in to have your cholesterol checked and if you were fearful of the doctor's office, if you felt anxious and out of control, or if you, like millions of others, were afraid at the prospect of having a needle stuck in your arm and having blood taken out, then just in the time that it took to walk into the doctor's office, to wait, and to have the nurse or physician draw blood, your blood cholesterol, which may have been 200 originally might have risen to 300 — and your doctor might decide to put you on a low-cholesterol diet. Whereas if you were in a better state of mind, if you were not anxious or fearful, then you might have received a much more realistic cholesterol reading. There are probably thousands of people walking around today who had normal cholesterol levels prior to having it checked, were under anxious or stressful conditions when they had it read, and because of their anxiety and stress were put on diets that deprive them of food otherwise nourishing and necessary for good health.

Your blood cholesterol fluctuates widely throughout the day. Even moderate exercise affects cholesterol levels. Dr. Meyer Friedman of San Francisco points out that too often, high cholesterol levels are blamed on dietary factors rather than behavioral patterns. Dr. Kenneth Rose of the University of Nebraska conducted a series of experiments that support this view. When his team tested animals under very stressful conditions, they found out this caused an increase in cholesterol levels.

If you have a kidney problem, as many Americans do (it's the fourth leading cause of disease in the U.S.), you may not have a normal cholesterol level. If you consume caffeine, whether in coffee, in carbonated beverages, in over-the-counter medications, or in herbal or ordinary teas, the caffeine can adversely affect your serum cholesterol level. Alcohol affects your cholesterol level and excessive alcohol affects it excessively. Closet drinkers who don't tell their physician they drink may be advised to severely alter their diet, when in fact changing their drinking habits is what is necessary to lower their cholesterol levels. If you have irregular sleeping habits, if you are pregnant, if you are on a low-protein diet, if you are a long-distance runner, too, you may have irregular cholesterol levels. In fact, the cholesterol levels of anyone who is catabolizing (breaking down) more muscle tissue than what is considered normal will be affected.

Exercise and Cholesterol

Right now ninety million Americans are involved in a regular exercise program or sports. They might play softball in the summertime, swim at their local Y, hike, bicycle, run, jog, play tennis or basketball. That's nearly 35 to 40 percent of the total American population. Of these, about one-third are involved in some sort of aerobic exercise on a regular basis. Those who are overindulging in an effort to be more competitive or to maintain ideal body weight should be aware that they are burning up protein (lean muscle tissue) as well as fat reserves. When you start catabolizing the protein in the body you will almost always have an altered cholesterol level. This is not necessarily dangerous. But it is important to let your physician know what type of and how much exercise you're doing so he or she doesn't think you are malnourished.

Other factors that can affect cholesterol levels include gallstones, infections, malnutrition, pancreatic irregularities, and diabetes. When you consider how many people suffer from various levels of subclinical malnutrition, when you consider how many diabetics there are in the U.S., then you have an idea of why it would be very easy to take any random group of Americans, check their cholesterol levels, and come out with irregularities when in fact the people's heart conditions could be normal.

How to Lower Cholesterol

From a dietary point of view, we know that sucrose (white sugar) also increases cholesterol levels. You should be just as apprehensive about consuming a white sugar product as a saturated fatty food if you are worried about your cholesterol levels.

There are other measures, short of cutting out eggs, dairy products, and organ meats, that can be taken to maintain a healthy blood cholesterol level. Vitamin C lowers cholesterol. Phospholipids such as lecithin will allow a better utilization of cholesterol in the body, where it acts as an emulsifying agent. (It does not unclog your arteries. It does not eat away cholesterol. But it does allow cholesterol to be more properly utilized.) Interestingly, the egg yolk, which does contain cholesterol, also includes substantial lecithin.

Cholesterol is Superseded

In the years since the Framingham study, other more important risk factors than cholesterol levels have been discovered. Other blood fractions are better predictors of heart disease than cholesterol: low density lipoproteins (fat-carrying proteins) are dangerous if their levels are too high; but high-density lipoproteins (HDLs) seem to offer protection against heart attack. You can increase your HDL levels by exercising regularly and by consuming lecithin in your diet.

Polyunsaturates

Polyunsaturated fats have been widely touted as an alternative to cholesterol-laden, high-saturated fats. However, ads for polyunsaturated fats are misleading. Besides, it is dangerous to sharply increase your intake of polyunsaturated fats.

Polyunsaturated fats are those that are liquid at room temperature such as salad oils and fish oils. Margarine is *not* polyunsaturated: while it may be made from what started off as 100 percent polyunsaturated oil, it is hardened by hydrogenation — which leaves it a saturated fat. Margarine is no different in its fat content than butter. Therefore, it is better to use the oil itself rather than the margarine.

But don't overdo it. It has not been shown that polyunsaturates will prevent heart disease. To the contrary, we have found that polyunsaturates for many individuals can result in the destruction of vitamin E, vital to a healthy heart. Polyunsaturates can also cause hair loss and diarrhea, and can affect our capillaries and prematurely age the cell, because they generate free radicals which can burn out the cell, that is, if you do not have adequate vitamin E and adequate antioxidants in the blood. The cells are protected by a fatty membrane which is adversely affected by the peroxides that can occur in the presence of polyunsaturated oil. The liver, too, has much more difficulty detoxifying the body with excess polyunsaturates. People who have had an increase in polyunsaturates in their diet have been shown to suffer a greater percentage of liver damage. Polyunsaturates have been associated with a condition known as sludging, in which red blood cells stick together in clumps. When this occurs, your blood simply is unable to travel through the blood vessels at a rate consistent with the oxygen needs of your body cells. This could also affect the lungs. Dr. Denham Harmon of the University of Nebraska School of Medicine has shown that if we use too much polyunsaturated oil in our diet — he included margarine products — it could also potentiate cancer, atherosclerosis, and other diseases. Taking too much can prematurely age the cells and in effect limit our life-span. Breast cancer has been shown to increase in women who eat high levels of polyunsaturated fats. Dr. Daniel Melnick showed an increase in breast cancer in laboratory animals when he fed them a diet of heated oil. Dr. David Kritchevesky of the Wistar Institute also fed animals heated corn oil and found that it helped to induce the development of atherosclerosis. Yet we eat so many polyunsaturates in the form of corn oils, heating it to make french fries, fried fish, chicken, and tempura foods. When heated, polyunsaturates become chemically unstable and the atoms begin to react. Polyunsaturates are oxidized by the heat of normal cooking; oxidation of polyunsaturates produces toxic lipid peroxides capable of converting normal cells into seroid pigments or dead cells with a burned appearance. The accumulation of these can cause premature aging. Heating of oil also increases the toxicity of polyunsaturates by converting them into polymers, the chemical compounds that are used to make shellac, varnish, and plastics. The longer the polyunsaturated fat is heated, the greater potential for toxic reactions. Remember that the next time you decide to have a tempura dish, french fries, fried chicken, onion rings, or some other fried foods. Thus, the three to six tablespoons per day of polyunsaturates that many of us are consuming to avoid cholesterol is probably dangerously excessive, especially if it is taken in cooked form. If you want polyunsaturated oil and essential fatty acids such as linoleic, linolenic, oleic acid, and carbonic acid, some will be synthesized naturally by the body from other compounds, and some will come specifically from foods such as avocados, olives, and various legumes and grains. Avocados and unsalted olives are two excellent sources of the unsaturated (essential) fatty acids.

The cholesterol scare has chased people away from nutritious foods, and it has given them false confidence that just by eliminating cholesterol from their diet they can prevent heart disease. Finally, it has distracted them from the need to focus on other factors, such as life-style, which could provide them with more optimal all-round health.

The unit value for cholesterol is given in milligrams.

Where the symbol N. A. appears in the calorie column, the information was not available.

All figures are based on an edible portion equaling 100 grams, or approximately 3 ounces. In the case of some of the foods listed, one would not consume 100 grams in one serving. Calculations should be adjusted accordingly.

Cholesterol

FOOD ITEM	CALS.	UNITS
Dried eggs commercial	592	1900.00
Egg yolks	664	1480.00
Kidneys beef	252	804.00
Chicken liver simmered	165	746.00
Eggs whole, cooked with nothing added	163	504.00
Eggs scrambled	173	411.00
Omelets with milk and fat	173	411.00
Ladyfinger cookies	360	356.00
Caviar (sturgeon), granular	262	300.00
Butter	716	250.00
Sponge cake homemade	297	246.00
Lobster Newburg	194	182.00
Lemon chiffon pie	313	169.00
Popovers homemade	224	147.00
Cream puffs with custard filling, commercial	233	144.00
Heavy whipping cream	352	133.00
Sardines canned in oil, solids and liquids	311	120.00
Cream cheese	374	111.00
Whole milk dry	502	109.00
Custard baked	115	105.00
Mackerel (Atlantic), broiled	236	101.00
Turkey all classes, dark meat, roasted	203	101.00
Crab all varieties, steamed	N.A.	100.00
Swiss cheese (domestic), unprocessed	370	100.00
Cheddar cheese unprocessed	398	99.00

FOOD ITEM	CALS.	UNITS
Limburger cheese	345	98.00
Herring canned, solids and liquid	208	97.00
Tapioca cream pudding	134	97.00
Lard	902	95.00
Parmesan cheese	393	95.00
Beef composite of all cuts	327	94.00
Lemon meringue pie commercial	255	93.00
Camembert cheese	299	92.00
Chicken (fryer), drumstick, fried	235	91.00
Low-fat milk (2% fat)	59	91.00
American cheese pasturized, processed	370	90.00
Brick cheese	370	90.00
Pork composite of all cuts, lean	410	88.00
Blue cheese	368	87.00
Chicken cooked, flesh and skin only	136	87.00
Lobster meat only, cooked	95	85.00
Brownies with nuts, homemade	485	83.00
Chicken breast cooked	203	80.00
Turkey all classes, light meat, roasted	176	77.00
Chicken a la king homemade	191	76.00
Pancakes from mix, made with eggs and milk	225	74.00
American cheese food pasteurized, processed	323	72.00
Cornbread homemade from degermed cornmeal	224	70.00
Mayonnaise salad dressing commercial	718	70.00
Light cream	211	66.00
Potato salad homemade with mayonnaise and eggs	145	65.00
Tuna canned in oil, drained solids	197	65.00
Bread pudding with raisins, commercial	187	64.00
Tuna canned in water, solids and liquid	127	63.00
Frankfurters	304	62.00
Pumpkin pie commercial	211	61.00
Waffles from mix, made with eggs and milk	356	60.00
Ice cream fat content 16%	222	57.00
Tuna canned in oil, solids and liquid	288	55.00
Muffins plain, homemade	294	53.00
Scallops muscle only, steamed	112	53.00
Tartar sauce regular	531	51.00
Margarine two thirds animal fat, one third vegetable fat	720	50.00
Dark fruitcake homemade	379	45.00
Yellow cake with chocolate frosting, homemade	365	44.00

FOOD ITEM	CALS.	UNITS
Chocolate cake with chocolate frosting, homemade	369	43.00
Half-and-half cream	134	43.00
Corn pudding commercial	104	42.00
Chicken fricassee homemade	161	40.00
Ice cream 10% fat content	193	40.00
Chicken chow mein without noodles, homemade	102	31.00
Chicken potpie homemade	235	31.00
Egg noodles enriched, cooked	125	31.00
Evaporated milk canned, unsweetened	137	31.00
Turkey potpie homemade	237	31.00
Welsh rarebit	179	31.00
Green peppers stuffed with beef and bread crumbs	170	30.00
Spaghetti with meatballs in tomato sauce, commercial	103	30.00
Beef and vegetable stew homemade with lean beef chunk	89	26.00
Oyster stew 1 part oysters to 2 parts milk, homemade	97	26.00
Oyster stew 1 part oysters to 3 parts milk, homemade	86	24.00
Nonfat dry milk instant	359	22.00
Beef potpie homemade, baked	246	21.00
Macaroni and cheese baked, homemade	215	21.00
Ice milk	152	20.00
Cottage cheese creamed, 4% fat, large or small curd	106	19.00
Potatoes au gratin made with milk and cheese, commercial	145	15.00
Beef and vegetable stew canned	79	14.00
Vanilla pudding homemade	111	14.00
Whole milk	65	14.00
Chocolate pudding from mix	124	12.00
Chow mein noodles canned	489	12.00
Rice pudding with raisins, commercial	146	11.00
Low-fat milk (2% fat)	59	9.00
Buttermilk made from liquid nonfat milk	36	2.00
Skim milk	36	2.00

Fiber

$$\left(\,5\,\right)$$

Fiber is the catchword of nutrition for the eighties. For years, it used to be considered a useless by-product of food processing, fit only to be fed to animals. It was Surgeon T.L. Cleave of the British Royal Navy who discovered that by including fiber in the diet of his crews aboard ship, he could largely prevent digestive problems and also improve overall attitude of crews at sea for lengthy periods of time.

Subsequently, Dr. Denis Burkitt, who practiced medicine in Africa for twenty years and who collected statistics on the health of native societies, demonstrated that those groups who consumed a high-fiber diet almost never suffered from colon-rectal cancer, appendicitis, or diverticulitis. They also had an extremely low incidence of coronary heart disease, high blood pressure, diabetes, and obesity. Some critics might have attributed this good fortune entirely to a high level of exercise (the groups he studied included cow herders who commonly walk ten to fifteen miles a day following their herds and visiting neighbors), or to a low-calorie diet. However, their diet was adequate in calories, and other athletic groups who consume less fiber do suffer from those diseases. So adequate amounts of simple nonnutritive food fiber were the one factor that could explain their excellent health.

What Is Fiber?

Fiber is the indigestible food matter present in grains, legumes, vegetables, and fruits. It supplies virtually no known nutrients. However, it is extremely important to our health, as it aids elimination by adding bulk to the feces.

It consists of the hard, outer husk of plants and seeds, and it is the material that enables plants to stand upright and maintain their shape. It is also known as roughage, residue, husk, or skin.

Benefits of Fiber in the Diet

Following Cleave and Burkitt's discoveries, dozens of books, magazines, and newspapers began touting the advantages of adding fiber to the diet. One easy way to do so is to add a teaspoon or two of miller's bran per day to cereal, soups, or salads. Hopping on the bandwagon, cereal manufacturers began adding bran — the outer part of the wheat — to breakfast cereals, and selling it as a food supplement. Doctors noted that the addition of a small amount of bran to the diet could help soften stools, allowing matter to pass more easily and more rapidly through the intestines. Bran, they found, could decrease transit time, the time required to digest and eliminate food, by almost one-third. This has great health benefits, since the longer food stays in the intestine, the greater the probability of combinations of chemical reactions occurring that can establish a disease state, whether irritable bowel syndrome, diverticulitis, appendicitis, toxic reactions, cancer, or other problems. With constipation and an impacted bowel comes straining, which can lead to hemorrhoids, varicose veins, and overall poor health, including heart problems.

Dr. Burkitt's studies in Africa confirmed this rule. He observed that hemorrhoids were virtually nonexistent among those groups who obtained most of their protein from high-fiber complex carbohydrates. However, as individuals migrated to the towns, their tastes became more "sophisticated" and they shifted to a diet high in animal protein and refined carbohydrate. Incidence of hemorrhoids — as well as that of the other problems listed above — then rose dramatically.

It is estimated that nearly one-half of all illnesses originate, at least in part, in the intestines. The health of the intestines is crucial to the health of the body. For years, the natural hygiene movement has espoused raw, live, enzyme-rich and fiber-rich foods, to keep the intestines clean.

High-Fiber Foods

The foods that are naturally richest in fiber, as the following list indicates, are whole grains and legumes. The fibers that seem to have the greatest water-holding capacity, that is, the capacity to stimulate peristalsis, are the cellulose fibers found in grains. Bran, which is wheat fiber, is one example.

Fruit fibers, found in the skin and seeds of fruits such as apples and grapes, are also nondigestible fiber. Fruit fiber provides pectin or alginates, which have the capacity to gel the matter in the intestines. Much as a plumber cleans out a pipe, this gelling action cleanses the walls of the intestines, picking off particles of undigested debris and helping to sweep it through. Fruit fiber does not, however, have the same water-holding or stool-softening capacity as grain fiber.

The use of wheat bran has perhaps been overemphasized by the cereal industry. It is inexpensive to produce. In fact, it is a by-product of the refining of flour. It stores easily, has hardly any taste, can be mixed with water, juice or cereals, and has a noticeable effect in overcoming constipation. Therefore, it has been widely extolled as a good fiber supplement. However, many people are allergic to all wheat products, including bran. (They may use rice bran as an alternative.) More to the point, if you consume a diet high in fiber-rich complex carbohydrates, it is unlikely that you will suffer from constipation, impacted intestines, or the diseases they can cause. You will most likely find you have no need to add bran to your diet if you eat whole grains instead of refined, since whole grains include the bran portion.

Too Much Fiber

If you take too much bran, as some people have a tendency to do, the phytates in grain may bind calcium and even zinc, and pull these important minerals out of the system. If you eat a diet high in whole grains already, and especially if you add fiber on top of that, make sure that you are getting adequate calcium and zinc in your diet by taking a small zinc supplement and by consuming either dairy or soy products for calcium.

Loss of Fiber from Our Foods

Bread was once so nutritious that our ancestors dubbed it the staff of life.

Today, nearly all the fiber has been refined out of the grains we eat, for the convenience and profit of the manufacturers. When the germ is also removed, as it normally is in food processing, we lose the natural vitamin, mineral, protein, and enzyme content of whole grains as well. Refined flour — because of its lack of essential nutrients, its lifelessness — can be easily and indefinitely stored: mice, and even most microorganisms, leave it alone. Pressure from consumers led to manufacturers' "enriching" this dead flour with a few minerals and synthetic vitamins, but not in the amounts removed. The fiber, protein, enzymes, and most nutrients are still missing from the mountains of white bread and pasta made from refined flour that most people still prefer. Even "whole wheat" and "rye" bread are usually just refined, bleached white flour, with dark coloring or enough rye flour added to provide a slight change in color and flavor. The grains included are still refined, and the product is missing the bran, germ, and enzymes of the whole grain. If you want to purchase ready-made, real whole wheat bread, look for the words "stone-ground whole wheat flour" on the ingredients list as the sole type of flour used. ("Enriched flour" just means the refined flour you are trying to avoid.) To save money, bake your own.

Rice, too, for reasons of status and convenience, is milled to remove the fibrous brown hull and make it white. Like white flour, white rice is almost pure starch.

Lacking fiber's bulk, refined carbohydrates are more profitable than whole, because you have to eat so much more in order to feel full. Consumers readily gulp down large quantities because soft, nonfibrous refined carbohydrates hardly need to be chewed in order to be swallowed. Manufacturers can thus sell larger quantities of products made from refined grain than from whole grains, not only because it keeps longer on store shelves, but because consumers eat more of it.

Refined Carbohydrates and Obesity

What's good for General Foods isn't necessarily good for America. The ease with which refined carbohydrates are swallowed without chewing is probably a major factor in the obesity so common in this country. Lengthy chewing — necessary when you eat fiber-rich foods — stimulates the secretion of quarts of digestive juices by the mouth and stomach at each meal. The longer you chew, the more liquid is secreted. These juices, mixed with your food, add to the feelings of satiety after a meal. Refined carbohydrates thus deny you that full feeling both because they lack bulk, and because they fail to stimulate the production of a large volume of digestive juices. No wonder overweight people complain that they never really feel full, even after a meal much higher in calories than would be provided by one including fiber foods.

Preparing and Eating

It is a good idea to switch to a high-fiber diet. When you do, you can no longer make a habit of grabbing a bite on the run. Remind yourself, as you boil your brown rice for the thirty minutes it takes to set the table, prepare your salad, and wash and steam your vegetables (instead of throwing one-minute rice into the pot just as you serve), that the extra time and effort invested will pay off in better health for yourself and your family.

Because of their fiber content, complex carbohydrates are only partly digested. The protein in dried legumes, for example, is only 78 percent digestible; in contrast, animal protein, which does not contain plant fiber, is 97 percent digestible. Cereal grains and fruits are about 85 percent digestible, vegetables about 83 percent. If you want to obtain most of your protein from plant sources, you may need to eat a bit more than you do of animal protein.

Cooking grains and legumes helps break down the cell walls and aids digestion. Indeed, legumes should always be well cooked since they contain certain toxins that are neutralized by heat. Sprouting is another method for adding to the digestibility of grains, seeds, or legumes. (See Protein section.) Sprouting also adds to the nutrient density of these valuable foods.

It is important to chew high-fiber foods well in order to obtain their full nutritional value. Otherwise, the fiber surrounding plant cells can insulate from your digestive enzymes the protein, starch, vitamins, and minerals inside the plant cells, and you won't obtain full benefit from the foods. But prepared correctly and chewed at leisure, high-fiber foods are your best health insurance.

The unit value for fiber is given in grams. Any food having less than .1 gram of fiber per 100-gram portion is considered to have a trace fiber content and is listed as having .00 for its unit value.

Where the symbol N.A. appears in the calorie column, the information was not available.

All figures are based on an edible portion equaling 100 grams, or approximately 3 ounces. In the case of some of the listed foods, one would not consume 100 grams in one serving. Calculations should be adjusted accordingly.

Fiber

FOOD ITEM	CALS.	UNITS
Rice bran	276	11.50
Buckwheat whole grain	335	9.90
Wheat bran crude, commercially milled	213	9.10
Bran sugar and malt extract added	240	7.80
Carob flour	180	7.70
Safflower seed meal partially defatted	355	7.40
Elderberries raw	72	7.00
Kelp raw	N.A.	6.80
Sesame seeds dry, whole	563	6.30
Dried pears uncooked	268	6.20
Cocoa powder low fat	187	5.80
Dried figs	274	5.60
Guavas whole, raw	62	5.60
Black raspberries raw	73	5.10
Sunflower seed flour partially defatted	339	4.60
Cocoa powder high fat	299	4.30
Blackberries raw	58	4.10
Coconut meat shredded, dried, sweetened	548	4.10

FOOD ITEM	CALS.	UNITS
Coconut meat fresh	346	4.00
Coconut meat dried, unsweetened	662	3.90
Dried sunflower seed kernels	560	3.80
Greek olives	338	3.80
Kumquats raw	65	3.70
Torula yeast	277	3.30
Millet whole grain	327	3.20
Brazil nuts	654	3.10
Dried peaches uncooked	262	3.10
Dried apricots uncooked	260	3.00
Filberts (hazelnuts)	634	3.00
Loganberries raw	62	3.00
Red raspberries raw	57	3.00
Dried pears cooked, no added sugar	126	2.90
Blackberries canned in water, with or without artificial sweetener, fruit and liquid	40	2.80
Blackberries canned in juice, fruit and liquid	54	2.70
Blackberries canned in light syrup, fruit and liquid	72	2.70
Boysenberries frozen, unsweetened	48	2.70
Peanut flour defatted	371	2.70
Peanuts with skins, roasted	582	2.70
Almonds dried	598	2.60
Almonds roasted and salted	627	2.60
Blackberries canned in extra-heavy syrup, fruit and liquid	110	2.60
Blackberries canned in heavy syrup, fruit and liquid	91	2.60
Baking chocolate	505	2.50
Bitter chocolate	505	2.50
Chestnuts dried	377	2.50
Macadamia nuts	691	2.50
Wheat germ raw, commercially milled	363	2.50
Artichokes (globe or French), raw	47	2.40
Artichokes (globe or French), boiled, and drained	47	2.40
Black currants raw	54	2.40
Sesame seeds dry, hulled	582	2.40
Whole wheat crackers commercial	403	2.40
Almond meal partially defatted	408	2.30
Dates (domestic), dry	274	2.30
Lemon peel candied	316	2.30
Miso (fermented soybean product)	171	2.30
Pecans	687	2.30

FOOD ITEM	CALS.	UNITS
Shredded wheat (cereal)	354	2.30
Soybean flour defatted	326	2.30
Whole wheat flours from hard wheat	333	2.30
Popcorn popped, plain	386	2.20
Red raspberries frozen, sweetened	98	2.20
Rye wafers whole grain	344	2.20
Irish moss (seaweed), raw	N.A.	2.10
Walnuts	651	2.10
Banana powder	340	2.00
Green peas boiled and drained	71	2.00
Lima bean flour	343	2.00
Parsnips raw	76	2.00
Parsnips boiled and drained	66	2.00
Puffed wheat (cereal) added nutrients, without salt	363	2.00
Baby lima beans frozen, boiled and drained	118	1.90
Boysenberries canned in water, and liquid with or without artificial sweetener	36	1.90
Gooseberries raw	39	1.90
Green peas frozen, boiled and drained	68	1.90
Hickory nuts	673	1.90
Peanuts without skins, raw	568	1.90
Pistachio nuts	594	1.90
Pumpkin and squash seed kernels dried	553	1.90
Bran muffins homemade from enriched flour	261	1.80
Cowpeas (including black-eyed peas), boiled and drained	108	1.80
Green chili peppers hot, pods, without seeds, raw	37	1.80
Lima beans boiled and drained	111	1.80
Winter squash baked	63	1.80
Black walnuts	628	1.70
Brewer's yeast debittered	283	1.70
Bulgur from club wheat, dry, commercial	359	1.70
Cowpeas (including black-eyed peas), young pods with seeds, boiled and drained	34	1.70
Lima beans dry, boiled and drained	138	1.70
Red peppers (sweet), mature, raw	31	1.70
Wheat germ toasted	391	1.70
Avocados raw	167	1.60
Brussels sprouts boiled and drained	36	1.60
Brussels sprouts raw	45	1.60
Cornmeal whole ground, white or yellow, unbolted	55	1.60

FOOD ITEM	CALS.	UNITS
Dandelion greens raw	45	1.60
Dried prunes uncooked	255	1.60
Lima beans frozen, boiled and drained	99	1.60
Potato flour	351	1.60
Prickly pears raw	42	1.60
Soybeans dry, cooked	130	1.60
Wheat flakes (cereal)	354	1.60
Whole wheat bread commercial, made with 20% nonfat dry milk	243	1.60
Whole wheat rolls commercial	257	1.60
Blueberries raw	62	1.50
Broccoli spears, boiled and drained	26	1.50
Broccoli spears, raw	32	1.50
Garlic cloves raw	137	1.50
Green peas (Alaska), canned, regular pack, solids and liquid	66	1.50
Oatmeal (baby food)	375	1.50
Parsley raw	44	1.50
Peas and carrots frozen, boiled and drained	53	1.50
Persimmons native, raw	127	1.50
Potato sticks	544	1.50
Red beans dry, boiled and drained	118	1.50
Cashew nuts	561	1.40
Cranberries raw	46	1.40
Dried lichees	277	1.40
Green peas (sweet), canned, regular pack, solids and liquid	57	1.40
Green peppers (sweet), boiled and drained	18	1.40
Green peppers (sweet), raw	22	1.40
Lemon candied	314	1.40
Pears with skin, raw	61	1.40
Winter squash raw	50	1.40
Beet greens raw	24	1.30
Brown mustard prepared	91	1.30
Celeriac root, raw	40	1.30
Dandelion greens boiled and drained	33	1.30
Green olives pickled, canned or bottled	116	1.30
Green peas (Alaska), canned, low sodium, solids and liquid	55	1.30
Green peas (sweet), canned, low sodium, solids and liquid	47	1.30
Kale stems and leaves, raw	38	1.30
Leeks bulb and lower-leaf portion, raw	52	1.30
Lima beans canned, regular, solids and liquid	71	1.30

FOOD ITEM	CALS.	UNITS
Pumpkin canned	33	1.30
Strawberries raw	37	1.30
Brussels sprouts frozen, boiled and drained	33	1.20
Figs raw	80	1.20
Lentils whole, dry, cooked	106	1.20
Lima beans canned, low sodium, solids and liquid	70	1.20
Mixed vegetables (carrots, corn, peas, green snap beans, and lima beans), frozen, boiled and drained	64	1.20
Winter squash frozen, cooked	38	1.20
Apple butter	186	1.10
Beet greens boiled and drained	18	1.10
Blueberries canned in water, with or without artificial sweetener, fruit and liquid	40	1.10
Broccoli chopped, frozen, boiled and drained	26	1.10
Chestnuts fresh	194	1.10
Chives raw	28	1.10
Frankfurters and beans canned	144	1.10
Garden cress raw	32	1.10
Ginger root fresh	49	1.10
Graham crackers plain	384	1.10
Kale leaves and stems, boiled and drained	28	1.10
Mustard greens raw	31	1.10
Pumpernickel bread commercial	246	1.10
Rutabagas raw, boiled and drained	35	1.10
Rutabagas raw	46	1.10
Yellow snap beans cut, frozen, boiled and drained	27	1.10
Apples freshly harvested, with skin, raw	58	1.00
Carrots boiled and drained	31	1.00
Carrots raw	42	1.00
Cauliflower boiled and drained	22	1.00
Cauliflower raw	27	1.00
Collards frozen, boiled and drained	30	1.00
Cowpeas (including black-eyed peas), dry, cooked	76	1.00
Dried peaches cooked, without added sugar, fruit and liquid	82	1.00
French fried potatoes	274	1.00
Green snap beans raw	32	1.00
Green snap beans boiled and drained	25	1.00
Green snap beans frozen, boiled and drained	25	1.00
Jams and preserves	272	1.00
Kohlrabi raw	29	1.00

FOOD ITEM	CALS.	UNITS
Kohlrabi raw	29	1.00
Mustard greens frozen, boiled and drained	20	1.00
Okra boiled and drained	29	1.00
Okra cuts and pods, frozen, boiled and drained	38	1.00
Red cabbage raw	31	1.00
Rye flour medium	350	1.00
Turnip greens frozen, boiled and drained	23	1.00
Yellow mustard prepared	75	1.00
Yellow snap beans boiled and drained	22	1.00
Yellow snap beans raw	27	1.00
Blueberries canned in extra-heavy syrup, fruit and liquid	101	.90
Collards leaves and stems, raw	40	.90
Dried peaches cooked, sugar added, fruit and liquid	119	.90
Eggplant boiled and drained	19	.90
Endive (curly endive and escarole), raw	20	.90
Garden cress boiled and drained	23	.90
Horseradish prepared	38	.90
Kale frozen, boiled and drained	31	.90
Mangoes raw	66	.90
Mustard greens boiled and drained	23	.90
Papayas raw	39	.90
Pine nuts	552	.90
Raisins	289	.90
Red beans dry, canned, solids and liquid	90	.90
Succotash frozen, boiled and drained	93	.90
Swamp cabbage boiled and drained	21	.90
Sweet potatoes with skin, baked	141	.90
Tomato paste canned	82	.90
Turnips boiled and drained	23	.90
Turnips raw	30	.90
Asparagus cuts and tips, frozen, boiled and drained	22	.80
Asparagus spears, frozen, boiled and drained	23	.80
Bread stuffing mix dry	371	.80
Cabbage raw	24	.80
Cabbage shredded, boiled and drained	20	.80
Cauliflower frozen, boiled and drained	18	.80
Chard, Swiss raw	25	.80
Chicory greens raw	20	.80
Chop suey with meat, canned	62	.80
Collards leaves and stems, boiled and drained	33	.80

FOOD ITEM	CALS.	UNITS
Corn sweet, yellow, whole kernel, canned, regular pack, solids and liquid	83	.80
Dried prunes cooked, no added sugar	119	.80
Green beans (baby food), commmercial	22	.80
Hash-browned potatoes	229	.80
Hot chocolate from mix	392	.80
Jerusalem artichokes raw, freshly harvested	7	.80
Mushrooms raw	28	.80
Pears canned in juice, fruit and liquid	46	.80
Pineapple candied	316	.80
Purslane leaves and stems, boiled and drained	15	.80
Red beets raw or boiled and drained	32	.80
Rhubarb frozen, cooked, sugar added	143	.80
Soybean sprouts boiled and drained	38	.80
Soybean sprouts raw	46	.80
Spinach chopped, frozen, boiled and drained	23	.80
Turnip greens leaves and stems, raw	28	.80
Water chestnuts raw	79	.80
Agar (seaweed), raw	N.A.	.70
Asparagus spears, raw	26	.70
Asparagus spears, boiled and drained	20	.70
Bamboo shoots raw	27	.70
Blueberry pie piecrust made with unenriched flour	242	.70
Brownies with nuts, homemade from enriched flour	485	.70
Chard, Swiss boiled and drained	18	.70
Chayote raw	28	.70
Coleslaw made with salad dressing	99	.70
Corn flour	368	.70
Corn on the cob (sweet, white and yellow), boiled and drained	91	.70
Corn on the cob (sweet), frozen, boiled and drained	94	.70
Cornflakes	386	.70
Cowpeas (including black-eyed peas), canned, solids and liquid	70	.70
Figs canned in water, with or without artificial sweetener, fruit and liquid	48	.70
Figs canned in light syrup, fruit and liquid	65	.70
Figs canned in heavy syrup, fruit and liquid	84	.70
Gingerroot (candied)	340	.70
Lettuce (cos and romaine), raw	18	.70

FOOD ITEM	CALS.	UNITS
Light fruit cake homemade	389	.70
Mung bean sprouts boiled and drained	28	.70
Mung bean sprouts raw	35	.70
New Zealand spinach raw	19	.70
Pears canned in water, with or without artificial sweetener, fruit and liquid	32	.70
Pears canned in light syrup, fruit and liquid	61	.70
Radishes (Oriental, including daikon and Chinese), raw	19	.70
Rhubarb raw	16	.70
Sauerkraut canned, solids and liquid	18	.70
Spinach canned, regular, solids and liquid	19	.70
Spinach canned, low sodium, solids and liquid	21	.70
Sweet potatoes with skin, boiled	114	.70
Tomato chili sauce bottled	104	.70
Turnip greens leaves and stems, boiled and drained	20	.70
Turnip greens leaves and stems, canned, solids and liquid	18	.70
Watercress leaves and stems, raw	19	.70
Apples freshly harvested, pared, raw	54	.60
Applesauce canned, unsweetened or artificially sweetened	41	.60
Apricots raw	51	.60
Baked potatoes with skin	93	.60
Barbecue sauce	91	.60
Brownies with nuts and chocolate frosting, frozen	419	.60
Carrots (baby food), commercial	29	.60
Carrots canned, regular, solids and liquid	28	.60
Carrots canned, low sodium, solids and liquid	22	.60
Celery (green and yellow varieties), boiled and drained	14	.60
Celery (green and yellow varieties), raw	17	.60
Chili con carne with beans, canned	133	.60
Chinese cabbage raw	14	.60
Corn (sweet, white and yellow), canned, regular pack, solids and liquid	66	.60
Crabapples raw	68	.60
Cucumbers with skin, raw	15	.60
Dark fruitcake homemade	379	.60
Figs canned in extra-heavy syrup, fruit and liquid	103	.60
Grapes (American), raw	69	.60
Green snap beans canned, regular, solids and liquid	18	.60
Green snap beans canned, low sodium, solids and liquid	16	.60
Honeydew melon	33	.60

FOOD ITEM	CALS.	UNITS
Mushrooms canned, solids and liquid	17	.60
Oats with toasted wheat germ and soy (cereal), cooked	62	.60
Onions boiled and drained	29	.60
Onions raw	38	.60
Peaches raw	38	.60
Pears canned in heavy syrup, fruit and liquid	76	.60
Pears canned in extra-heavy syrup, fruit and liquid	92	.60
Pimientos canned, solids and liquid	27	.60
Puffed rice and rice flakes (cereal)	390	.60
Rhubarb cooked, sugar added	141	.60
Shredded corn (cereal)	389	.60
Spinach boiled and drained	23	.60
Spinach raw	26	.60
Squash (summer), raw	19	.60
Summer squash boiled and drained	14	.60
Summer squash frozen, boiled and drained	21	.60
Sweet potatoes candied	168	.60
Sweet potatoes canned in syrup, solids and liquid	114	.60
Tomatoes ripe, boiled	26	.60
Yellow snap beans canned, regular, solids and liquid	19	.60
Yellow snap beans canned, low sodium, solids and liquid	15	.60
Applesauce canned, sweetened	91	.50
Applesauce (baby food), commercial	72	.50
Asparagus spears, canned, regular, solids and liquid	18	.50
Asparagus spears, canned, low sodium, solids and liquid	16	.50
Bananas raw	85	.50
Barley pearled, light	349	.50
Cherries candied	339	.50
Chop suey with meat, homemade	120	.50
Corn (sweet, white and yellow), canned, low sodium, solids and liquid	57	.50
Corn sweet, frozen, boiled and drained	79	.50
Corn fritters commercial	377	.50
Corn muffins homemade from whole-ground cornmeal	288	.50
Corn pudding commercial	104	.50
Cornbread homemade from whole-ground cornmeal	207	.50
Corned beef hash with potatoes, canned	181	.50
Cracked wheat bread commercial	263	.50
Creamed corn (sweet, white and yellow), canned, regular pack, solids and liquid	82	.50

FOOD ITEM	CALS.	UNITS
Dried apples cooked, no sugar added	78	.50
Dried apples cooked, sugar added	112	.50
Fennel leaves, raw	28	.50
Frosting (chocolate fudge), from mix, made with water and tablefat	378	.50
Fruit salad canned in water, with or without artificial sweetener, fruit and liquid	35	.50
Grapes (European), raw	67	.50
Lettuce (Boston and Bibb), raw	13	.50
Limes raw	28	.50
Oranges raw	49	.50
Pecan pie commercial	418	.50
Pickles (dill)	11	.50
Pickles (sour)	10	.50
Potatoes with skin, boiled	76	.50
Pumpkin pie commercial	211	.50
Red beets canned, regular, solids and liquid	34	.50
Red beets canned, low sodium, solids and liquid	32	.50
Rice cereal (baby food), commercial	371	.50
Spanish rice homemade	87	.50
Tangerines	46	.50
Tomato catsup bottled	106	.50
Apple pie commercial	256	.40
Apricots canned in water, with or without artificial sweetener, fruit and liquid	38	.40
Apricots canned in juice, fruit and liquid	54	.40
Apricots canned in light syrup, fruit and liquid	66	.40
Apricots canned in heavy syrup, fruit and liquid	86	.40
Apricots canned in extra-heavy syrup, fruit and liquid	101	.40
Buckwheat pancakes and waffles from mix, made with eggs and milk	200	.40
Cherries (sweet), raw	70	.40
Chicken potpie homemade	235	.40
Chocolate chip cookies homemade from enriched flour	516	.40
Chocolate chip cookies commercial	471	.40
Chocolate syrup (fudge)	330	.40
Corn flakes cereal	386	.40
Corn flakes and puffed corn (cereal), sugar coated	386	.40
Fruit cocktail canned in water, with or without artificial sweetener, fruit and liquid	37	.40

FOOD ITEM	CALS.	UNITS
Fruit cocktail canned in light syrup, fruit and liquid	60	.40
Fruit cocktail canned in heavy syrup, fruit and liquid	76	.40
Fruit cocktail canned in extra-heavy syrup, fruit and liquid	92	.40
Fruit salad canned in light syrup, fruit and liquid	59	.40
Fruit salad canned in heavy syrup, fruit and liquid	75	.40
Fruit salad canned in extra-heavy syrup, fruit and liquid	90	.40
Gluten flour	378	.40
Lemons peeled, raw	27	.40
Marmalade citrus	257	.40
Mashed potatoes milk added	65	.40
Mashed potatoes frozen, heated	93	.40
Milk chocolate candy plain	520	.40
Nectarines raw	64	.40
Peaches canned in water, with or without artificial sweetener, fruit and liquid	31	.40
Peaches canned in juice, fruit and liquid	45	.40
Peaches canned in light syrup, fruit and liquid	58	.40
Peaches canned in heavy syrup, fruit and liquid	78	.40
Peaches canned in extra-heavy syrup, fruit and liquid	97	.40
Peas dry, cooked	115	.40
Pineapple raw	52	.40
Plantain (baking banana), raw	119	.40
Plums raw, prune-type	75	.40
Potato salad homemade with salad dressing and seasonings	99	.40
Puffed corn cereal	399	.40
Raisins cooked, sugar added, fruit and liquid	213	.40
Red bananas raw	90	.40
Rye bread (American), commercial	243	.40
Saltine crackers	433	.40
Split pea soup canned, condensed	118	.40
Tomato puree canned, regular or low sodium	39	.40
Tomatoes ripe, canned, regular, solids and liquid	21	.40
Tomatoes canned, low sodium, solids and liquid	20	.40
Turkey potpie homemade	237	.40
Apple pie frozen	254	.30
Beef and vegetable stew canned	79	.30
Beef noodle dinner (baby food), commercial	48	.30
Blueberry muffins homemade from enriched flour	281	.30
Bread crumbs dry, grated	392	.30
Cantaloupe	30	.30

FOOD ITEM	CALS.	UNITS
Cherries (sweet), canned in water, with or without artificial sweetener, fruit and liquid	48	.30
Cherries (sweet), canned in light syrup, fruit and liquid	65	.30
Cherries (sweet), canned in heavy syrup, fruit and liquid	81	.30
Cherries (sweet), canned in extra-heavy syrup, fruit and liquid	100	.30
Chicken chow mein without noodles, canned	38	.30
Chicken chow mein without noodles, homemade	102	.30
Chocolate cake with chocolate frosting, homemade	369	.30
Creamed corn (sweet, white and yellow), canned, low sodium, solids and liquid	82	.30
French salad dressing commercial, regular	410	.30
French salad dressing commercial, low calorie (low fat)	96	.30
Fruit pudding (baby food), commercial	96	.30
Lichees raw	64	.30
Manhattan clam chowder canned, condensed	66	.30
Maraschino cherries bottled, fruit and liquid	116	.30
Mashed potatoes dehydrated, flakes without milk	93	.30
Oat and wheat cereal cooked	65	.30
Pear nectar canned	52	.30
Pineapple all kinds except crushed, canned in water, with or without artificial sweetener	39	.30
Pineapple canned in juice, fruit and liquid	58	.30
Pineapple canned in light syrup, fruit and liquid	59	.30
Pineapple canned in heavy syrup, fruit and liquid	74	.30
Pineapple canned in extra-heavy syrup, fruit and liquid	90	.30
Pizza with sausage, homemade	234	.30
Pizza frozen	245	.30
Plums (purple), canned in water, with or without artificial sweetener, fruit and liquid	46	.30
Plums canned in light syrup, fruit and liquid	63	.30
Plums canned in heavy syrup, fruit and liquid	83	.30
Plums canned in extra-heavy syrup, fruit and liquid	102	.30
Pretzels	390	.30
Russian salad dressing commercial, regular	494	.30
Shredded rice (cereal)	392	.30
Spaghetti with meatballs in tomato sauce, homemade	134	.30
Sweet potatoes canned in liquid, solids and liquid, unsweetened	46	.30
Tartar sauce regular	531	.30

FOOD ITEM	CALS.	UNITS
Tartar sauce low calorie	224	.30
Thousand Island salad dressing commercial, regular	502	.30
Thousand Island salad dressing commercial, low calorie	180	.30
Vegetable juice cocktail canned	17	.30
Watermelon raw	26	.30
Wheat flour enriched and unenriched	365	.30
Zwieback	423	.30
Apricot nectar canned	57	.20
Beef with vegetables (baby food), commercial	87	.20
Biscuits homemade from enriched flour	369	.20
Biscuits from mix, made with milk	325	.20
Cake or pastry flour	364	.20
Cheese crackers commercial	479	.20
Chicken with vegetables (baby food), commercial	100	.20
Chocolate pudding homemade	148	.20
Corn muffins from mix, made with eggs and milk	324	.20
Corn muffins homemade from enriched degermed cornmeal	314	.20
Cornbread from mix, made with eggs and milk	233	.20
Custard pudding (baby food), commercial	100	.20
French bread enriched or unenriched, commercial	290	.20
Fruit dessert with tapioca (baby food), commercial	84	.20
Grapefruit raw	41	.20
Grapefruit segments, canned in water, with or without artificial sweetener,fruit and liquid	30	.20
Grapefruit segments, canned in light syrup, fruit and liquid	70	.20
Hard rolls enriched, commercial	312	.20
Ice cream cones	377	.20
Italian bread enriched or unenriched, commercial	276	.20
Pastry plain, homemade from enriched or unenriched flour	500	.20
Pea soup from mix	50	.20
Piecrust homemade from enriched or unenriched flour	500	.20
Piecrust from mix	464	.20
Pomegranate pulp, raw	63	.20
Potatoes canned, solids and liquid	44	.20
Red cherries (sour), raw	58	.20
Red cherries (sour), frozen, sweetened	112	.20
Rolls from mix	299	.20
Rolls and buns homemade	339	.20
Rolls and buns plain, commercial	298	.20

FOOD ITEM	CALS.	UNITS
Soybean milk powder	429	.20
Spaghetti with cheese in tomato sauce, homemade	104	.20
Spaghetti with cheese in tomato sauce, canned	76	.20
Sweet rolls commercial	316	.20
Tomato juice canned or bottled, regular or low sodium	19	.20
Tomato juice cocktail canned or bottled	21	.20
Tomato soup canned, condensed	36	.20
Tomato soup canned, condensed, prepared with milk	69	.20
White bread made with 1% - 2% nonfat dry milk	269	.20
White cake with chocolate frosting from mix, made with egg whites	351	.20
Assorted cookies commercial	480	.10
Beef broth, bouillon, and consomme canned, condensed	26	.10
Blue and Roquefort cheese salad dressing commercial, regular	504	.10
Bread pudding with raisins, commercial	187	.10
Chicken noodle dinner (baby food), commercial	49	.10
Chicken noodle soup canned, condensed	53	.10
Corn grits degermed, enriched, cooked	51	.10
Corn muffins from mix, made with eggs and water	297	.10
Cornmeal (white or yellow), degermed, enriched, cooked	50	.10
Cornstarch	362	.10
Danish pastry commercial	422	.10
Doughnuts cake type	391	.10
Egg noodles enriched, cooked	125	.10
Gingerbread homemade from enriched flour	317	.10
Hot chocolate homemade	95	.10
Macaroni enriched or unenriched, cooked until tender	111	.10
Muffins plain, homemade from enriched or unenriched flour	294	.10
Orange juice fresh	45	.10
Orange juice canned, sweetened or unsweetened	48	.10
Orange juice concentrate, prepared with water	46	.10
Orange juice canned, sweetened	52	.10
Pancakes homemade from enriched or unenriched flour	231	.10
Pancakes from mix, made with eggs and milk	225	.10
Peach nectar canned	48	.10
Pie (cherry), piecrust made with unenriched flour, commercial	261	.10
Pineapple juice frozen concentrate, unsweetened	52	.10
Pineapple juice canned, unsweetened	55	.10
Plain cake or cupcakes homemade from enriched flour	364	.10

FOOD ITEM	CALS.	UNITS
Popovers baked, commercial	224	.10
Pound cake homemade from enriched flour	473	.10
Pudding from mix, made with milk	131	.10
Red cherries (sour), canned in water, fruit and liquid	43	.10
Red cherries (sour), canned in light syrup, fruit and liquid	74	.10
Red cherries (sour), canned in heavy syrup, fruit and liquid	89	.10
Red cherries (sour), canned in extra-heavy syrup, fruit and liquid	112	.10
Rice pudding with raisins, commercial	146	.10
Salad dressing (blue cheese and Roquefort cheese), commercial, low calorie	76	.10
Spaghetti enriched, cooked until tender	111	.10
Spaghetti with meatballs in tomato sauce, canned	103	.10
Strained bananas (baby food), commercial	84	.10
Tofu (soybean curd)	72	.10
Tomato vegetable soup with noodles from mix	27	.10
Waffles homemade from enriched or unenriched flour	279	.10
Waffles from mix, made with enriched or unenriched flour	225	.10
White rice (fully milled or polished), long grain	106	.10
Angel food cake from mix	259	.00
Beef noodle soup from mix	28	.00
Chicken and noodles homemade	153	.00
Chicken noodle soup from mix	22	.00
Cranberry juice cocktail bottled	65	.00
Eclairs with custard filling and chocolate frosting, commercial	239	.00
Farina enriched, regular, cooked	42	.00
Grape drink canned	54	.00
Grape juice canned or bottled	66	.00
Grape juice frozen concentrate, sweetened	53	.00
Grapefruit juice	39	.00
Grapefruit juice canned, sweetened	53	.00
Grapefruit juice frozen concentrate, sweetened	47	.00
Grapefruit juice canned, unsweetened	41	.00
Grapefruit juice frozen concentrate, unsweetened	41	.00
Italian salad dressing commercial, regular	552	.00
Italian salad dressing commercial, low calorie	50	.00
Lemon juice canned or bottled, unsweetened	23	.00
Lemonade frozen concentrate	44	.00
Lime juice canned or bottled, unsweetened	26	.00
Limeade frozen concentrate	41	.00

FOOD ITEM	CALS.	UNITS
Malt extract dried	367	.00
Mayonnaise commercial, regular or low calorie	718	.00
Orange juice frozen concentrate, unsweetened	45	.00
Oysters fried	239	.00
Prune juice canned or bottled	77	.00
Rice cereal cooked	50	.00
Tangelo juice	41	.00
Tea instant	2	.00
Vanilla pudding homemade	111	.00

Sodium

We're going to take a look at an old nutrient. Just imagine this situation. You go into your favorite restaurant, order the soup du jour — a bowl of minestrone, vegetable, or sweet and sour lentil soup, perhaps — the waitress serves the soup and, before taking a spoonful, what happens? Does your hand automatically reach for the salt shaker and give it one or two shakes — or more likely, three, four, or five? Do you bother even to taste first to see whether the soup would satisfy your craving and taste for sodium without the added salt?

Or say you go into a fast food operation and order a hamburger with pickles on it. You might have some mustard, some french fries with ketchup, and a cola drink. It might taste good — but have you any idea how much sodium you are consuming? Perhaps you prepared fried chicken from a mix last night; or ordered steak tartare with mushroom sauce the last time you went out to a fine restaurant. Have you ever considered how much sodium you might have consumed at these meals?

Any number of foods you might have eaten today probably included extra sodium. To the sodium used in processing, packaging, and preparation, you've probably added more table salt than you realize. At the end of the day, you may feel that you have been conscientious concerning your dietary habits. But there is much more sodium in our foods than most of us are aware of. And every time you consume more sodium than your body needs, you have increased your chance of developing one of America's most formidable opponents — the silent killer, high blood pressure.

It is estimated that more than thirty million Americans suffer from chronic hypertension. If you're over sixty-five, your chances of having high blood pressure are one in two. The problem with high blood pressure is that it can be a symptomless disease: unless you have it checked, you may not be aware you have it. We've all heard stories about apparently healthy people who went out for a jog one day, and suddenly ended up with a heart attack. You may have wondered how that is possible. But someone who never had a problem with heart disease as such may still have had the silent killer all the time. That's why it is so important to have your blood pressure checked regularly, and to understand how it gets elevated and how to keep it normal.

Since overconsumption of sodium is implicated in high blood pressure, let's reexamine some of the foods we eat during the day to see how sodium gets into our food, why we need it, how much is the right amount, and what we can do to maintain normal levels. Suppose when you salted your food you added a teaspoon of salt. During the course of a meal this would not be difficult, especially if you shake without tasting at each course, or if you usually eat so much salt your taste buds are no longer sensitive to it. Well, with that one teaspoon, you've consumed 1,900 milligrams (mg.) of sodium. If you ate at a fast food restaurant and you had a McDonald's Big Mac, you consumed 1,500 mg. of sodium. If you had breakfast there, it would have been 900 mg. Let's say you cut up a pickle and put it on a grilled cheese sandwich, a pita bread sandwich, or a hamburger: that large Heinz pickle gave you 1,100 mg. of sodium. Did you make yourself an instant lunch in the form of broth? One serving of Herbox instant broth contains 800 mg. of sodium. Or perhaps you're on a diet. Even people who think that their diet is very carefully monitored because they are on one of the Weight Watchers' programs should examine a little more carefully what they are consuming; Weight Watchers' frozen eggplant parmigiana contains 1,049 mg. of sodium. Even a simple 4-ounce serving of cottage cheese, a dieter's special which seems to represent for many a move toward a less toxic, more healthful diet, could contain 460 mg. of sodium. So it is not difficult to understand how the average American can consume two and one-half teaspoons of salt every day — 4,750 mg. of sodium. These figures appeared in a report published by the Center for Science in the Public Interest showing the sodium content of average servings of packaged and fast foods. It's not hard to imagine how much sodium your child will be consuming by eating that fast food meal — one such meal can easily add 3,000 to 4,000 mg.

You might ask, "What is the problem? That's not a lot of sodium. Americans consume from 10,000 to 15,000 mg. of sodium a day." That's true, but it presupposes that to be average is to be healthy. If the average American consumes above 5,000 mg. of sodium a day, he or she is consuming more than twelve times what the body actually requires. The FDA has informed us that it is not unusual to consume more than twenty-five to thirty-five times the amount of sodium that we need. Although there is no recommended daily allowance for sodium consumption, the estimates of our needs are far lower than the reality of what we take. We need no more than about 400 mg. of sodium a day; and some people require as little as 200 mg. When you compare our needs to our average intake, you start to realize the average situation is not a healthy state of affairs.

Some of our common misconceptions about sodium help maintain the status quo of overconsumption. One myth is that people who live in hot climates have always used extra salt to overcome the effects of perspiration. That is not true. In fact, epidemiological studies of natives of Africa, South America, and other tropical climates show that their diet has a lower sodium content than ours. Not coincidentally, they do not suffer from the high degree of hypertension that we do; nor do they have the same degree of kidney failure. (The kidneys help to maintain normal blood pressure and normal mineral balance.) Many of our athletes and long distance runners still believe in this shibboleth, and take salt tablets prior to a sporting event. In the summertime, when the temperature is up around 85 or 90 and the humidity is 60 to 90 percent, you'll see heavily padded and uniformed football players taking one, two, or sometimes even three sodium tablets containing as much as 1,000 mg. of sodium chloride per tablet. Not only is that unhealthy, but it could cause serious problems, because it is not lack of sodium that causes fatigue, irritability, and exhaustion after sweaty exertion. It is dehydration and consequent loss, not of sodium, but of potassium.

Loss of potassium can cause severe side effects. Instead of replacing the sodium after a heavy workout, you should be replacing potassium. A piece of fruit, or a tall, cool glass of juice, is more than adequate for this purpose, and is preferable to a sodium tablet, which might cause imbalances in other nutrients. Apricots, bananas, celery juice, carrot juice, and prune juice are good sources of potassium. If you find you are still deficient, potassium ascorbate, a source of vitamin C, is on the market now, supplying extra potassium to the cells. But, it is better to obtain these nutrients first from your diet.

Let's take a look at sodium's role in the body, both positive and negative. Sodium helps our body maintain a homeostasis, or balance, of fluid levels in the body. Normally, sodium ions (in the form of positively charged particles) are found in the fluid surrounding each cell. They are also found in the aquasolution in the blood. Potassium ions, on the other hand, are usually inside the cells. This sodium/potassium balance is maintained, and allows communication between the cells to take place. Impulses travel along the nerves in a smooth, even manner because of the exchange of sodium and potassium through nerve cell membranes. The sodium/potassium balance also allows the muscles to contract. Every time you make a fist, or move a muscle, sodium is playing a part in the ability of that muscle to contract. (Calcium is also important here.) This is true also of the contracting and releasing of the heart muscle. Because the right concentration of sodium is so important to these vital body functions, and to every cell, your body maintains that balance no matter how much or little you consume. However, overconsumption can tax the organs that maintain the balance. You need adequate sodium, but you do not need excess sodium. It is entirely possible to get all the sodium you need from fresh vegetables and juices.

What happens when we have too much sodium? We end up harming the kidneys, which are the regulating mechanisms for the fluid levels in the body. The kidneys have to remove the sodium or dilute it by keeping extra water in the body. When you are retaining too much water because of excess sodium, this not only places a strain on the kidneys, but it can cause edema — fluid buildup — which can strain your heart.

Suppose the kidneys can't get rid of all the sodium you consume fast enough. Sodium works in your body much as it does in cooking: it draws water from areas where it is less concentrated. That's one of the reasons sodium was used as a preserving agent to preserve ham. The ham would be soaked in a brine (salt) solution to draw out the moisture. Unfortunately, salt does something similar to your cells when you have too much of it circulating in your body fluids. The excess sodium in the fluid surrounding the cells draws water out of your cells. Now you have the water that was in the cell outside the cell. This increases the total volume of water in the blood. With the increased volume, you create greater pressure in the veins. In addition, because of this expanded volume of blood, the pull of gravity tends to keep the fluid in the peripheral areas such as the leg, foot, calf, hands, and arms. So the heart has to pump harder to make it circulate. The expanded volume of blood also courses faster through your arteries and veins than normal, and the cells that normally would be nourished by the blood cannot absorb enough nutrients from it. As a result, many cells in the body become deficient in certain nutrients. Thus, this expanded volume of blood, which causes the heart to beat harder and faster to get the blood circulating against the pull of gravity, deprives the cells of the nutrients that they need. The problem is probably exacerbated by a weakened capillary system to begin with, especially in older people. High blood pressure can thus cause various states of mineral and vitamin deficiency (though these may be at subclinical levels) hard to detect. Mineral deficiencies in themselves can cause the arteries to further deteriorate.

The kidneys are the fail-safe organs. They're the ones that have to stop this vicious cycle created by overconsumption of salt. The kidneys try to lower the blood pressure by extracting some of the fluid, and excrete the extra salt to redevelop a balance between the salt and the fluid. The kidneys can handle that strain occasionally — but what happens when it occurs all the time? We destroy the kidneys. Add on to that all the distress in our lives that activates our nervous system, which can also precipitate high blood pressure, and you'll realize that many of us are walking around in a rather dangerous state.

There are many individuals who are sincere in trying to avoid sodium. They wouldn't dream of picking up the salt shaker or the soy sauce, but they would think nothing of popping a Rolaids tablet — which contains 50 mg. of sodium. Maybe they miscombine their foods or overeat, as many millions of Americans do, get an upset stomach, and take an antacid such as Bromo Seltzer — 700 mg. of sodium in each and every glass — or Alka Seltzer — over 500 mg. of sodium. Even the soft water we consume has a high sodium content. Almost all communities in the U.S. except some rural ones use water-softening agents, and sodium is a primary means of precipitating the hard minerals out of the water. Now 8 ounces of tap water contain 12 mg. of sodium. If you consume the amount of water that you should — eight 8-ounce glasses a day — that's almost 100 mg. of sodium right there, or one-fourth of your total requirements of sodium.

Of course, these instances are almost incidental compared to some of the major hidden sources of sodium in our foods. There is sodium benzoate, used as a preservative in hundreds of foods; sodium nitrite, added to processed meat such as bacon, salami, bologna, and even steaks, hamburgers, and hot dogs; sodium bisulfate, used as an antioxidant instead of the more natural vitamin E; and of course, sodium bicarbonate, baking soda, used in almost all baked goods.

What about the individuals who take 3,000 to 10,000 mg. a day of sodium ascorbate, a commonly used form of vitamin C? They are consuming a substantial amount of sodium. They may consciously restrict and monitor their diet so as not to include salt other than that which occurs naturally in food, and yet in an effort to be healthy take sodium ascorbate and end up raising their blood pressure because of excess sodium, all because they failed to note the word "sodium" on their vitamin label. It takes careful reading of all food labels to make sure the products you consume do not supply you with excess sodium.

The world of processed foods is a nutritional mine field: you have to walk gingerly and be extremely selective in the foods you consume. This is especially so with canned foods; sodium has been used as a preservative in canned vegetables for years, along with sugar. The problem is we acquire a taste for sodium, as we do for sugar. By constantly ingesting any food, whether it's salty or sugary, overtolerance for it builds up and we develop a desire for still larger quantities of it. Manufacturers have played a part in developing these taste preferences. For years, baby food manufacturers added salt and MSG — *monosodium glutamate* — (along with sugar) into baby food to entice the taste buds of the parents — even though the babies would have enjoyed the foods just as much without those chemical additives. As a result, all those children grew up with preferences for salty (and sweet) foods.

Salt is added to many highly processed foods to cover up the loss of taste due to processing. Oils, for example, are removed from grains, along with the germ, because they can go bad. The food's unique taste is usually locked into the oils. When you eliminate the oil you are basically left with a tasteless product. Then it is further altered so it won't go bad; it won't mold; it'll stay a certain color, texture, and consistency; it will have a certain flowability out of a box or can. There will be antifungus and antibacterial agents. Hundreds of additives can be used without being specifically named on the label. In fact, manufacturers don't even have to tell you how much sodium is in a particular food. As a result, you can be sitting down to what you think is a relatively healthy serving of canned peas — and indeed, if those peas were in a natural form, they would have a small amount of sodium — but canned they may have more than 200 times more sodium than fresh peas. You wouldn't know that, because it's not on the menu and not on the label.

In order to return the flavor to a tasteless processed food, sugar and salt are added in substantial quantities. Look how many products containing cornstarch used MSG as a flavor "enhancer." (Manufacturers only have to enhance what they have dulled.) So be wary. Processed foods that contain sodium could pose a major threat to your health if consumed over a period of time and if they trigger a reaction that raises your blood pressure level.

All diets have advantages and drawbacks. It is a mistake to adopt any dietary regimen without scrutinizing it for weaknesses. Some Americans have embraced a Japanese or Oriental diet. There are many benefits to such a diet. Orientals have cultivated a wide variety of vegetables; their cuisine emphasizes combining vegetable sources of protein, such as rice and soy, with animal proteins used almost as condiments; it includes plenty of fiber; it is high in B-vitamins and vitamin C. But its shortcoming is a predilection for sodium. This is because at one time famine was a more frequent threat, and people had to pickle or dry their food using salt as a preservative because they couldn't be sure when they would next be able to obtain fresh fish, produce, vegetables, or pork. Those customs, like many dietary traditions, were beneficial and useful once but have lost their significance and become counterproductive. Epidemiological studies show that the Japanese have among the highest, if not the highest, incidence of high blood pressure in the world. This is directly attributable to their use of sodium (salt) in soy sauces and in the pickling and processing of their foods.

If you want to wean yourself away from overconsumption of salt, but fear that food may seem tasteless without it, there are a number of spices and salt substitutes you can use to enliven the taste of foods. Potassium chloride is an excellent salt substitute. It tastes salty, yet it's beneficial to you because it's potassium. However, too much potassium can be dangerous to kidney patients. A full spectrum of salt-free substitutes are found in health food stores. Some natural flavor enhancers you may enjoy include lemon, chives, cumin, curry powder, onions, and garlic. (Garlic has the added advantage of lowering blood pressure and purifying the blood naturally if taken raw.) There are also parsley, mustard, thyme, and the vinegars, including rice vinegar and apple cider vinegar.

It may take some time to train your taste buds to enjoy the natural flavors of foods seasoned with herbs and spices instead of salt; but it is well worth the effort in terms of increasing your chances of enjoying good health and longevity.

The unit value for sodium is given in milligrams. Any food having less than 1 milligram of sodium per 100-gram portion is considered to have a trace sodium content and is listed as having 0 for its unit value.

Where the symbol N. A. appears in the calorie column, the

information was not available.

All figures are based on an edible portion equaling 100 grams, or approximately 3 ounces. In the case of some of the listed foods, one would not consume 100 grams in one serving. Calculations should be adjusted accordingly.

Sodium

FOOD ITEM	CALS.	UNITS
Salt	0	38758
Bouillon cubes or powder	120	24000
Baking powder	109	10953
Soy sauce	68	7325
Pickled olives canned or bottled	338	3288
Kelp raw	N.A.	3007
Miso (fermented soybean product)	171	2950
Irish moss (seaweed), raw	N.A.	2892
Green olives pickled, canned or bottled	116	2400
Caviar (sturgeon), granular	262	2200
Italian salad dressing commercial, regular	552	2092
Corned beef medium fat content, cooked	372	1740
Pretzels	390	1680
Pickles (dill)	11	1428
French salad dressing commercial, regular	410	1370
Pickles (sour)	10	1353
Tomato chili sauce bottled	104	1338
Bread stuffing mix dry	371	1331
Brown mustard prepared	91	1307
Bologna	304	1300
Yellow mustard prepared	75	1252
American cheese pasteurized, processed	370	1136
Blue and Roquefort cheese salad dressing commercial, regular	504	1108
Blue and Roquefort cheese salad dressing commercial, low calorie	76	1094
Wheat flour self rising, enriched	352	1079
Bran sugar and malt extract added	240	1060
Puffed corn (cereal)	399	1060
Tomato catsup bottled	106	1042
Cheese crackers commercial	479	1039
Wheat flakes (cereal)	354	1032

FOOD ITEM	CALS.	UNITS
Bacon cured, broiled or fried, drained	611	1021
Cornflakes	386	1005
Crab canned	101	1000
Shredded corn (cereal)	389	988
Butter	716	987
Margarine	720	987
Rice flakes (cereal)	390	987
Biscuits from mix, made with enriched flour and milk	325	973
Pork sausage links or bulk, cooked	476	958
Rye wafers whole grain	344	882
Russian salad dressing commercial, regular	494	868
Shredded rice (cereal)	392	846
Chicken noodle soup canned, condensed	53	816
Barbecue sauce	91	815
Pie crust from mix	464	813
Tuna canned in oil, solids and liquid	288	800
French salad dressing commercial, low calorie	96	787
Italian salad dressing commercial, low calorie	50	787
Cornflakes sugar coated	386	775
Split pea soup canned, condensed	118	767
Manhattan clam chowder canned, condensed	66	766
Sauerkraut canned, solids and liquid	18	747
Cornbread from mix, made with eggs and milk	233	744
Bread crumbs dry, grated	392	736
Parmesan cheese	393	734
Pizza with sausage, homemade	234	729
Pickle relish (sweet), commercial	138	712
Swiss cheese (domestic), unprocessed	370	710
Tartar sauce regular	531	707
Tartar sauce low calorie	224	707
Pizza homemade, with cheese	236	702
Cheddar cheese unprocessed	398	700
Thousand Island salad dressing commercial, regular	502	700
Thousand Island salad dressing commercial, low calorie	180	700
Graham crackers plain	384	670
Beef broth, bouillon, and consomme' canned, condensed	26	652
Pizza frozen, with cheese	245	647
Waffles frozen, commercial	253	644
Blueberry muffins homemade from enriched flour	281	632
Cornbread homemade from whole-ground cornmeal	207	628

FOOD ITEM	CALS.	UNITS
Biscuits homemade from enriched flour	369	626
Hard rolls commercial, enriched	312	625
Piecrust and plain pastry made with enriched or unenriched flour, commercial, baked	464	611
Peanut butter salt added	581	607
Mayonnaise	718	597
Italian bread enriched or unenriched	276	585
French bread enriched or unenriched	290	580
Pumpernickel bread	246	569
Pancakes from mix, made with eggs and milk	225	564
Whole wheat rolls commercial	257	564
Weakfish broiled	208	560
Rye bread (American), commercial	243	557
Chop suey with meat, canned	62	551
Whole wheat crackers commercial	403	547
Corn beef hash with potatoes, canned	181	540
Frankfurters and beans canned	144	539
Skim milk dry, regular	363	532
Chili con carne with beans, canned	133	531
Rice cereal (baby food), commercial	371	530
Cracked wheat bread commercial	263	529
Potato salad homemade with cooked salad dressing	99	528
Whole wheat bread commercial	243	527
Sardines (Atlantic), canned in oil, solids and liquid	311	510
White bread made with 1% - 2% nonfat dry milk	269	507
Rolls and buns plain, commercial	398	506
Doughnuts cake type	391	501
Corn muffins homemade from whole-ground cornmeal	288	495
Spaghetti with meatballs in tomato sauce, canned	103	488
Corn muffins homemade from enriched degermed cornmeal	314	481
Corn muffins from mix, made with eggs and milk	324	479
Corn fritters commercial	377	477
Buckwheat pancakes from mix, made with eggs and milk	200	475
Waffles homemade	279	475
Bran muffins homemade	261	448
Muffins plain, homemade	294	441
Oatmeal (baby food), commercial	375	437
Corn pudding commercial	104	436
Tomato vegetable soup with noodles from mix	27	427
Pancakes homemade from enriched or unenriched flour	231	425

FOOD ITEM	CALS.	UNITS
Tomato soup canned, condensed, prepared with milk	69	422
Chop suey with meat, homemade	120	421
Beef and vegetable stew canned	79	411
Spaghetti with meatballs in tomato sauce, homemade	134	407
Whole milk dry	502	405
Chocolate chip cookies commercial	471	401
Mushrooms canned, solids and liquid	17	400
Sardines (Pacific), canned in tomato sauce, solids and liquid	197	400
Tomato puree canned, regular	39	399
Tomato soup canned, condensed	36	396
Sweet rolls commercial	316	389
Manhattan clam chowder canned, condensed	33	383
Hot chocolate from mix	392	382
Spaghetti with cheese in tomato sauce, canned	76	382
White sauce medium	162	379
White rice fully milled or polished, enriched	109	374
Danish pastry commercial	422	366
Assorted cookies commercial	480	365
Mashed potatoes frozen	93	359
White rice fully milled or polished, enriched, long grain	106	358
Chocolate chip cookies homemade from enriched flour	516	348
Corn muffins from mix	297	346
Eggs fried	216	338
Welsh rarebit	179	332
Pea soup from mix	50	325
White cake homemade	375	323
Gelatin dessert powder	371	318
Spanish rice homemade	87	316
Rolls from mix	299	313
Beef dinner with vegetables (baby food), commercial	87	304
Cherry pie commercial	261	304
Gingerbread from mix	276	304
Apple pie commercial	256	301
Mashed potatoes milk added	65	301
Cake and cupcake (plain), homemade	364	300
Hash browned potatoes frozen, cooked	224	299
Chicken noodle dinner (baby food), commercial	49	297
Oat cereal with toasted wheat germ and soy	62	292
Chicken chow mein without noodles, canned	38	290
Cottage cheese uncreamed, large or small curd	86	290

FOOD ITEM	CALS.	UNITS
Lemon candied	314	290
Chicken chow mein without noodles, homemade	102	287
Angel food cake homemade	269	283
Brown rice cooked	119	282
Rolls and buns homemade	339	279
Eggs poached	163	271
Beef noodle dinner (baby food), commercial	48	269
Blueberry pie piecrust made with unenriched flour	242	268
Chicken with vegetables (baby food), commercial	100	265
Scallops (bay and sea), steamed	112	265
Eggs scrambled	173	257
Omelets	173	257
Beef kidneys braised	252	253
Brownies with nuts, homemade from enriched flour	485	251
Chicken and noodles homemade	153	250
Cream cheese unprocessed	374	250
Zwieback	423	250
Chicken noodle soup from mix	22	241
Flounder baked	202	237
Gingerbread homemade from enriched flour	317	237
Alaska green peas canned, regular, solids and liquid	66	236
Asparagus spears, canned, regular, solids and liquid	18	236
Carrots canned, regular, solids and liquid	28	236
Corn (sweet, yellow), canned, vacuum pack, solids and liquid	83	236
Corn (sweet, white and yellow), whole kernel, canned, regular pack, solids and liquid	66	236
Cowpeas (including black-eyed peas), canned, solids and liquid	70	236
Creamed corn (sweet, white and yellow), canned, regular pack, solids and liquid	82	236
Green peas (sweet), canned, regular, solids and liquid	57	236
Green snap beans canned, regular, solids and liquid	18	236
Lima beans canned, regular, solids and liquid	71	236
Red beets canned, regular, solids and liquid	34	236
Spinach canned, regular, solids and liquid	19	236
Turnip greens leaves and stems, canned, solids amd liquid	18	236
Yellow snap beans canned, regular, solids and liquid	19	236
Chocolate cake with chocolate frosting, homemade	369	235
Ice cream cones	377	232

FOOD ITEM	CALS.	UNITS
Mashed potatoes dehydrated, flakes without milk	93	231
Cottage cheese creamed	106	229
White cake with chocolate frosting made from mix	351	227
Caramels plain or chocolate	399	226
Pecan pie commercial	418	221
Popovers baked	224	220
Pumpkin pie commercial	211	214
Green beans (baby food), commercial	22	213
Lobster (Northern), canned or fresh	95	210
Tomato juice canned, concentrate	20	209
Oysters fried	239	206
Corn grits degermed, cooked	51	205
Bread pudding with raisins, commercial	187	201
Brownies with nuts and chocolate icing, frozen	419	200
Tomato juice cocktail canned or bottled	21	200
Almonds roasted and salted	627	198
Whitefish (lake), stuffed, baked	215	195
Light fruitcake homemade	389	193
French fried shrimp	225	186
Haddock fried	165	177
Rice cereal cooked, added nutrients	50	176
Beef noodle soup from mix	28	175
Carrots (baby food), commmercial	29	169
Oat and wheat cereals cooked	65	168
New Zealand spinach raw	19	159
Dark fruitcake homemade	379	158
Frosting (chocolate fudge), from mix, made with water and table fat	378	156
Ocean perch (Atlantic), fried	227	153
Custard pudding (baby food), commercial	100	150
Chard (Swiss), raw	25	147
Farina enriched, regular, cooked	42	144
Halibut (Atlantic and Pacific), broiled	171	134
Beet greens raw	24	130
Buttermilk cultured, made from skim milk	36	130
Tomatoes ripe, canned, regular, solids and liquid	21	130
Baby lima beans frozen, boiled and drained	118	129
Pudding from mix, made with milk	125	129
Fruit pudding (baby food), commercial	96	128
Celery (green and yellow varieties), raw	17	126

FOOD ITEM	CALS.	UNITS
Lobster salad	110	124
Eggs hard-boiled	163	122
Brewer's yeast debittered	283	121
Evaporated milk canned, unsweetened	137	118
Salmon cooked, broiled or baked	182	116
Green peas frozen, boiled and drained	68	115
Condensed milk canned, sweetened	321	112
Creamed pollack	128	111
Cod broiled	170	110
Cornmeal (white and yellow), degermed, cooked	50	110
Pound cake homemade	473	110
Sturgeon steamed	160	108
Bluefish baked or broiled	159	104
Lima beans frozen, boiled and drained	99	101
Celeriac root, raw	40	100
Blackstrap molasses	213	96
Horseradish prepared	38	96
Milk chocolate plain	520	94
New Zealand spinach boiled and drained	13	92
Celery (green and yellow varieties), boiled and drained	14	88
Chard (Swiss), boiled and drained	18	86
Chicken all classes, dark meat, roasted, without skin	176	86
Peas and carrots frozen, boiled and drained	53	84
Eclairs with custard filling and chocolate frosting, commercial	239	82
Malt extract dried	367	80
Custard baked, commercial	115	79
Shad baked	201	79
Beet greens boiled and drained	18	76
Dandelion greens raw	45	76
Kale leaves and stems, raw	38	75
Roe (cod and shad), baked or broiled	126	73
Beef tripe commercial	100	72
Coffee instant, powder	129	72
Rice pudding with raisins, commercial	146	71
Spinach raw	26	71
Corn syrup (light and dark)	290	68
Ice milk	152	68
Butterscotch candy	397	66
Vanilla pudding homemade	111	65
Chicken all classes, light meat, roasted, without skin	166	64

FOOD ITEM	CALS.	UNITS
Beef tongue medium fat content, braised	244	61
Red beets raw	43	60
Sesame seeds dry, whole	563	60
Chocolate pudding homemade	148	56
Sunflower seed flour partially defatted	339	56
Fruit dessert with tapioca (baby food), commercial	84	53
Mixed vegetables (carrots, corn, peas, green snap beans, and lima beans), frozen, boiled and drained	64	53
Chocolate syrup (thin)	245	52
Skim milk	36	52
Spinach chopped, frozen, boiled and drained	23	52
Watercress leaves and stems, raw	19	52
Hot cocoa homemade	97	51
Tamarinds	239	51
Yogurt made from partially skimmed milk	50	51
Spinach boiled and drained	23	50
Whole milk	66	50
Turnips raw	30	49
Hot chocolate homemade	95	48
Sweet potatoes canned in syrup, solids and liquid	114	48
Carrots raw	42	47
Hamburger regular ground, cooked	286	47
Yogurt made from whole milk	62	47
Half-and-half cream	134	46
Red beets canned, low sodium, solids and liquid	32	46
Parsley raw	44	45
Dandelion greens boiled and drained	33	44
Collards leaves and stems, raw	40	43
Kale leaves and stems, boiled and drained	28	43
Red beets boiled and drained	32	43
Sweet potatoes candied	168	42
Tuna canned in water, solids and liquid	127	41
Black-eyed peas frozen, boiled and drained	130	39
Carrots canned, low sodium, solids and liquid	22	39
Cowpeas boiled and drained	130	39
Succotash frozen, boiled and drained	93	38
Tomato paste canned	82	38
Light whipping cream	300	36
Dried figs	274	34
Goat's milk	67	34

FOOD ITEM	CALS.	UNITS
Potato flour	351	34
Spinach canned, low sodium, solids and liquid	21	34
Turnips boiled and drained	23	34
Carrots boiled and drained	31	33
Heavy whipping cream	352	32
Mustard greens raw	31	32
Artichokes (globe or French), boiled and drained	44	30
Brown sugar beet or cane	373	30
Sunflower seed kernels dried	560	30
Raisins uncooked	289	27
Dried apricots uncooked	260	26
Red cabbage raw	31	26
Collards leaves and stems, boiled and drained	29	25
Chinese cabbage raw	14	23
Coconut meat fresh	346	23
Kale frozen, boiled and drained	31	21
Cabbage raw	24	20
Chinese water chestnuts raw	79	20
Garlic cloves raw	137	19
Cowpeas (including black-eyed peas), dry, cooked	76	18
Mustard greens boiled and drained	23	18
Radishes raw	17	18
Jellies	273	17
Turnip greens leaves and stems, frozen, boiled and drained	23	17
Collards frozen, boiled and drained	30	16
Dried peaches uncooked	262	16
Broccoli spears, raw	32	15
Broccoli chopped, frozen, boiled and drained	26	15
Cashew nuts	561	15
Mushrooms raw	28	15
Torula yeast	277	15
Brussels sprouts raw	45	14
Brussels sprouts frozen, boiled and drained	33	14
Cabbage shredded, boiled and drained	20	14
Endive (curly endive and escarole), raw	20	14
Garden cress raw	32	14
Maple sugar	348	14
Marmalade (lemon or orange)	720	14
Cauliflower raw	27	13
Green peppers (sweet), raw	22	13

FOOD ITEM	CALS.	UNITS
Raisins cooked, sugar added, fruit and liquid	213	13
Split peas cooked	115	13
Cantaloupe	30	12
Chestnuts dried	377	12
Honeydew melon	33	12
Jams and preserves	272	12
Parsnips raw	76	12
Shallots bulbs, raw	72	12
Sweet potatoes with skin, baked	141	12
Sweet potatoes canned, in liquid, solids and liquid, unsweetened	46	12
Broccoli spears, boiled and drained	26	10
Brussels sprouts boiled and drained	36	10
Cauliflower frozen, boiled and drained	18	10
Maple syrup	252	10
Mustard greens frozen, boiled and drained	20	10
Onions mature, raw	38	10
Orange sherbet	134	10
Sweet potatoes with skin, boiled	114	10
Cauliflower boiled and drained	22	9
Green peppers (sweet), boiled and drained	18	9
Lettuce (Boston and bibb), raw	14	9
Peanut flour defatted	371	9
Wheat bran crude, commercially milled	213	9
Dried prunes uncooked	255	8
Kohlrabi thickened bulb-like stems, raw	29	8
Parsnips boiled and drained	66	8
Almond meal partially defatted	408	7
Beer	42	7
Chicory (endive), raw	15	7
Dried pears	268	7
Green snap beans raw	32	7
Kumquats raw	65	7
Mangoes raw	66	7
Onions boiled and drained	29	7
Tofu (soybean curd)	72	7
Yellow snap beans raw	27	7
Applesauce (baby food), commercial	72	6
Chestnuts fresh	194	6

FOOD ITEM	CALS.	UNITS
Cocoa powder high fat	299	6
Cocoa powder low fat	187	6
Cucumbers with skin, raw	15	6
French fried potatoes	274	6
Ginger root fresh	49	6
Kohlrabi thickened bulb-like stems, boiled and drained	24	6
Lemon peel	N.A.	6
Nectarines raw	64	6
Pecans	687	6
Tomato puree canned, low sodium	39	6
Dried peaches cooked without sugar, fruit and liquid	82	5
Fruit cocktail canned in water, fruit and liquid with or without artificial sweetener	37	5
Fruit cocktail canned in light syrup, fruit and liquid	60	5
Fruit cocktail canned in heavy syrup, fruit and liquid	76	5
Fruit cocktail canned in extra-heavy syrup, fruit and liquid	92	5
Honey	304	5
Leeks bulb and lower leaf, raw	52	5
Mung bean sprouts raw	35	5
Peanuts without skins, raw	568	5
Peanuts with skins, roasted	582	5
Plantains (baking bananas), raw	119	5
Rutabagas raw	46	5
Wine	85	5
Almonds dried	598	4
Avocados raw	167	4
Baked potatoes with skin	93	4
Baking chocolate	505	4
Banana powder	340	4
Bitter chocolate	505	4
Dried prunes cooked, without added sugar	119	4
Dried prunes cooked, no added sugar	119	4
French fried potatoes frozen, heated	220	4
Grapefruit canned in water, with or without artificial sweetener, fruit and liquid	30	4
Guavas whole, raw	62	4
Lima beans canned, low sodium, solids and liquid	70	4
Mung bean sprouts boiled and drained	28	4
Puffed wheat (cereal)	363	4
Rutabagas boiled and drained	35	4

FOOD ITEM	CALS.	UNITS
Tomatoes ripe, boiled	26	4
Asparagus spears, canned, low sodium, solids and liquid	16	3
Barley pearled, light	349	3
Black currants (European), raw	54	3
Black walnuts	628	3
Cowpeas (including black-eyed peas), with seeds, boiled and drained	34	3
Dried pears cooked, with added sugar, fruit and liquid	151	3
Dried pears cooked without added sugar, fruit and liquid	126	3
Grapes (American), raw	69	3
Grapes (European), raw	67	3
Green peas (Alaska), low sodium, solids and liquid	55	3
Green peas (sweet), canned, low sodium, solids and liquid	47	3
Lichees dried	277	3
Lychees raw	64	3
Papayas raw	39	3
Pomegranate pulp, raw	63	3
Potatoes with skin, boiled	76	3
Red beans canned, solids and liquid	90	3
Rhubarb frozen, cooked, sugar added	143	3
Shredded wheat (cereal)	354	3
Summer squash (yellow crookneck), frozen, boiled and drained	21	3
Tomato juice canned or bottled, low sodium	19	3
Tomatoes ripe, raw	22	3
Tomatoes ripe, canned, low sodium, solids and liquid	20	3
Wheat germ raw, commercially milled	363	3
Whole wheat flour	333	3
Yellow snap beans boiled and drained	22	3
Apple butter	186	2
Applesauce canned, sweetened	91	2
Applesauce canned, unsweetened or artificially sweetened	41	2
Asparagus spears, raw	26	2
Bread flour enriched or unenriched	365	2
Cake or pastry flour	364	2
Corn sweet, (white and yellow), canned, low sodium, solids and liquid	57	2
Cranberries raw	46	2
Creamed corn (sweet, white and yellow), canned, low sodium, solids and liquid	82	2

FOOD ITEM	CALS.	UNITS
Egg noodles enriched, cooked	125	2
Figs raw	80	2
Figs canned in water, with or without artificial sweetener, fruit and liquid	48	2
Figs canned in light syrup, solids and liquid	65	2
Figs canned in heavy syrup, fruit and liquid	84	2
Figs canned in extra-heavy syrup, fruit and liquid	103	2
Filberts (hazelnuts)	634	2
Grape juice canned or bottled	66	2
Green snap beans canned, low sodium, solids and liquid	16	2
Lemons peeled, raw	27	2
Lima beans dry, boiled and drained	138	2
Limes raw	28	2
Okra boiled and drained	29	2
Okra cuts and pods, frozen, boiled and drained	38	2
Peaches canned in water or juice, with or without artificial sweetener, fruit and liquid	31	2
Peaches canned in light syrup, fruit and liquid	57	2
Peaches canned in heavy syrup, fruit and liquid	78	2
Peaches canned in extra-heavy syrup, fruit and liquid	97	2
Pears with skin, raw	61	2
Plums purple, canned in water, with or without artificial sweetener, fruit and liquid	46	2
Prickly pears raw	42	2
Prune juice canned or bottled	77	2
Puffed rice (cereal), added nutrients	399	2
Pumpkin canned	33	2
Red cherries (sour), canned in water, solids and liquid	43	2
Red cherries (sour), frozen, sweetened	712	2
Rhubarb cooked, sugar added	141	2
Rhubarb raw	16	2
Soybeans dry, cooked	130	2
Tangerines	46	2
Walnuts	651	2
Yellow snap beans canned, low sodium, solids and liquid	15	2
Alcoholic beverages gin, rum, vodka, and whiskey	231	1
Apples freshly harvested, with skin, raw	58	1
Apples freshly harvested, without skin, raw	54	1
Apricots raw	51	1
Apricots canned in water, with or without artificial sweetener, fruit and liquid	38	1

FOOD ITEM	CALS.	UNITS
Apricots canned in juice, fruit and liquid	54	1
Apricots canned in light syrup, fruit and liquid	66	1
Apricots canned in heavy syrup, fruit and liquid	86	1
Apricots canned in extra-heavy syrup, fruit and liquid	101	1
Asparagus spears, boiled and drained	20	1
Asparagus cuts and tips, frozen, boiled and drained	22	1
Black raspberries raw	73	1
Blackberries raw	62	1
Blackberries canned in water, with or without artificial sweetener, fruit and liquid	40	1
Blackberries canned in juice, fruit and liquid	54	1
Blackberries canned in light syrup, fruit and liquid	72	1
Blackberries canned in heavy syrup, fruit and liquid	91	1
Blackberries canned in extra-heavy syrup, fruit and liquid	110	1
Blueberries raw	62	1
Blueberries canned in extra-heavy syrup, fruit and liquid	101	1
Blueberries canned in water, with or without artificial sweetener, fruit and liquid	39	1
Boysenberries	36	1
Brazil nuts	654	1
Cherries (sweet), canned in water, with or without artificial sweetener, fruit and liquid	48	1
Cherries (sweet), canned in light syrup, fruit and liquid	65	1
Cherries (sweet), canned in heavy syrup, fruit and liquid	81	1
Cherries (sweet), canned in extra-heavy syrup, fruit and liquid	100	1
Cider vinegar	14	1
Coffee instant	1	1
Corn (sweet), whole kernels, boiled and drained	79	1
Corn on the cob boiled and drained	94	1
Cowpeas (including black-eyed peas), boiled and drained	108	1
Cranberry juice cocktail bottled	65	1
Cranberry sauce canned, sweetened, strained	146	1
Dates (domestic), dry	274	1
Dried apples cooked, sugar added	112	1
Dried apples cooked, no sugar added	78	1
Eggplant boiled and drained	19	1
Fruit salad canned in water, with or without artificial sweetener, fruit and liquid	35	1
Fruit salad canned in light syrup, fruit and liquid	59	1

FOOD ITEM	CALS.	UNITS
Fruit salad canned in heavy syrup, fruit and liquid	75	1
Fruit salad canned in extra-heavy syrup, fruit and liquid	90	1
Gooseberries raw	39	1
Grape drink canned	54	1
Grape juice frozen concentrate, sweetened	53	1
Grapefruit raw	41	1
Grapefruit canned in juice, sweetened, fruit and liquid	53	1
Grapefruit canned in syrup, fruit and liquid	70	1
Grapefruit canned in juice, unsweetened, fruit and liquid	41	1
Grapefruit juice	39	1
Grapefruit juice frozen concentrate, sweetened	47	1
Grapefruit juice frozen concentrate, unsweetened	41	1
Green peas immature, boiled and drained	71	1
Green snap beans boiled and drained	25	1
Green squash (zucchini and cocozelle), raw or boiled and drained	12	1
Lemon juice canned or bottled, unsweetened	23	1
Lima beans boiled and drained	111	1
Lime juice canned or bottled, unsweetened	26	1
Macaroni enriched or unenriched, cooked until tender	111	1
Orange drink from mix	46	1
Orange juice fresh, commercial	45	1
Orange juice canned, sweetened or unsweetened	52	1
Orange juice frozen concentrate, unsweetened	45	1
Orange juice canned, unsweetened	45	1
Oranges peeled, raw	49	1
Peach nectar canned	48	1
Peaches raw	38	1
Pear nectar canned	52	1
Pears canned in water, with or without artificial sweetener, fruit and liquid	32	1
Pears canned in juice, fruit and liquid	46	1
Pears canned in light syrup, fruit and liquid	61	1
Pears canned in heavy syrup, fruit and liquid	76	1
Pears canned in extra-heavy syrup, fruit and liquid	92	1
Persimmons (native), raw	127	1
Pineapple raw	52	1
Pineapple canned in water, with or without artificial sweetener, fruit and liquid	39	1
Pineapple canned in juice, fruit and liquid	58	1

FOOD ITEM	CALS.	UNITS
Pineapple canned in light syrup, fruit and liquid	59	1
Pineapple canned in heavy syrup, fruit and liquid	74	1
Pineapple canned in extra-heavy syrup, fruit and liquid	90	1
Pineapple juice canned, unsweetened	55	1
Pineapple juice frozen concentrate, unsweetened	52	1
Plums (prune type), raw	75	1
Plums canned in light syrup, fruit and liquid	63	1
Plums canned in heavy syrup, fruit and liquid	83	1
Plums canned in extra-heavy syrup, fruit and liquid	102	1
Potatoes canned, solids and liquid	44	1
Red bananas raw	90	1
Red cherries canned in light syrup, fruit and liquid	74	1
Red cherries canned in heavy syrup, fruit and liquid	89	1
Red cherries canned in extra-heavy syrup, fruit and liquid	112	1
Red raspberries raw	57	1
Red raspberries frozen, sweetened	98	1
Soybean flour defatted	326	1
Spaghetti enriched, cooked until tender	111	1
Strawberries raw	37	1
Strawberries canned in water, with or without artificial sweetener, fruit and liquid	22	1
Sugar (beet or cane), granulated	385	1
Sugar (beet or cane), powdered	385	1
Summer squash raw or boiled and drained	14	1
Tangerine juice fresh	43	1
Tangerine juice canned, sweetened	50	1
Tangerine juice frozen concentrate, unsweetened	46	1
Tangerine juice canned, unsweetened	43	1
Watermelon raw	26	1
Winter squash boiled	38	1
Winter squash baked	63	1
Winter squash raw	37	1
Yellow snap beans frozen, boiled and drained	27	1
Corn on the cob (sweet, white and yellow), boiled and drained	91	0
Lemonade frozen concentrate	44	0
Lime ice	78	0
Limeade frozen concentrate	41	0
Rice bran	276	0

Vitamins

$$\bigcirc 7$$

A vitamin is an organic compound necessary for sustaining life. Vitamins are one of the six classes of essential nutrients, along with protein, fats, carbohydrates, minerals, and water. As with minerals, we need certain vitamins only in tiny quantities, and others, in larger amounts. For example, we need only a few micrograms — millionths of a gram — of vitamin B_{12} each day. Other vitamins are required in larger amounts, measured in milligrams, that can add up to several grams.

The best sources of vitamins are dark green leafy vegetables, yellow vegetables, grains, legumes, nuts and seeds, and animal products. Refined foods are not good sources. Not only are they depleted of vitamins, but their digestion and utilization saps the body's stores of certain vitamins.

Vitamins are divided into two categories, oil-soluble and water-soluble. The oil-soluble vitamins are A, D, E, and K. They require oil to be absorbed and stored by the body, and are usually found in nature in oily sources such as the germ of grains, or in fish liver. Because they can be stored for longer lengths of time in the body than the water-soluble vitamins, the amount stored can accumulate. Hence, there is a possibility with certain of them of a toxic reaction, when too much builds up in the body's tissues. These include vitamin D, which is added to our milk and can also be produced by the body in the presence of sunlight, and vitamin A, also produced by the body from precursors found in the yellow pigments of plants, and found in fish liver oils. You would need to take 50,000 to 100,000 units of vitamin A for a number of weeks in order to obtain too much, and much has been made of the fact that toxicity reactions do occasionally occur. (In addition, sometimes the skin of people who drink large quantities of carrot juice becomes jaundiced; however, this quickly reverses when they cut back on their consumption of the yellow pigment carotene.) The fact remains that most Americans are deficient in vitamin A — an indication of the inadequacy of the typical American diet, since vitamin A is so easily obtained from foods.

The most obvious symptoms of vitamin A deficiency include night blindness, in which the eye takes a long time to adjust from bright to dim lighting (and which no doubt takes its toll in nighttime automobile accidents), and retarded growth in children. Vitamin A is necessary for healthy epithelial tissues — that is, the skin, the lining of the hollow organs of the respiratory, urinary, and digestive systems, and the tissues of the body. A deficiency can lead to degeneration of these tissues, leaving you susceptible to infections of the eye, ear, nose, respiratory and urinary tracts. Still more important, vitamin A is essential for maintaining the body's immune response: it is the anti-infective vitamin. Vitamin C has gained all the publicity in this respect, but in fact vitamin A is equal to C in its importance in helping the body fight infection. Adequate amounts of the two vitamins together in the diet are a good source of protection against infections.

Vitamin D is important to healthy bones and teeth, since it regulates the absorption of calcium and phosphorus from the digestive tract, and controls the deposit of calcium in bones and teeth.

Vitamin E has been much maligned. For years, physicians believed that it was irresponsible to show that there was a correlation between diet and health, or that any food supplement or food might have the ability to begin to reverse a degenerative condition such as heart disease, varicose veins, diabetes, or kidney disease. Yet that is exactly what Drs. Evan and Wilfred Shute, two pioneers in the clinical use of vitamin E, were accomplishing, with tens of thousands of patients. The controversy that surrounded their efforts and that of other researchers on vitamin use — notably Linus Pauling, with his discovery of the beneficial effect of vitamin C on the body's immune response to illnesses from the common cold to cancer — discouraged many people from taking vitamins. The result of reliance on the basic four food groups to supply all the body's nutrients is that most Americans are vitamin deficient, grossly so in the case of vitamins C and A. It is only recently that medicine has been evolving into acceptance of therapeutic and preventive usage of, for example, antistress formulas to protect the heart, combining vitamins C, E, and zinc. The medical establishment is now attempting to claim credit for "discoveries" that were popularized in the 1950s, '60s, and '70s among the 3 percent of the population that supported the health food industry. In the meantime, the blind eye of the established medical and nutrition community has allowed ignorance to result in needless suffering and sickness.

Vitamin E helps to maintain healthy muscles and red blood cells, and is involved to a degree in protecting women against miscarriage and premature birth, as well as improving the quality of sperm. Most significant is its effect as an antioxidant; as such, it may slow down the aging process, at the same time keeping usable oxygen available to the tissues for increased energy, stamina, and endurance. It seems to promote healing, particularly of burns. As an anticoagulant, its special quality is that it does not, conversely, produce hemorrhaging; it is these properties that make it effective in the treatment of heart disease, rheumatic fever, varicose veins, thrombophlebitis, and hemorrhoids (according to Drs. Shute and Alton Ochsner).

While vitamin E is not toxic in large doses like vitamins A and D, there have been several studies showing that it can produce weakness and fatigue in large doses (over 300 International Units), and people with high blood pressure, hyperthyroidism, or chronic rheumatic heart disease are cautioned against taking large amounts.

Vitamin K, usually synthesized by bacteria in the lower intestinal tract (except in the presence of sulfa drugs or antibiotics), helps stimulate production of the proteins which promote blood clotting, and is often recommended as a food supplement prior to surgery. The best source is alfalfa.

The Water-Soluble Vitamins

The B-vitamins form a complex that when combined play a vital role in the metabolic processes of all cells. B_1, thiamine, is important in carbohydrate metabolism and in oxidation in the cells, and for the nerves. Without enough, people become irritable, jumpy, and tired, and children have difficulty learning. Alcoholics are usually deficient in this vitamin, both because of poor diet and because the amount they do consume is used up in metabolizing alcohol. Beriberi is its deficiency disease.

Vitamin B_2, riboflavin, is vital to general health. The gastrointestinal tract cannot function without it, nor can iron be assimilated efficiently by the body. Alcohol, fats, and minerals tend to deplete the body's supply — one more reason for moderation in the intake of alcohol and fats. A deficiency is signaled by cracked lips, purplish tongue, dry and burning eyes, light sensitivity, hair loss, eczema, spinal pain, or weight loss, and deficiency may damage the central nervous system.

Niacin (nicotinic acid — not to be confused with the nicotine present in tobacco) is necessary to prevent pellagra, which was once a prevalent cause of skin and gastrointestinal problems, mental illness, and death in the U.S. Pellagra is no longer common here, since most people obtain enough of the amino acid tryptophan, from which the body produces niacin in the presence of vitamin B_6.

Vitamin B_6, pyridoxine, is necessary in the metabolism of amino acids. Deficiency has been linked to multiple sclerosis and retardation in children, and to depression in women taking oral contraceptives. Supplements are therefore recommended for those on birth control pills, and for pregnant women, since adequate vitamin B_6 is crucial to proper brain development of fetuses.

Pantothenic acid, present in every living cell, is involved in the metabolism of carbohydrates, fats, and proteins, and in the synthesis of cholesterol, steroid hormones, hemoglobin, and the phospholipids. It is involved in the body's production of all the other B-vitamins. Recently discovered, pantothenic acid is believed to prevent fatigue, depression, and low resistance to infection, and to aid recovery from many illnesses.

Biotin is a micronutrient which is synthesized by intestinal bacteria. It is involved in the synthesis of fatty acids and in the oxidation of carbohydrates. Because so little is needed by the body, deficiency is rare. It is sometimes used in the treatment of eczema.

Choline, found in all living cells, metabolizes and transports fats from the liver and is central to the transmission of nerve impulses. Deficiency leads to muscle weakness and excessive scarring, but it is rare, since the body produces its own supply in the presence of protein and other B-vitamins. It has been used in treating hepatitis and hyperthyroid conditions.

Like choline, inositol is found in lecithin. It is involved in lecithin production in the body, and helps to lower cholesterol levels, and prevent blood sugar disorders.

Para-aminobenzoic acid, PABA, is necessary for the body's production of folic acid. Sulfa drugs may cause a deficiency; their side effects include digestive problems, nervousness, and depression. It is an effective sun-screening agent.

Vitamin B_{12}, cyanocobalamin, is important in the functioning of the cells of the gastrointestinal tract, nervous system, and bone marrow. Deficiencies are rarely caused by poor diet, except in the case of vegans who fail to eat seaweed or tempeh (a soy food), or take supplements. Rather, faulty absorption is sometimes a problem. Deficiency can cause a form of psychosis, and therefore doctors are urged to test the blood of mental patients for B_{12} deficiency.

Folic acid is more easily destroyed by heat and light than the other B-vitamins. It prevents anemia by aiding the growth of red blood cells, and is necessary for the manufacture of DNA and RNA and for the conversion of amino acids. While it is synthesized by certain intestinal bacteria, lack of protein impairs its utilization, and deficiencies are not uncommon among older people with poor diets, pregnant women, and infants whose intake of either folic or ascorbic acid is low. Brewer's yeast, dark green leafy vegetables, wheat germ, oysters, salmon, and chicken all contain folic acid.

Because the B-vitamins are found together in nature, and interact in the body, Adelle Davis popularized the concept that the B-vitamins should all be taken at the same time, and in certain specific proportions. She pointed out that they form a natural tranquilizer, because of their importance to the functioning of of the nerves and central nervous system. While the latter is true, her idea of taking all of them at the same time is being challenged by researchers who find that different people need each vitamin in different, specific amounts. Only a blood chemistry work-up can tell your doctor or nutritionist of which B-vitamins you may need supplements.

In the last five years, megavitamin therapy has become popular, and the vitamin manufacturers have competed to produce higher and higher "antistress" B-complex formulas. However, very large doses of B-vitamins, instead of acting as a tranquilizer can, by causing imbalances, actually bring on depression, anxiety, and other nervous symptoms. The B-vitamins are biochemically active substances, and your body usually does not need megadoses. Doses smaller than ten milligrams of vitamins B_1, B_2, and B_6 are generally effective in alleviating any symptoms caused by deficiencies, except in certain special cases of dependency.

Different B-vitamins are prevalent in various B-complex-rich foods. The best source of B-complex as a group is brewer's yeast. Other foods high in B-vitamins include whole grains, wheat germ, legumes, nuts, egg yolk, green vegetables, fruit, and organ meats.

Vitamin C, like vitamin E, has engendered enormous controversy. Some doctors still hold that ascorbic acid is merely a preventative for scurvy, since it is essential in the formation of collagen, the gelatinous substance that holds together connective tissue, cartilage, and bone. However, the discovery of vitamin C as a detoxicant, able to combat the effects of air pollution, smoking, heavy metals such as mercury, and various drugs and bacteria, has generated considerable excitement. It also may prove to be a weapon against arteriosclerosis: those groups most prone to coronary thrombosis, such as smokers, men, and older people, have lower levels of vitamin C in their system. Vitamin C also seems to make pregnancy and labor more comfortable and shorter.

Vitamin C should be taken after meals in order to avoid irritating the gastrointestinal tract. Aspirin hinders its effectiveness. Any kind of stress increases the body's need for vitamin C: fever, surgery, alcohol, smoking, poor diet, illness, anxiety, even strenuous exercise. As much as three grams daily have not been shown to be harmful in any way, as long as the vitamin is not oxidized. Unlike other animals, human beings do not produce vitamin C in their bodies. Fresh citrus juice, alfalfa, kale, turnip greens, green peppers, broccoli, strawberries, tomatoes, and cantaloupe are some good sources. Natural sources of C also provide bioflavonoids, for good capillary health. However, beware of allergies to citrus fruits and other acidic foods. An allergic reaction, like any stress, uses up vitamin C. Allergies to citrus fruits are quite common. For those people with such allergies, citrus fruits will not help them to obtain vitamin C.

How Do You Know If You Are Getting Enough Vitamins?

For years, Americans adopted a false notion of health: we assumed that if we were not sick in a hospital bed, we were well. But there are levels and degrees of health: a sudden heart attack, or a sudden diagnosis of cancer, is the result of years of slowly deteriorating health. Clinicians were taught to look for the classical, clinical symptoms of the vitamin deficiency diseases — scurvy, pellagra, etc. — but not for signs of subclinical deficiencies such as allergies, nasal congestion, menstrual cramps, hot flashes during menopause, depression, skin problems, etc. Now, we are becoming aware of the subtle biochemical changes that subclinical deficiencies, or special dependencies resulting in the need for megadoses of particular vitamins for particular people, can produce. Today, specialists in clinical ecology, preventive medicine, and nutrition are learning how to test for the vitamin and mineral deficiencies and other chemical imbalances that can result in a wide variety of very specific symptoms, and are achieving dramatic results that are revolutionizing the very concept of disease. Most important, they are developing the ability to prescribe the particular nutrients in the particular amounts that will rebalance a person's individual, unique biochemistry.

The unit value for Vitamin A is given in International Units. Any food having less than 10 International Units of Vitamin A per 100-gram portion is considered to have a trace Vitamin A content and is listed as having 0 for its unit value. Vitamins B_1, B_2, B_6, B_{12}, C, and E have unit values given as milligrams. Any food having less than .01 milligram B_1 or B_2 or less than 1 milligram of vitamin C is considered to have a trace content for that vitamin and is listed as having .00 for its unit value.

Where the symbol N. A. appears in the calorie column, the information was not available.

All figures are based on an edible portion equaling 100 grams, or approximately 3 ounces. In the case of some of the listed foods, one would not consume 100 grams in one serving. Calculations should be adjusted accordingly.

Vitamin A

FOOD ITEM	CALS.	UNITS
Carrots dried	341	100000
Lamb liver broiled	261	74500
Beef liver fried	229	53400
Calf liver fried	261	32700
Carrots canned, regular, drained solids	30	15000
Carrots canned, low sodium, drained solids	25	15000
Dandelion greens raw	45	14000
Chicken liver simmered	165	12300
Dandelion greens boiled and drained	33	11700
Carrots raw	42	11000
Dried apricots uncooked	260	10900
Carrots boiled and drained	31	10500
Carrots canned, regular, solids and liquid	28	10000
Carrots canned, low sodium, solids and liquid	22	10000
Mustard spinach (tendergreen), raw	22	9900
Red chili peppers (hot), canned in sauce	21	9590
Collards leaves, raw	45	9300
Garden cress	32	9300
Peas and carrots frozen, boiled and drained	53	9300
Kale leaves and stems, raw	38	8900
Parsley raw	44	8500
Kale frozen, boiled and drained	31	8200
Mustard spinach (tendergreen), boiled and drained	16	8200
Spinach raw	26	8100
Spinach boiled and drained	23	8100
Spinach leaves, frozen, boiled and drained	24	8100
Sweet potatoes with skin, baked	141	8100
Spinach canned, low sodium, drained solids	26	8000

FOOD ITEM	CALS.	UNITS
Spinach chopped, frozen, boiled and drained	23	7900
Sweet potatoes with skin, boiled	114	7900
Collards leaves, boiled and drained	33	7800
Garden cress boiled and drained	23	7700
Turnip greens leaves and stems, raw	28	7600
Kale leaves and stems, boiled and drained	28	7400
Mustard greens raw	31	7000
Turnip greens leaves and stems, frozen, boiled and drained	23	6900
Collards frozen, boiled and drained	30	6800
Braunschweiger	319	6530
Liverwurst smoked	319	6530
Liverwurst	307	6530
Collards leaves and stems, raw	40	6500
Butternut squash baked	68	6400
Pumpkin canned	33	6400
Sweet potatoes candied	168	6300
Turnip greens leaves and stems, boiled and drained	23	6300
Beet greens raw	24	6100
Mustard greens frozen, boiled and drained	20	6000
Chives raw	28	5800
Mustard greens boiled and drained	23	5800
Chicken (giblets), fried	252	5760
Spinach canned, regular, solids and liquid	19	5500
Spinach canned, low sodium, solids and liquid	21	5500
Butternut squash mashed, boiled	41	5400
Chard Swiss, boiled and drained	18	5400
Collards leaves and stems, cooked	29	5400
Beet greens boiled and drained	18	5100
Creamed spinach (baby food), commercial	43	5000
Sweet potatoes canned in syrup, solids and liquid	114	5000
Sweet potatoes canned, unsweetened, solids and liquid	46	5000
Mixed vegetables (carrots, corn, peas, green snap beans, and lima beans), frozen, boiled and drained	64	4950
Watercress leaves and stems, raw	19	4900
Hubbard squash baked	50	4800
Mangoes raw	66	4800
Red peppers (sweet), raw	31	4450
Winter squash baked	63	4200
Hubbard squash boiled, mashed	30	4100

FOOD ITEM	CALS.	UNITS
Butter oil or dehydrated	876	4080
Chicory greens raw	20	4000
Green onions (bunching variety), young, tops, raw	27	4000
Dried peaches uncooked	262	3900
Fennel leaves, raw	28	3500
Winter squash boiled, mashed	38	3500
Cantaloupe	30	3400
Butter	716	3300
Endive (curly endive and escarole), raw	20	3300
Margarine salted	720	3300
Tomato paste canned	82	3300
Spoon cabbage boiled	4	3100
Spoon cabbage raw	16	3100
Apricots cooked, without added sugar, fruit and liquid	85	3000
Persimmons (Japanese or kaki), raw	77	2710
Apricots canned in juice, fruit and liquid	54	2700
Apricots cooked, sugar added, fruit and liquid	122	2600
Broccoli chopped, frozen, boiled and drained	26	2600
Broccoli spears, raw	32	2500
Broccoli spears, boiled and drained	26	2500
Purslane leaves and stems, raw	21	2500
Vegetable beef broth canned, condensed	64	2500
Pumpkin pies piecrust made with unenriched flour, commercial	211	2470
Squash (baby food), commercial	25	2400
Pimientos canned, solids and liquid	27	2300
Vegetarian vegetable soup canned, condensed	64	2300
Vegetables and lamb with cereal (baby food), commercial	58	2200
Crab steamed	93	2170
Swordfish broiled	174	2050
Green onions (bunching variety), young, raw	36	2000
Whitefish (lake), cooked, stuffed, baked	215	2000
Broccoli spears, frozen, boiled and drained	26	1900
Egg yolk and bacon dinner (baby food), commercial	208	1900
Lettuce (cos and romaine), raw	18	1900
Apricots canned in water, with or without artificial sweetner, fruit and liquid	38	1830
Chicken vegetable soup canned, condensed	62	1800
Apricots canned in light syrup, fruit and liquid	66	1780
Apricots canned in heavy syrup, fruit and liquid	86	1740
Apricots canned in extra-heavy syrup, fruit and liquid	101	1720

FOOD ITEM	CALS.	UNITS
Nectarines raw	64	1650
Dried prunes	255	1600
Tomato puree canned, regular or low sodium	39	1600
Cream cheese	374	1540
Heavy whipping cream	352	1540
Eggs fried	216	1420
Cowpeas (including black-eyed peas), boiled and drained	34	1400
Tomato catsup bottled	106	1400
Acorn squash baked	55	1330
Chicken potpie homemade	235	1330
Peaches raw	38	1330
Turkey potpie homemade	237	1330
American cheese pasteurized, processed	370	1310
Vegetable beef broth canned, condensed	32	1300
Light whipping cream	300	1280
Plums (purple), canned in water, with or without artificial sweetener,fruit and liquid	46	1250
Blue or Roquefort cheese	368	1240
Brick cheese	370	1240
Plums (purple), canned in light syrup, fruit and liquid	63	1230
American cheese pasteurized, processed	370	1220
Peaches cooked, without added sugar, fruit and liquid	82	1220
Plums (purple), canned in heavy syrup, fruit and liquid	83	1210
Vegetarian vegetable soup canned, condensed	32	1200
Eggs hard-boiled	163	1180
Plums (purple), canned in extra-heavy syrup, fruit and liquid	102	1180
Eggs poached	163	1170
Limburger cheese	345	1140
Whole milk dry	502	1130
Beef with vegetables (baby food), commercial	87	1100
Swiss cheese pasteurized, processed	355	1100
Vegetable with beef soup canned, condensed	32	1100
Eggs scrambled	173	1080
Omelets	173	1080
Dried peaches cooked, sugar added, fruit and liquid	119	1070
Parmesan cheese	393	1060
Camembert cheese	299	1010
Chicken with vegetables (baby food), commercial	100	1000
Red cherries (sour), raw	58	1000
Strained tomato soup (baby food), commercial	54	1000

FOOD ITEM	CALS.	UNITS
Tomatoes ripe, boiled	26	1000
Turkey with vegetables (baby food), commercial	86	1000
Vegetables and chicken with cereal (baby food), commercial	52	1000
Vegetables and ham with cereal (baby food), commercial	64	1000
American cheese food pasteurized, processed	323	980
Beef and vegetable stew homemade with lean beef chuck	89	980
Lettuce (Boston and bibb), raw	14	970
Minestrone soup canned, condensed	43	960
Orange juice canned concentrate, unsweetened	200	960
Apricot nectar canned	57	950
Asparagus boiled and drained	20	900
Asparagus spears, raw	21	900
Tomato juice canned, concentrate	20	900
Tomatoes ripe, canned, low sodium, solids and liquid	20	900
Tomatoes ripe, canned, regular, solids and liquid	21	900
Cheese fondue homemade	265	880
American cheese spread pasteurized, processed	288	870
Tomato juice dehydrated, (crystals), prepared with water	20	860
Asparagus cuts and tips, frozen, boiled and drained	22	850
Light cream	211	840
Beef potpie homemade	246	820
Chicken (fryers), with skin and giblets, fried	249	820
Asparagus spears, canned, low sodium, drained solids	20	800
Asparagus spears, canned, regular, drained solids	21	800
Cheese souffle homemade	218	800
Chicken noodle dinner (baby food), commercial	49	800
Tomato juice canned or bottled, regular or low sodium	19	800
Tomato juice cocktail canned or bottled	21	800
Veal with vegetables (baby food), commercial	63	800
Chicken (roaster), with skin and giblets	242	790
Asparagus spears, frozen, boiled and drained	23	780
Green chili peppers (hot), pods without seeds, raw	37	770
Bananas dried or powdered	340	760
Dried prunes cooked, without added sugar	119	750
Charlotte russe with ladyfingers and whipped cream filling	286	740
Peach pie commercial	255	730
Ground cherries raw	53	720
Manhattan clam chowder canned, condensed	33	710
Passion fruit pulp and seeds, raw	90	700
Vegetable juice cocktail canned	17	700

FOOD ITEM	CALS.	UNITS
Green peas canned, low sodium, solids and liquid	55	690
Green peas (sweet), canned, low sodium, drained solids	55	690
Russian salad dressing commercial, regular	494	690
Halibut (Atlantic and Pacific), broiled	171	680
Red cherries (sour), canned in water, fruit and liquid	43	680
Peaches canned in juice, fruit and liquid	45	670
Frozen custard fat content 16%	222	660
Ice cream fat content 16%	222	660
Red cherries (sour), canned in light syrup, fruit and liquid	74	660
Spanish rice homemade	87	660
Bread stuffing from mix, made with water and table fat	358	650
Butter cookies rich, thin	457	650
Red cherries (sour), canned in heavy syrup, fruit and liquid	89	650
Green peas raw	84	640
Spaghetti with meatballs in tomato sauce, homemade	134	640
Pizza with cheese topping, homemade	236	630
Red cherries (sour), canned in extra-heavy syrup, fruit and liquid	112	630
Beef noodle dinner (baby food), commercial	48	620
Green chili peppers (hot), pods without seeds, canned, solids and liquid	25	610
Applesauce and apricots (baby food), commercial	86	600
Elderberries raw	72	600
Green peas (sweet), frozen, boiled and drained	68	600
Green snap beans raw	32	600
Kumquats raw	65	600
Split peas with ham or bacon (baby food), commercial	80	600
Watermelon raw	26	590
Rutabagas raw	46	580
Snap beans cut, frozen, boiled and drained	25	580
Brussels sprouts frozen, boiled and drained	33	570
White sauce thick	198	570
Pizza with sausage, homemade	236	560
Rutabagas boiled and drained	35	550
Green peas boiled and drained	71	540
Green snap beans boiled and drained	25	540
Mackerel (Atlantic), broiled in butter or margarine	236	530
Brussels sprouts boiled and drained	36	520
Cream substitutes dried	509	520
Frozen custard fat content 12%	207	520

FOOD ITEM	CALS.	UNITS
Ice cream fat content 12%	207	520
Pork and bean soup canned, condensed	134	520
Asparagus spears, canned, low sodium, solids and liquid	16	510
Asparagus spears, canned, regular, solids and liquid	18	510
Cornmeal (white or yellow), whole ground, unbolted	355	510
Macaroni, tomatoes, meat, and cereal (baby food), commercial	67	500
Peaches (baby food), commercial	81	500
Strained peas (baby food), commercial	54	500
Okra boiled and drained	29	490
Salad dressing cooked, homemade	164	490
Cornmeal (white or yellow), nearly whole grain, bolted	362	480
Half-and-half cream	134	480
Okra cuts and pods, frozen, boiled and drained	38	480
Tomato soup canned, condensed, prepared with milk	69	480
Fruit salad canned in water, with or without artificial sweetener, fruit and liquid	35	470
Green snap beans canned, low sodium, drained solids	22	470
Green snap beans canned, regular, drained solids	24	470
Chicken a la king homemade	191	460
Fruit salad canned in light syrup, fruit and liquid	59	460
White sauce medium	162	460
Cornmeal (white or yellow), self-rising, without added wheat flour	347	450
Fruit dessert with tapioca (baby food), commercial	84	450
Fruit salad canned in extra-heavy syrup, fruit and liquid	92	450
Fruit salad canned in heavy syrup, fruit and liquid	76	450
Green peas (Alaska), canned, low sodium, solids and liquid	55	450
Green peas (sweet), canned, low sodium, solids and liquid	47	450
Green peas canned, regular, solids and liquid	66	450
Green peas (Alaska), canned, regular, solids and liquid	66	450
Green peas (sweet), canned, regular, solids and liquid	57	450
Peaches canned in water, with or without artificial sweetener, fruit and liquid	31	450
Shad creole	152	450
Sponge cake homemade	297	450
Oysters fried	239	440
Peaches canned in light syrup, fruit and liquid	58	440
Mackerel (Atlantic), canned, solids and liquid	183	430

FOOD ITEM	CALS.	UNITS
Peach nectar canned	48	430
Peaches canned in heavy syrup, fruit and liquid	78	430
Spaghetti with cheese in tomato sauce, homemade	104	430
Green peppers (sweet), raw	22	420
Peaches canned in extra-heavy syrup, fruit and liquid	97	420
Tangerine juice canned, sweetened	50	420
Tangerine juice fresh	43	420
Tangerine juice canned, unsweetened	43	420
Tangerines raw	46	420
Sapotes (marmalade plums), raw	125	410
Tangerine juice frozen concentrate, unsweetened	46	410
Tomato soup canned, condensed	36	410
Corn fritters commercial	377	400
Corn on the cob (white and yellow), boiled and drained	91	400
Green beans (baby food), commercial	22	400
Red bananas raw	90	400
Spaghetti with meatballs in tomato sauce, canned	103	400
Summer squash boiled and drained	14	390
Spaghetti with cheese in tomato sauce, canned	76	370
Barbecue sauce	91	360
Cheese crackers commercial	479	360
Condensed milk canned, sweetened	321	360
Split pea soup canned, condensed	118	360
Corn (sweet, yellow), regular, solids and liquid	53	350
Cowpeas (including black-eyed peas), boiled and drained	108	350
Custard baked, commercial	115	350
Corn flour	368	340
Eclairs with custard filling and chocolate frosting, commercial	239	340
Creamed corn (sweet, white and yellow), canned, regular pack, solids and liquid	82	330
Lettuce (iceberg), raw	13	330
Waffles homemade	279	330
Evaporated milk canned, unsweetened	137	320
Thousand Island salad dressing commercial, regular	502	320
Thousand Island salad dressing commercial, low calorie	180	320
Corn muffins homemade from whole-ground cornmeal	288	310
Danish pastry commercial	422	310
Black walnuts	628	300

FOOD ITEM	CALS.	UNITS
Bread pudding with raisins, commercial	187	300
Corn muffins homemade from enriched degermed cornmeal	314	300
Green olives pickled, canned or bottled	116	300
Plums (prune-type)	75	300
Summer squash (zucchini and cocozelle), boiled and drained	12	300
Gooseberries raw	39	290
Green snap beans canned, regular, solids and liquid	18	290
Green snap beans canned, low sodium, solids and liquid	16	290
Tuna salad	170	290
Guavas whole, raw	62	280
Lima beans boiled and drained	111	280
Mayonnaise	718	280
Pound cake homemade	473	280
Corn (sweet, white and yellow), canned, wet pack, solids and liquid	82	270
Cornbread from mix, made with eggs and milk	233	270
Creamed corn (sweet, white and yellow), canned, low sodium, solids and liquid	82	270
Frosting chocolate fudge, from mix, made with water and table fat	378	270
Milk chocolate plain	520	270
Corn pudding commercial	104	260
Cucumbers with skin, raw	15	250
Pancakes from mix, made with eggs and milk	225	250
Yellow snap beans raw	27	250
Celery (green and yellow varieties), raw	17	240
Chop suey with meat, homemade	120	240
Corn muffins from mix, made with eggs and milk	324	240
Black currants (European), raw	54	230
Bran muffins homemade	261	230
Celery (green and yellow varieties), boiled and drained	14	230
Lima beans frozen, boiled and drained	99	230
Pistachio nuts	594	230
Salmon (sockeye), canned, solids and liquid	171	230
Yellow snap beans boiled and drained	22	230
Baby lima beans frozen, boiled and drained	118	220
Blueberry muffins homemade	281	220
Tartar sauce regular	531	220
Tartar sauce regular or low calorie	224	220

FOOD ITEM	CALS.	UNITS
Ice milk	152	210
Blackberries raw	58	200
Brownies with nuts, homemade from enriched flour	485	200
Gooseberries canned in water, with or without artificial sweetener, fruit and liquid	26	200
Orange juice canned, sweetened	52	200
Orange juice fresh, commercial	45	200
Orange juice canned, unsweetened	48	200
Orange juice frozen concentrate, unsweetened	45	200
Orange juice (crystals)	46	200
Oranges raw	49	200
Tomato vegetable soup with noodles from mix	27	200
Bananas raw	85	190
Gooseberries canned in heavy syrup, fruit and liquid	90	190
Chicken and noodles homemade	153	180
Cod broiled	170	180
Gooseberries canned in extra-heavy syrup, fruit and liquid	117	180
Sardines (Atlantic), canned in oil, solids and liquid	311	180
Black-eyed peas frozen, boiled and drained	130	170
Blue cheese and Roquefort salad dressing commercial, low calorie	76	170
Plain cake or cupcakes homemade, without icing	364	170
Hot cocoa homemade	97	160
Pecan pie commercial	418	160
Salmon broiled or baked	182	160
Vanilla pudding homemade	111	160
Blackberries canned in juice, fruit and liquid	54	150
Chicken all classes, dark meat, roasted, without skin	176	150
Chinese cabbage raw	14	150
Chocolate cake homemade, without icing	366	150
Chocolate pudding homemade	148	150
Coleslaw made with salad dressing	99	150
Corn muffins from mix, made with eggs and water	297	150
Cornbread homemade from whole-ground cornmeal	207	150
Fruit cocktail canned in water, with or without artificial sweetener, fruit and liquid	37	150
Blackberries canned in water, with or without artificial sweetener, fruit and liquid	40	140
Butterscotch candy	397	140

FOOD ITEM	CALS.	UNITS
Fruit cocktail canned in light syrup, fruit and liquid	60	140
Fruit cocktail canned in heavy syrup, fruit and liquid	76	140
Fruit cocktail canned in extra-heavy syrup, fruit and liquid	92	140
Hot chocolate homemade	95	140
Pickles fresh	73	140
Potato salad homemade	99	140
Summer squash (yellow crookneck), frozen, boiled and drained	21	140
Whole milk 3.5% fat	65	140
Yogurt made from whole milk	62	140
Blackberries canned in light syrup, fruit and liquid	72	130
Blackberries canned in heavy syrup, fruit and liquid	91	130
Blackberries canned in extra-heavy syrup, fruit and liquid	110	130
Boysenberries canned in water, with or without artificial sweetener, fruit and liquid	36	130
Cabbage shredded, boiled and drained	20	130
Frankfurters and beans canned	144	130
Lima beans canned, low sodium, solids and liquid	70	130
Lima beans canned, regular, solids and liquid	71	130
Mashed potatoes dehydrated, flakes without milk	93	130
Pudding from mix, prepared with milk	124	130
Red raspberries raw	57	130
Beef noodle soup from mix, dehydrated	387	120
Chocolate chip cookies commercial	471	120
Dark fruitcake homemade	379	120
Pancakes homemade from enriched or unenriched flour	231	120
Cherries (sweet), raw	70	110
Chicken chow mein without noodles, homemade	102	110
Chocolate chip cookies homemade from enriched flour	516	110
Rice pudding with raisins, commercial	146	110
Wheat germ toasted	391	110
Blueberries raw	62	100
Cashew nuts	561	100
Custard pudding (baby food), commercial	100	100
Fruit pudding (baby food), commercial	96	100
Grapes (American), raw	69	100
Muffins plain, homemade from enriched or unenriched flour	294	100
Pickles (dill)	11	100
Pickles (sour)	10	100
Rhubarb raw	16	100

FOOD ITEM	CALS.	UNITS
Yellow snap beans cut, frozen, boiled and drained	27	100
Apples freshly harvested with skin, raw	58	90
Gingerbread homemade from enriched flour	317	90
Pickles (sweet)	146	90
Tuna canned in oil, solids and liquid	288	90
Assorted cookies commercial	480	80
Doughnuts cake type	391	80
Dried figs	274	80
Grapefruit raw	41	80
Grapefruit juice	38	80
Rhubarb cooked,sugar added	141	80
Rolls and buns homemade with milk and enriched flour	339	80
Soybean sprouts raw	46	80
Soybean sprouts boiled and drained	38	80
Dried pears cooked	268	70
Egg noodles enriched, cooked	125	70
Light fruitcake homemade	389	70
Pineapple raw	52	70
Pumpkin and squash seed kernels dried	553	70
Sweet rolls commercial	316	70
Yogurt made from partially skimmed milk	50	70
Baking chocolate	505	60
Bitter chocolate	505	60
Cauliflower raw	27	60
Cauliflower boiled and drained	22	60
Cherries (sweet), canned in light syrup, fruit and liquid	65	60
Cherries (sweet), canned in water, with or without artificial sweetener, fruit and liquid	48	60
Cherries (sweet), canned in heavy syrup, fruit and liquid	81	60
Chicken all classes, light meat, roasted, without skin	166	60
Chicken chow mein without noodles, canned	38	60
Chili con carne with beans, canned	133	60
Corn grits degermed, enriched, cooked	51	60
Cornmeal (white or yellow), degermed, enriched, cooked	50	60
Cottonseed flour	356	60
Cowpeas (including black-eyed peas), canned, solids and liquid	70	60
Orange sherbet	134	60
Pineapple canned in juice, fruit and liquid	58	60
Prickly pears raw	42	60

FOOD ITEM	CALS.	UNITS
Strawberries raw	37	60
White cake with chocolate frosting, from mix	351	60
Yellow snap beans canned, regular, solids and liquid	19	60
Bluefish baked or broiled	159	50
Cherries (sweet), canned in extra-heavy syrup, fruit and liquid	100	50
Lemon peel raw	N.A.	50
Pineapple canned in light syrup, fruit and liquid	59	50
Pineapple all styles except crushed, canned in water, with or without artificial sweetener	39	50
Pineapple canned in heavy syrup, fruit and liquid	74	50
Pineapple juice canned, unsweetened	55	50
Sauerkraut canned, solids and liquid	18	50
Sunflower seed kernels dried	560	50
Whey dried	349	50
Apples freshly harvested, pared, raw	54	40
Applesauce canned, unsweetened or artificially sweetened	41	40
Applesauce canned, sweetened	91	40
Applesauce (baby food), commercial	72	40
Beef chuck cuts, choice grade, braised or pot roasted	327	40
Blueberries canned in water, with or without artificial sweetener, fruit and liquid	39	40
Blueberries canned in extra-heavy syrup, fruit and liquid	101	40
Cranberries raw	46	40
Hamburger regular ground, cooked	286	40
Honeydew melon	33	40
Leeks bulk and lower leaf, raw	52	40
Miso (fermented soybean product)	171	40
Onions raw	38	40
Onions boiled and drained	29	40
Pineapple canned in extra-heavy syrup, fruit and liquid	90	40
Red cabbage raw	31	40
Soybean flour defatted	326	40
Soybean milk fluid	33	40
Split peas cooked	115	40
Strawberries canned in water, with or without artificial sweetener, fruit and liquid	22	40
Strawberry pie piecrust made with unenriched flour, commercial	198	40
Zwieback	423	40

FOOD ITEM	CALS.	UNITS
Blueberry pie commercial	242	30
Casaba	27	30
Cauliflower frozen, boiled and drained	18	30
Chicken noodle soup canned, condensed	53	30
Chop suey with meat, canned	62	30
Dried pears cooked, with added sugar, fruit and liquid	151	30
Dried pears cooked, without added sugar, fruit and liquid	126	30
Figs canned in light syrup, fruit and liquid	65	30
Figs canned in heavy syrup, fruit and liquid	84	30
Figs canned in water, with or without artificial sweetener, fruit and liquid	48	30
Figs canned in extra-heavy syrup, fruit and liquid	103	30
Mackerel (Pacific), canned, solids and liquid	180	30
Parsnips boiled and drained	66	30
Sardines (Pacific), canned in tomato sauce, solids and liquid	197	30
Sesame seeds dry, whole	563	30
Shad baked	201	30
Skim milk dry, regular	363	30
Soybeans dry, cooked	130	30
Walnuts	651	30
White cake homemade, without icing	375	30
Bamboo shoots raw	27	20
Chicken noodle soup from mix	22	20
Cranberry sauce canned, sweetened, strained	146	20
Green pea soup from mix	50	20
Jerusalem artichokes raw, freshly harvested	7	20
Kohlrabi thickened bulb-like stems, raw	29	20
Kohlrabi thickened bulb-like stems, boiled and drained	24	20
Lemon juice canned or bottled, sweetened	25	20
Lemon juice fresh	23	20
Lemons peeled, raw	27	20
Lentils whole, dry, cooked	106	20
Mashed potatoes milk added	65	20
Mung bean sprouts raw	35	20
Mung bean sprouts boiled and drained	28	20
Pears with skin, raw	61	20
Raisins	289	20
Red beets raw	43	20
Red beets boiled and drained	32	20
Beef noodle soup from mix	28	10

FOOD ITEM	CALS.	UNITS
Caramels plain or chocolate	399	10
Cocoa powder low fat	187	10
Cowpeas (including black-eyed peas), dry, cooked	76	10
Eggplant boiled and drained	19	10
Ginger root fresh	49	10
Grapefruit canned, sweetened	53	10
Grapefruit canned in water, with or without artificial sweetener, fruit and liquid	30	10
Grapefruit canned in syrup, fruit and liquid	70	10
Grapefruit canned in juice, unsweetened	41	10
Grapefruit juice frozen concentrate, sweetened	47	10
Grapefruit juice frozen concentrate, unsweetened	41	10
Grapefruit juice frozen concentrate, sweetened	47	10
Jams and preserves	272	10
Jellies	273	10
Lime juice fresh	26	10
Lime juice canned or bottled, unsweetened	26	10
Limes raw	28	10
Pineapple juice frozen concentrate, unsweetened	52	10
Radishes (Oriental, including daikon and Chinese), raw	19	10
Raisins cooked, sugar added, fruit and liquid	213	10
Red beets canned, low sodium, solids and liquid	32	10
Red beets canned, regular, solids and liquid	32	10
Figs raw	80	0
Baker's yeast (active), dry	282	0
Beef broth, bouillon, and comsomme canned, condensed	13	0
Biscuits homemade from enriched flour	369	0
Biscuits from mix, with enriched flour, prepared with milk	325	0
Black raspberries raw	73	0
Brazil nuts	654	0
Bread stuffing mix, dry, commercial	371	0
Breadcrumbs dry, grated	392	0
Brewer's yeast debittered	283	0
Buttermilk cultured	36	0
Chicory raw	15	0
Chocolate syrup (thin)	245	0
Cranberry juice cocktail bottled	65	0
Devil's food cake from mix	339	0
Garlic cloves raw	137	0
Hard rolls enriched, commercial	312	0

FOOD ITEM	CALS.	UNITS
Ice cream cones	377	0
Italian salad dressing commercial, regular	552	0
Italian salad dressing commercial, low calorie	50	0
Lemonade frozen concentrate	44	0
Limeade frozen concentrate	41	0
Mushrooms raw	28	0
Mushrooms canned, solids and liquid	17	0
Pear nectar canned	52	0
Pears canned in light syrup, fruit and liquid	61	0
Pears canned in heavy syrup, fruit and liquid	76	0
Pears canned in water, with or without artificial sweetener, fruit and liquid	32	0
Pears canned in juice, fruit and liquid	46	0
Pears canned in extra-heavy syrup, fruit and liquid	92	0
Pomegranate pulp, raw	63	0
Potato chips	568	0
Potato flour	351	0
Potato sticks	544	0
Potatoes french-fried	274	0
Potatoes in skin, boiled	76	0
Potatoes with skin, baked	93	0
Potatoes (hash browned)	229	0
Potatoes canned, solids and liquid	44	0
Red beans dry, boiled and drained	118	0
Red beans canned, solids and liquid	90	0
Rolls from mix	299	0
Shallots bulbs, raw	72	0
Skim milk	36	0
Torula yeast	277	0
Turnips boiled and drained	23	0
Whole wheat rolls commercial	257	0

Vitamin B$_1$

FOOD ITEM	CALS.	UNITS
Brewer's yeast debittered	283	15.61
Torula yeast	277	14.01
Eggs whole, fresh	163	11.00
Barley cereal (baby food), commercial	348	3.71
High-protein cereal (baby food), commercial	357	3.67

FOOD ITEM	CALS.	UNITS
Shredded oats (cereal)	379	3.53
Rice cereal (baby food), commercial	371	2.56
Yeast dry (active)	282	2.33
Rice bran	276	2.26
Wheat germ raw, commercially milled	363	2.01
Sunflower seed kernels dried	560	1.96
Rice polish	265	1.84
Rice cereal with casein	382	1.70
Cornflakes with protein concentrate	378	1.65
Wheat germ toasted	391	1.65
Pine nuts	635	1.28
Peanuts with skins, raw	564	1.14
Pork loin fat class, separable lean, broiled	270	1.13
Pork loin medium fat content, separable lean, roasted	270	1.13
Pork loin thin class, separable lean, broiled	270	1.13
Safflower seed meal partially defatted	355	1.12
Soybean flour defatted	326	1.09
Pork loin thin class, separable lean, roasted	254	1.08
Puffed oats (cereal), sugar coated	396	1.03
Pork loin thin class, all edible parts, broiled (77% lean, 23% fat)	359	1.00
Peanuts without skins, raw	568	.99
Puffed corn (cereal), presweetened, fruit flavored	395	.99
Puffed oats (cereal)	397	.98
Sesame seeds whole, dry	563	.98
Brazil nuts	654	.96
Pork fresh, loin, trimmed, medium fat class, broiled	391	.96
Pork fresh, loin, trimmed, thin class, roasted	333	.96
Canadian bacon broiled or fried, drained	277	.92
Pork fresh, loin, trimmed, fat class, broiled	418	.92
Soybean flour high fat	380	.89
Pork fresh, loin, trimmed, fat class, roasted	387	.88
Puffed corn (cereal), added nutrients	399	.88
Pecans	687	.86
Soybean flour full fat	421	.85
Soybean flour low fat	356	.83
Puffed corn (cereal), presweetened, cocoa flavored, added nutrients	390	.79
Wheat bran crude, commercially milled	213	.72
Baker's yeast compressed	86	.71

FOOD ITEM	CALS.	UNITS
Flaked oats (cereal)	397	.71
Pistachio nuts	594	.67
Wheat flakes (cereal)	354	.64
Pine nuts	552	.62
Puffed wheat (cereal)	363	.55
Whole wheat flour	333	.55
Bacon cured, boiled or fried, drained	611	.51
Whey dried	349	.50
Filberts (hazelnuts)	634	.46
Boiled ham (luncheon meat)	234	.44
Bread flour enriched	365	.44
Bread flour self-rising	358	.44
Puffed rice (cereal)	399	.44
Cashew nuts	561	.43
Cornflakes (cereal)	386	.43
Rye whole grain	334	.43
Potato flour	351	.42
Shredded corn (cereal)	389	.42
Cornflakes (cereal), sugar coated	386	.41
Cowpeas (including black-eyed peas), boiled and drained	130	.40
Shredded rice (cereal)	392	.39
Cornmeal (white or yellow), whole ground, unbolted	355	.38
Malt extract dried	367	.36
Rice flakes (cereal)	390	.35
Skim milk dry, regular	363	.35
Macadamia nuts	691	.34
Whole wheat rolls commercial	257	.34
Walnuts	651	.33
Almond meal partially defatted	408	.32
Chestnuts dried	377	.32
Peanuts with skins, roasted	582	.32
Rye wafers whole grain	344	.32
Bulgur dry, commercial, from club wheat	359	.30
Cowpeas (including black-eyed peas), boiled and drained	108	.30
Rye flour medium	350	.30
Italian bread enriched	276	.29
Whole milk	502	.29
French bread enriched or unenriched	290	.28
Green peas boiled and drained	71	.28
Rolls and buns plain, commercial	298	.28

FOOD ITEM	CALS.	UNITS
Biscuits from mix, prepared with milk	325	.27
Green peas frozen, boiled and drained	68	.27
Hard rolls enriched, commercial	312	.26
Whole wheat bread	243	.26
Garlic cloves raw	137	.25
Rolls and buns homemade, with milk and enriched flour	339	.25
Salami cooked	311	.25
White bread enriched, made with 1% - 2% nonfat dry milk	269	.25
Almonds dried	598	.24
Pumpernickel bread	246	.23
Soybean sprouts raw	46	.23
Black walnuts	628	.22
Breadcrumbs dry, grated, commercial	392	.22
Chestnuts fresh	194	.22
Peas (edible-podded) boiled and drained	43	.22
Shredded wheat (cereal)	354	.22
Baking powder biscuits homemade from enriched flour	369	.21
Potato chips	568	.21
Potato sticks	544	.21
Soybeans dry, cooked	130	.21
Collards leaves and stems, raw	40	.20
Corn flour	368	.20
Corn muffins homemade from enriched degermed cornmeal	314	.20
Jerusalem artichokes raw, freshly harvested	7	.20
Liverwurst	307	.20
Pastry plain, made with enriched flour	500	.20
Piecrust made with enriched flour, commercial	500	.20
Split pea soup canned, condensed	118	.20
Tomato paste canned	82	.20
Brownies with nuts, homemade from enriched flour	485	.19
Dandelion greens raw	45	.19
Peas and carrots frozen, boiled and drained	53	.19
Asparagus spears, raw	26	.18
Banana powder	340	.18
Corn muffins from mix, made with eggs and milk	324	.18
Dried bananas	340	.18
Lima beans boiled and drained	111	.18
Rye bread (American), commercial	243	.18
Sesame seeds dry, hulled	582	.18
Corn muffins homemade from whole-ground cornmeal	288	.17

FOOD ITEM	CALS.	UNITS
Muffins plain, homemade from enriched flour	294	.17
Oysters fried	239	.17
Pancakes homemade from enriched flour	231	.17
Waffles homemade from enriched flour	279	.17
Asparagus spears, boiled and drained	20	.16
Asparagus spears, frozen, boiled and drained	22	.16
Blueberry muffins homemade from enriched flour	281	.16
Bologna	304	.16
Corn fritters	377	.16
Cowpeas (including black-eyed peas), dry, cooked	76	.16
Crab steamed	93	.16
Doughnuts cake type	391	.16
Oat cereal with toasted wheat germ and soy grits, cooked	62	.16
Pecan pie piecrust made with unenriched flour, commercial	418	.16
Salmon broiled or baked	182	.16
Soybean sprouts boiled and drained	38	.16
Bamboo shoots raw	27	.15
Frankfurters	304	.15
Mackerel (Atlantic), broiled with butter or margarine	236	.15
Split peas cooked	115	.15
Turnip greens leaves and stems, boiled and drained	20	.15
Asparagus cuts and tips, frozen, boiled and drained	22	.14
Bran muffins homemade from enriched flour	261	.14
Chinese water chestnuts raw	79	.14
Collards leaves and stems, boiled and drained	29	.14
Corn on the cob (sweet), frozen, boiled and drained	94	.14
Egg noodles enriched, cooked	125	.14
French fried potatoes frozen	220	.14
Lamb leg, prime grade, roasted	319	.14
Macaroni enriched, cooked until tender	111	.14
Okra cuts and pods, frozen, boiled and drained	38	.14
Popovers homemade	224	.14
Spaghetti enriched, cooked until tender	111	.14
Spaghetti with cheese in tomato sauce, canned	76	.14
Cane syrup	263	.13
Cornbread homemade from whole-ground cornmeal	207	.13
Dandelion greens boiled and drained	33	.13
Dark fruitcake homemade from enriched flour	379	.13
French fried potatoes	274	.13
Lima beans dry, boiled and drained	138	.13

FOOD ITEM	CALS.	UNITS
Mung bean sprouts raw	35	.13
Peanut butter	581	.13
Shad baked	201	.13
Abalone canned	80	.12
Corn muffins from mix, prepared with eggs and water	297	.12
Corn on the cob (sweet, white and yellow), boiled and drained	91	.12
Cracked wheat bread	263	.12
Gingerbread homemade from enriched flour	317	.12
Mixed vegetables (carrots, corn, peas, green snap beans, and lima beans), frozen, boiled and drained	64	.12
Parsley raw	44	.12
Avocados raw	167	.11
Blackstrap molasses cane	213	.11
Bluefish baked or broiled	159	.11
Cauliflower raw	27	.11
Chocolate chip cookies homemade from enriched flour	516	.11
Chop suey with meat, homemade	120	.11
Green peas (sweet), regular, solids and liquid	57	.11
Green peas (sweet), low sodium, solids and liquid	47	.11
Leeks bulbs and lower leaf, raw	52	.11
Mustard greens raw	31	.11
Raisins unsulfured	289	.11
Red beans dry, boiled and drained	118	.11
White rice fully milled or polished, enriched, cooked	109	.11
Whitefish (lake), stuffed, baked	215	.11
Baked potatoes with skin	93	.10
Beet greens raw	24	.10
Bran (cereal), sugar and malt extract added	240	.10
Broccoli spears, raw	32	.10
Brussels sprouts raw	45	.10
Dried figs uncooked	274	.10
Eggs fried	216	.10
Light fruitcake homemade from enriched flour	389	.10
Lobster (northern), canned or cooked	95	.10
Mushrooms raw	28	.10
Ocean perch (Atlantic), fried	227	.10
Oranges raw	49	.10
Pineapple chunks, canned in juice or syrup, fruit and liquid	58	.10
Spaghetti with cheese in tomato sauce, homemade	104	.10
Spaghetti with meatballs in tomato sauce, homemade	134	.10

FOOD ITEM	CALS.	UNITS
Spinach raw	26	.10
Weakfish broiled	208	.10
Baby lima beans frozen, boiled and drained	118	.09
Broccoli spears, boiled and drained	26	.09
Brown rice cooked	119	.09
Cauliflower boiled and drained	22	.09
Chicken with vegetables (baby food), commercial	100	.09
Corn (sweet), frozen, boiled and drained	79	.09
Cowpeas (including black-eyed peas), canned, solids and liquid	70	.09
Dates (domestic), unsulfured, dry	274	.09
Eggs hard-boiled	163	.09
Green chili peppers (hot), raw, pods without seeds	37	.09
Green peas (Alaska), canned, regular, solids and liquid	53	.09
Green peas (Alaska), canned, regular, solids and liquid	65	.09
Hamburger regular ground, cooked	286	.09
Italian bread unenriched, commercial	276	.09
Lobster salad	110	.09
Mung bean sprouts boiled and drained	28	.09
Oat and wheat cereal cooked	65	.09
Orange juice fresh, commercial	45	.09
Orange juice frozen concentrate, unsweetened	45	.09
Pineapple raw	52	.09
Pizza with sausage, homemade	234	.09
Potatoes with skin, boiled	76	.09
Prunes dried, uncooked	255	.09
Red cabbage raw	31	.09
Soybeans canned, solids and liquid	75	.09
Succotash frozen, boiled and drained	93	.09
Sweet potatoes with skin, boiled	114	.09
Sweet potatoes with skin, baked	141	.09
Tomato catsup bottled	106	.09
Tomato puree canned, regular or low sodium	39	.09
White bread unenriched, made with 1% - 2% nonfat dry milk	269	.09
Bread flour unenriched	365	.08
Brussels sprouts boiled and drained	36	.08
Brussels sprouts frozen, boiled and drained	33	.08
Chives raw	28	.08
Cod broiled	170	.08
Condensed milk canned, sweetened	321	.08

FOOD ITEM	CALS.	UNITS
Crab canned	101	.08
French bread unenriched, commercial	290	.08
Garden cress raw	32	.08
Green peppers (sweet), raw	22	.08
Green snap beans raw	32	.08
Hash-browned potatoes	229	.08
Kumquats raw	65	.08
Mashed potatoes milk added	65	.08
Mustard greens boiled and drained	23	.08
Orange juice dehydrated	46	.08
Parsnips raw	76	.08
Pineapple all styles except crushed, canned in water	39	.08
Pineapple all styles, canned in extra-heavy syrup, fruit and liquid	90	.08
Pineapple all styles, canned in light syrup, fruit and liquid	59	.08
Pineapple all styles, canned in heavy syrup, fruit and liquid	74	.08
Potato salad homemade with cooked salad dressing and seasonings	99	.08
Soybean milk	33	.08
Watercress leaves and stems, raw	19	.08
Yellow snap beans raw	27	.08
Artichokes (globe or French), boiled and drained	44	.07
Beef with vegetables (baby food), commercial	87	.07
Beet greens boiled and drained	18	.07
Chicken all classes, dark meat, roasted, without skin	176	.07
Danish pastry commercial	442	.07
Elderberries raw	72	.07
Endive (curley endive and escarole), raw	20	.07
Flounder baked	202	.07
Frankfurters and beans canned	144	.07
Green snap beans boiled and drained	25	.07
Green snap beans cut, frozen, boiled and drained	25	.07
Hash-browned potatoes frozen	224	.07
Lentils whole, dry, cooked	106	.07
Lima beans frozen, boiled and drained	99	.07
Natto (fermented soybean product)	167	.07
Orange juice canned, unsweetened	48	.07
Orange juice canned, sweetened	52	.07
Parsnips boiled and drained	66	.07
Pineapple juice frozen concentrate, unsweetened	52	.07

FOOD ITEM	CALS.	UNITS
Rutabagas raw	46	.07
Spinach boiled and drained	23	.07
Spinach chopped, frozen, boiled and drained	23	.07
Swamp cabbage raw	29	.07
Tomatoes ripe, boiled	26	.07
Yellow snap beans boiled and drained	22	.07
Yellow snap beans cut, frozen, boiled and drained	27	.07
Asparagus spears, canned, regular, solids and liquid	18	.06
Asparagus spears, canned, low sodium, solids and liquid	16	.06
Bread pudding with raisins, commercial	187	.06
Broccoli chopped, frozen, boiled and drained	26	.06
Carrots raw	42	.06
Chard, Swiss raw	25	.06
Chicory greens raw	20	.06
Coconut meat dried, unsweetened	662	.06
Collards frozen, boiled and drained	30	.06
Cornmeal (white or yellow), degermed, enriched, cooked	50	.06
Figs raw	80	.06
Finnan haddie (smoked haddock)	103	.06
Garden cress boiled and drained	23	.06
Green pea soup from mix	50	.06
Green peppers (sweet), boiled and drained	18	.06
Kale frozen, boiled and drained	31	.06
Lettuce (Boston and bibb), raw	14	.06
Mackerel (Atlantic), canned, solids and liquid	183	.06
Milk chocolate plain	520	.06
Miso (fermented soybean product)	171	.06
Pancakes from mix, made with eggs and milk	225	.06
Pizza with cheese, homemade	236	.06
Pizza frozen	245	.06
Plantains (baking bananas), raw	119	.06
Rice cereal cooked	50	.06
Rutabagas boiled and drained	35	.06
Shallots bulbs, raw	72	.06
Spaghetti with meatballs in tomato sauce, canned	103	.06
Summer squash (yellow crookneck), frozen, boiled and drained	21	.06
Sweet potatoes candied	168	.06
Tangerine juice fresh	43	.06
Tangerine juice frozen concentrate, unsweetened	46	.06

FOOD ITEM	CALS.	UNITS
Tangerines raw	46	.06
Tofu (soybean curd)	72	.06
Tomatoes ripe, raw	22	.06
Almonds roasted and salted	627	.05
Baking chocolate	505	.05
Beef chuck cuts, choice grade, braised or pot roasted	327	.05
Beef tongue braised, meduim	244	.05
Bitter chocolate	505	.05
Black currants (European), raw	54	.05
Cabbage raw	24	.05
Carrots boiled and drained	31	.05
Chinese cabbage raw	14	.05
Chop suey with meat, canned	62	.05
Coconut meat fresh	346	.05
Coleslaw made with salad dressing	99	.05
Eggplant boiled and drained	19	.05
Grapes (European), raw	67	.05
Guavas whole, raw	62	.05
Halibut (Atlantic and Pacific), broiled	171	.05
Ice cream cones	377	.05
Ice milk	152	.05
Lettuce (cos and romaine), raw	18	.05
Mangoes raw	66	.05
Pancakes homemade from unenriched flour	231	.05
Pineapple juice canned, unsweetened	55	.05
Pumpkin raw	26	.05
Red bananas raw	90	.05
Red beans canned, solids and liquid	90	.05
Red cherries (sour), raw	58	.05
Red cherries (sweet), raw	70	.05
Rockfish oven steamed	107	.05
Rolls from mix	299	.05
Russian salad dressing regular, commercial	494	.05
Summer squash raw or boiled and drained	19	.05
Swamp cabbage boiled and drained	21	.05
Tomato juice canned or bottled, regular or low sodium	19	.05
Tomato juice canned, concentrate	20	.05
Tomato juice cocktail canned or bottled	21	.05
Tomatoes ripe, canned, low sodium, solids and liquid	20	.05
Tomatoes ripe, canned, regular, solids and liquid	21	.05

FOOD ITEM	CALS.	UNITS
Winter squash raw or boiled and drained	63	.05
Zwieback	423	.05
Beef noodle soup from mix	28	.04
Buttermilk cultured, made from skim milk	36	.04
Cabbage shredded, boiled and drained	20	.04
Cantaloupe	30	.04
Cauliflower frozen, boiled and drained	18	.04
Chard, Swiss boiled and drained	18	.04
Chicken all classes, light meat, roasted, without skin	166	.04
Chocolate chip cookies commercial	471	.04
Coconut meat shredded, dried, sweetened	548	.04
Corn grits degermed, enriched, cooked	51	.04
Custard baked, commercial	115	.04
Eclairs with custard filling and chocolate frosting, commercial	239	.04
Evaporated milk canned, unsweetened	137	.04
Farina enriched, regular, cooked	42	.04
Frozen custard medium fat content	193	.04
Goat's milk	67	.04
Graham crackers plain	384	.04
Grape juice canned or bottled	66	.04
Grapefruit pulp, raw	41	.04
Grapefruit juice	39	.04
Grapefruit juice frozen concentrate, unsweetened	41	.04
Haddock fried	165	.04
Honeydew melon	33	.04
Hot cocoa homemade	97	.04
Ice cream fat content 10%	193	.04
Lemons peeled, raw	27	.04
Lima beans canned, low sodium, solids and liquid	70	.04
Lima beans canned, regular, solids and liquid	71	.04
Mashed potatoes dehydrated, flakes without milk	93	.04
Muffins (plain), homemade from unenriched flour	294	.04
New Zealand spinach raw	19	.04
Potatoes canned, solids and liquid	44	.04
Raisins cooked, sugar added, fruit and liquid	213	.04
Red cherries (sour), frozen, unsweetened	55	.04
Shrimp fried	225	.04
Skim milk	36	.04
Spanish rice homemade	87	.04
Swordfish broiled	174	.04

FOOD ITEM	CALS.	UNITS
Tomato soup canned, condensed, prepared with milk	69	.04
Tuna canned in oil, solids and liquids	288	.04
Tuna salad	170	.04
Welsh rarebit	179	.04
Winter squash boiled and mashed	38	.04
Yogurt made from partially skimmed milk	50	.04
Apples freshly harvested, without skin, raw	54	.03
Apples freshly harvested, with skin, raw	58	.03
Apricots raw	51	.03
Assorted cookies commercial	480	.03
Beef and vegetable stew canned	79	.03
Beef noodle dinner (baby food), commercial	49	.03
Blackberries raw	58	.03
Blue cheese or Roquefort cheese unprocessed	368	.03
Cake or pastry flour	364	.03
Caramels (plain or chocolate)	399	.03
Celery (green and yellow varieties), raw	17	.03
Chayote raw	28	.03
Cheddar cheese unprocessed	398	.03
Chicken chow mein without noodles, homemade	102	.03
Chicken noodle soup from mix	22	.03
Chili con carne with beans, canned	133	.03
Coconut milk	252	.03
Corn (sweet, white and yellow), whole kernel, regular or low sodium, solids and liquid	57	.03
Corn pudding	104	.03
Cottage cheese uncreamed	86	.03
Cottage cheese creamed	106	.03
Cranberries raw	46	.03
Creamed corn (sweet, white and yellow), canned, regular or low sodium, solids and liquid	82	.03
Creamed pollack	128	.03
Cucumbers with skin, raw	15	.03
Dried prunes cooked, without added sugar	119	.03
Dried prunes cooked, with added sugar	172	.03
Figs canned in water, with or without artificial sweetener, fruit and liquid	48	.03
Fruit pudding (baby food), commercial	96	.03
Gingerbread from mix, made with water	276	.03
Grapefruit canned in water, solids and liquid	30	.03

FOOD ITEM	CALS.	UNITS
Grapefruit juice frozen concentrate, sweetened	47	.03
Green chili peppers (hot), canned in chili sauce	20	.03
Green snap beans canned, regular, solids and liquid	18	.03
Green snap beans canned, low sodium, solids and liquid	16	.03
Half-and-half cream	134	.03
Lemon juice canned or bottled, unsweetened	23	.03
Lemon juice fresh	25	.03
Limes raw	28	.03
Mackerel (Pacific), canned, solids and liquid	180	.03
Mustard greens frozen, boiled and drained	20	.03
New Zealand spinach boiled and drained	13	.03
Onions boiled and drained	24	.03
Onions raw	38	.03
Pastry plain, made with unenriched flour	500	.03
Piecrust made with unenriched flour, commercial	500	.03
Piecrust from mix	464	.03
Plums (prune type), raw	75	.03
Pomegranate pulp, raw	63	.03
Pound cake homemade	473	.03
Pumpkin canned	33	.03
Pumpkin pie piecrust made with unenriched flour, commercial	211	.03
Purslane leaves and stems, raw	21	.03
Radishes (Oriental, including daikon and Chinese), raw	19	.03
Red beets boiled and drained	32	.03
Red beets raw	43	.03
Red cherries (sour), frozen, sweetened	112	.03
Red cherries (sour), canned in water, fruit and liquid	43	.03
Red cherries (sour), canned in light syrup, fruit and liquid	74	.03
Red cherries (sour), canned in heavy syrup, fruit and liquid	89	.03
Red cherries (sour), canned in extra-heavy syrup, fruit and liquid	112	.03
Red raspberries raw	57	.03
Rice pudding with raisins, commercial	146	.03
Sauerkraut canned, solids and liquid	18	.03
Strawberries raw	37	.03
Sweet potatoes canned in syrup, solids and liquid	114	.03
Sweet potatoes canned, in liquid, solids and liquid, unsweetened	46	.03
Vanilla pudding homemade	111	.03
Watermelon raw	26	.03

FOOD ITEM	CALS.	UNITS
Whole milk 3.5% fat	65	.03
Yellow snap beans canned, regular, solids and liquid	19	.03
Yellow snap beans canned, low sodium, solids and liquid	15	.03
Yogurt made from whole milk	62	.03
American cheese pasteurized, processed	370	.02
Applesauce canned, sweetened, artificially sweetened or un-sweetened	41	.02
Apricots canned in water, with or without artificial sweetener, fruit and liquid	38	.02
Apricots canned in light syrup, fruit and liquid	66	.02
Apricots canned in heavy syrup, fruit and liquid	86	.02
Apricots canned in extra-heavy syrup, fruit and liquid	101	.02
Beef noodle dinner (baby food), commercial	48	.02
Blackberries canned in juice, fruit and liquid	54	.02
Blackberries canned in water, with or without artificial sweeten-er, fruit and liquid	40	.02
Carrots canned, regular, solids and liquid	28	.02
Carrots canned, low sodium, solids and liquid	22	.02
Cherries (sweet), canned in water, with or without artificial sweetener,fruit and liquid	48	.02
Cherries (sweet), canned in light syrup, fruit and liquid	65	.02
Cherries (sweet), canned in heavy syrup, fruit and liquid	81	.02
Chicken and noodles homemade	153	.02
Chicken chow mein without noodles, canned	38	.02
Chicken gizzard all classes, simmered	148	.02
Chocolate pudding homemade	148	.02
Chocolate syrup (thin)	245	.02
Coconut cream	334	.02
Corned beef medium fat content	372	.02
Custard pudding (baby food), commercial	100	.02
Fruit cocktail canned in water, with or without artificial sweeten-er, fruit and liquid	37	.02
Fruit cocktail canned in heavy syrup, fruit and liquid	76	.02
Fruit cocktail canned in light syrup, fruit and liquid	60	.02
Ginger root fresh	49	.02
Grape juice frozen concentrate, sweetened	53	.02
Heavy whipping cream	352	.02
Light whipping cream	300	.02
Lime juice fresh, canned, or bottled, unsweetened	26	.02

FOOD ITEM	CALS.	UNITS
Marmalade (lemon or orange)	720	.02
Mayonnaise	718	.02
Mushrooms canned, solids and liquid	17	.02
Parmesan cheese	393	.02
Peaches raw	38	.02
Pears raw	61	.02
Pimientos raw, canned, solids and liquid	27	.02
Plums (purple), canned in water, with or without artificial sweetener,fruit and liquid	46	.02
Plums (purple), canned in light syrup, fruit and liquid	63	.02
Plums (purple), canned in heavy syrup, fruit and liquid	83	.02
Plums (purple), canned in extra-heavy syrup, fruit and liquid	102	.02
Pretzels	390	.02
Pudding from mix	124	.02
Purslane leaves and stems, boiled and drained	15	.02
Rhubarb frozen, cooked, sugar added	143	.02
Rose apples raw	56	.02
Sardines (Atlantic), canned in oil, solids and liquid	311	.02
Soy sauce	68	.02
Spinach canned, regular or low sodium, solids and liquid	19	.02
Spinach canned, low sodium, solids and liquid	21	.02
Strained bananas (baby food), commercial	84	.02
Thousand Island salad dressing commercial, regular	502	.02
Thousand Island salad dressing low calorie	180	.02
Tomato soup canned, condensed	36	.02
Tomato vegetable soup with noodles from mix	27	.02
Turnip greens leaves and stems, canned, solids and liquid	18	.02
Angel food cake homemade	269	.01
Apple butter	186	.01
Apple juice canned or bottled	47	.01
Applesauce (baby food), commercial	72	.01
Apricot nectar canned	57	.01
Barbecue sauce	91	.01
Blackberries canned in light syrup, fruit and liquid	72	.01
Blackberries canned in heavy syrup, fruit and liquid	91	.01
Blackberries canned in extra-heavy syrup, fruit and liquid	110	.01
Blueberries canned in extra-heavy syrup, fruit and liquid	101	.01
Brown sugar (beet or cane)	373	.01
Cheese crackers commercial	479	.01
Chicken noodle soup canned, condensed	53	.01

FOOD ITEM	CALS.	UNITS
Clams canned, solids and liquid	52	.01
Corned beef hash with potatoes, canned	181	.01
Cranberry juice cocktail	65	.01
Cranberry sauce canned, sweetened, strained	46	.01
Dried apricots sulfured, uncooked	260	.01
Dried pears	268	.01
Frosting (chocolate fudge), from mix, made with water and table fat	378	.01
Fruit cocktail canned in extra-heavy syrup, fruit and liquid	92	.01
Fruit salad canned in water, with or without artificial sweetener, fruit and liquid	37	.01
Grape drink canned	54	.01
Jams and preserves	272	.01
Macaroni unenriched, cooked until tender	111	.01
Manhattan clam chowder canned, condensed	33	.01
Orange sherbet	134	.01
Peach nectar canned	48	.01
Peaches canned in water, with or without artificial sweetener, fruit and liquid	31	.01
Peaches canned in juice, fruit and liquid	45	.01
Peaches canned in light syrup, fruit and liquid	58	.01
Peaches canned in heavy syrup, fruit and liquid	78	.01
Peaches canned in extra-heavy syrup, fruit and liquid	97	.01
Pears canned in light syrup, fruit and liquid	61	.01
Pears canned in heavy syrup, fruit and liquid	76	.01
Pears canned in extra-heavy syrup, fruit and liquid	92	.01
Prickly pears raw	42	.01
Red beets canned, regular, solids and liquid	34	.01
Red beets canned, low sodium, solids and liquid	32	.01
Salad dressing (blue cheese and Roquefort cheese), commercial, regular	504	.01
Sardines (Pacific), canned in tomato sauce, solids and liquid	197	.01
Strawberries canned in water, with or without artificial sweetener, fruit and liquid	22	.01
Swiss cheese (domestic), unprocessed	370	.01
Tartar sauce low calorie	224	.01
Tartar sauce regular	531	.01
Beef broth, bouillon, and consomme canned, condensed	13	.00
Blue cheese and Roquefort cheese commercial, low calorie	76	.00

FOOD ITEM	CALS.	UNITS
Coconut water	222	.00
Dried apples cooked, no sugar added	18	.00
Dried peaches cooked, no sugar added	82	.00
Dried pears cooked, no added sugar	126	.00
Honey	304	.00
Hot chocolate homemade	95	.00
Italian salad dressing commercial, regular	552	.00
Italian salad dressing commercial, low calorie	50	.00
Lemonade frozen concentrate	44	.00
Limeade frozen concentrate	41	.00
Pear nectar canned	48	.00
Pickles (dill)	11	.00
Pickles (sour)	10	.00
Pickles (sweet)	46	.00

Vitamin B$_2$

FOOD ITEM	CALS.	UNITS
Baker's yeast dry (active)	288	5.41
Torula yeast	277	5.06
Beef kidneys braised	252	4.82
Brewer's yeast debittered	283	4.28
Shredded oats (cereal)	261	4.23
Beef liver fried	227	4.19
Calf liver fried	261	4.17
Turkey giblets simmered	233	2.72
Chicken liver simmered	165	2.69
Whey dried	349	2.51
Rice cereal with wheat gluten	386	2.10
Turkey liver all classes, simmered	177	2.09
Strained liver (baby food), commercial	97	2.00
Strained liver and bacon (baby food), commercial	123	1.99
Skim milk dry, regular	363	1.80
Skim milk dry, instant	359	1.78
Buttermilk dry	387	1.72
Rice cereal with wheat gluten	386	1.70
Almond meal partially defatted	408	1.68
Cornflakes with protein concentrate	378	1.65
Whole milk dry	502	1.46

FOOD ITEM	CALS.	UNITS
Braunschweiger (luncheon meat)	319	1.44
Calf heart braised	208	1.44
Liverwurst smoked	319	1.44
Mixed cereal (baby food), precooked or dry, commercial	368	1.35
Red chili peppers (hot), pods, dried	321	1.33
Liverwurst	307	1.30
Rice cereal (baby food), commercial	371	1.24
Beef heart lean, braised	188	1.22
Barley cereal (baby food), precooked or dry, commercial	348	1.20
Cream substitutes with cream, and skim milk, dried, calcium reduced	508	1.17
Chili powder with added seasoning	340	1.13
Oatmeal (baby food), precooked or dry, commercial	375	1.05
Tea instant, powder, sugar added	294	.95
Almonds dried	598	.92
Chicken heart simmered	173	.92
Camembert cheese	299	.75
Cocoa powder with nonfat dry milk	359	.73
Parmesan cheese	393	.73
Fish flour from whole fish	336	.62
Blue cheese and Roquefort cheese	368	.61
Amercian cheese pasteurized, processed	323	.58
Chicken (fryers), with skin and giblets, fried	249	.57
Teething biscuits (baby food), commercial	378	.57
Malted milk powder	410	.54
Almonds chocolate-coated	569	.53
Limburger cheese	345	.50
Natto (fermented soybean product)	N.A.	.50
Chicken (fryers), thigh, fried	237	.48
Chicken (fryers), rib, fried	298	.47
Cocoa powder high fat	299	.46
Cocoa powder high fat, with alkali	295	.46
Cocoa powder medium fat, processed with alkali	261	.46
Cocoa powder low to medium fat	220	.46
Cocoa powder low to medium fat, processed with alkali	215	.46
Cocoa powder low fat	187	.46
Mushrooms raw	28	.46
Sunflower seed flour partially defatted	339	.46
Brick cheese	370	.45
Chicken (fryers), dark meat with skin, fried	263	.45

FOOD ITEM	CALS.	UNITS
Chicken (fryers), dark meat without skin, fried	220	.45
Cod dried, lightly salted	375	.45
Malt extract dried	367	.45
American cheese pasteurized, processed	370	.41
Chicken (fryers), skin only, fried	419	.41
Milk chocolate with almonds	532	.41
Chicken (fryers), drumstick, fried	235	.40
Safflower seed meal partially defatted	355	.40
Swiss cheese (domestic), unprocessed	370	.40
Swiss cheese pasteurized, processed	355	.40
Chestnuts dried	377	.38
Condensed milk canned, sweetened	321	.38
Proso millet whole grain	327	.38
Wheat bran crude, commercially milled	213	.35
Cocoa powder medium fat	265	.34
Evaporated milk canned, unsweetened	137	.34
Milk chocolate plain	520	.34
Pork sausage links or bulk	476	.34
Soybean flour defatted	326	.34
Breadcrumbs dry, grated	392	.30
Eggs fried	216	.30
Green chili peppers hot, canned in chili sauce	20	.30
Beef tongue medium fat content, braised	244	.29
Bran sugar and malt extract added	240	.29
Fried oysters	239	.29
Cottage cheese uncreamed	86	.28
Eggs whole, fresh	163	.28
Smoked herring kippered	211	.28
Sardines (Pacific), canned in tomato sauce, solids and liquid	197	.27
Dandelion greens raw	45	.26
Garden cress raw	32	.26
Parsley raw	44	.26
Rolls and buns homemade	339	.26
Shad baked	201	.26
Shrimp paste or lobster paste canned	180	.26
Wheat flour enriched	365	.26
Biscuits from mix, with enriched flour and milk	325	.25
Cashew nuts	561	.25
Cottage cheese creamed	106	.25
Eggs poached	163	.25

FOOD ITEM	CALS.	UNITS
Mushrooms canned, solids and liquid	17	.25
Popovers	224	.25
Rice bran (cereal)	276	.25
Soy sauce	68	.25
Waffles homemade	279	.25
Baking chocolate	505	.24
Bitter chocolate	505	.24
Bran muffins homemade from enriched flour	261	.24
Cream cheese	374	.24
Pancakes from mix, made with eggs and milk	225	.24
Salami cooked	311	.24
Sesame seeds dry, whole	563	.24
Turnip greens leaves and stems, boiled and drained	20	.24
Broccoli spears, raw	32	.23
Chicken all classes, dark meat, roasted, without skin	176	.23
Corn muffins homemade from enriched degermed cornmeal	314	.23
Hard rolls enriched, commercial	312	.23
Muffins (plain), homemade from enriched flour	294	.23
Puffed wheat (cereal)	376	.23
Sunflower seed kernels dried	560	.23
Welsh rarebit	179	.23
Beet greens raw	376	.22
Bologna	304	.22
Chestnuts fresh	194	.22
French bread enriched or unenriched	290	.22
Ice milk	152	.22
Mustard greens raw	31	.22
Pancakes homemade from enriched flour	231	.22
Peanut flour defatted	371	.22
Rye whole grain	334	.22
Baking powder biscuits homemade from enriched flour	369	.21
Chicken gizzard simmered	148	.21
Frozen custard fat content 10%	193	.21
Graham crackers plain	384	.21
Hamburger regular ground, cooked	286	.21
Ice cream fat content 10%	193	.21
Ice cream cones	377	.21
Asparagus spears, raw	26	.20
Avocados raw	167	.20
Beef chuck cuts, choice grade, braised or pot roasted	327	.20

FOOD ITEM	CALS.	UNITS
Blueberry muffins homemade from enriched flour	281	.20
Broccoli spears, boiled and drained	26	.20
Chinese water chestnuts raw	79	.20
Collards leaves and stems, boiled and drained	29	.20
Corn fritters	377	.20
Cornbread from mix, made with eggs and milk	233	.20
Frankfurters	304	.20
Italian bread enriched, commercial	276	.20
Pizza homemade with cheese topping	236	.20
Soybean sprouts raw	46	.20
Spinach raw	26	.20
Blackstrap molasses (cane)	213	.19
Bread pudding with raisins, commercial	187	.19
Corn muffins from mix, made with eggs and milk	324	.19
Cornbread homemade from whole-ground cornmeal	207	.19
Custard commercial	115	.19
Dried peaches uncooked	262	.19
Pumpkin and squash seed kernels dried	553	.19
Asparagus spears, boiled and drained	20	.18
Buttermilk cultured	36	.18
Corned beef medium fat content	372	.18
Hot cocoa homemade	97	.18
Puffed corn (cereal)	399	.18
Rolls and buns plain, commercial	298	.18
Shredded corn (cereal)	389	.18
Skim milk	36	.18
Yogurt made from partially skimmed milk	50	.18
Beef with vegetables (baby food), commercial	87	.17
Bran flakes (cereal)	303	.17
Caramels plain or chocolate	399	.17
Chard, Swiss raw	25	.17
Corn muffins homemade from whole-ground cornmeal	288	.17
Dried prunes uncooked	344	.17
New Zealand spinach raw	19	.17
Okra cuts and pods, frozen, boiled and drained	38	.17
Pizza frozen	245	.17
White bread enriched, made with 1% - 2% nonfat dry milk	369	.17
Whole milk sow's, 3.5% fat	65	.17
Buckwheat pancakes and waffles from mix, made with eggs and milk	200	.16

FOOD ITEM	CALS.	UNITS
Dandelion greens boiled and drained	33	.16
Doughnuts cake type	391	.16
Dried apricots uncooked	260	.16
Eclairs with custard filling and chocolate frosting, commercial	239	.16
Garden cress boiled and drained	23	.16
Half-and-half cream	134	.16
Hot chocolate homemade	95	.16
Sardines (Atlantic), canned in oil, solids and liquid	311	.16
Vanilla pudding homemade	111	.16
Watercress leaves and stems, raw	19	.16
Yogurt made from whole milk	62	.16
Beef tripe commercial	100	.15
Beet greens boiled and drained	18	.15
Chicken with vegetables (baby food), commercial	100	.15
Chop suey with meat, homemade	120	.15
Danish pastry commercial	422	.15
Kale frozen, boiled and drained	31	.15
Soybean sprouts boiled and drained	38	.15
Spinach chopped, frozen, boiled and drained	23	.15
Angel food cake homemade	269	.14
Asparagus spears, frozen, boiled and drained	22	.14
Brussels sprouts boiled and drained	36	.14
Chocolate pudding homemade	148	.14
Collards frozen, boiled and drained	30	.14
Dark fruitcake homemade	379	.14
Endive (curley endive and escarole), raw	20	.14
Muffins plain, homemade from unenriched flour	294	.14
Mustard greens boiled and drained	23	.14
Pancakes homemade from unenriched flour	231	.14
Pastry (plain), made with enriched flour	500	.14
Piecrust made with enriched flour	500	.14
Potato flour	351	.14
Prune whip	156	.14
Pumpernickel bread commercial	246	.14
Rice pudding with raisins, commercial	146	.14
Wheat flakes (cereal), added nutrients	354	.14
Asparagus cuts and tips, frozen, boiled and drained	22	.13
Chives raw	28	.13
Corn pudding commercial	104	.13
Creamed pollack	128	.13

FOOD ITEM	CALS.	UNITS
Mung bean sprouts raw	35	.13
Peanut butter fat and salt added	581	.13
Peanuts without skins, raw or roasted	568	.13
Pecans	687	.13
Sesame seeds dry, hulled	582	.13
Walnuts	651	.13
Whole wheat rolls and buns commercial	257	.13
Winter squash baked	63	.13
Brazil nuts	654	.12
Broccoli chopped, frozen, boiled and drained	26	.12
Brownies with nuts, homemade from enriched flour	485	.12
Corn muffins from mix, made with eggs and water	297	.12
Custard pudding (baby food), commercial	100	.12
Dried apples uncooked	275	.12
Green snap beans boiled and drained	25	.12
Light whipping cream	300	.12
Peas edible podded, raw	53	.12
Pizza with sausage, homemade	234	.12
Rockfish oven steamed	107	.12
Rolls from mix	299	.12
Rye flour medium	350	.12
Spaghetti with meatballs in tomato sauce, homemade	134	.12
Split pea soup canned, condensed	118	.12
Swamp cabbage raw	29	.12
Tomato paste canned	82	.12
Wheat whole grain, hard red spring or winter	330	.12
Wheat whole grain, white	335	.12
Whole wheat flour	333	.12
Black walnuts	628	.11
Black-eyed peas frozen, boiled and drained	130	.11
Chard, Swiss boiled and drained	18	.11
Chocolate chip cookies homemade from enriched flour	516	.11
Clams canned, solids and liquid	52	.11
Cod boiled	170	.11
Cornmeal (white or yellow), whole ground, unbolted	355	.11
Cowpeas boiled and drained	108	.11
Dark fruitcake homemade	379	.11
Gingerbread homemade from enriched flour	317	.11
Goat's milk	67	.11
Green peas boiled and drained	71	.11

FOOD ITEM	CALS.	UNITS
Heavy whipping cream	352	.11
Macadamia nuts	691	.11
Ocean perch (Atlantic), fried	227	.11
Peas edible podded, boiled and drained	43	.11
Shredded wheat (cereal)	354	.11
Spaghetti with cheese in tomato sauce, canned	76	.11
Tuna salad	170	.11
Wheat whole grain, soft red winter	326	.11
Whitefish (lake), stuffed, baked	215	.11
Yellow snap beans raw	27	.11
Blue cheese and Roquefort cheese salad commercial, regular	504	.10
Bluefish baked or broiled	159	.10
Boysenberries frozen, sweetened	96	.10
Brussels sprouts frozen, boiled and drained	33	.10
Bulgur (parboiled wheat), from club wheat, dry, commercial	359	.10
Cauliflower raw	27	.10
Cheese crackers	479	.10
Chicken all classes, light meat, roasted, without skin	166	.10
Chicory greens raw	20	.10
Chocolate cake with chocolate frosting, homemade	369	.10
Corn on the cob (sweet, white and yellow), boiled and drained	91	.10
Dates (domestic), natural, dry	274	.10
Dried figs uncooked	274	.10
Kumquats raw	65	.10
Lima beans boiled and drained	111	.10
Miso (fermented soybean product)	171	.10
Mung bean sprouts boiled and drained	28	.10
Mustard greens frozen, boiled and drained	20	.10
New Zealand spinach boiled and drained	13	.10
Peanut spread	601	.10
Pumpkin pie piecrust made with unenriched flour	211	.10
Purslane leaves and stems, raw	21	.10
Spinach canned, regular, solids and liquid	19	.10
Spinach canned, low sodium, solids and liquid	21	.10
Tomato soup canned, condensed, prepared with milk	69	.10
Tuna canned in water, solids and liquid	127	.10
Winter squash boiled, mashed	38	.10
Asparagus spears, canned, regular, solids and liquid	18	.09
Asparagus spears, canned, low sodium, solids and liquid	16	.09

FOOD ITEM	CALS.	UNITS
Chicken chow mein without noodles, homemade	102	.09
Corned beef hash canned	181	.09
Cracked wheat bread commercial	263	.09
Gingerbread from mix	276	.09
Green peas frozen, boiled and drained	68	.09
Green snap beans cut, frozen, boiled and drained	25	.09
Green snap beans boiled and drained	25	.09
Parsnips raw	76	.09
Pound cake old fashioned, homemade	473	.09
Red raspberries raw	57	.09
Soybeans canned, solids and liquid	75	.09
Soybeans dry, cooked	130	.09
Tuna canned in oil, solids and liquid	288	.09
Turnip greens leaves and stems, canned, solids and liquid	18	.09
Turnip greens leaves and stems, frozen, boiled and drained	23	.09
Yellow snap beans boiled and drained	22	.09
Brownies with nuts and chocolate frosting, frozen	419	.08
Cauliflower boiled and drained	22	.08
Cod canned	85	.08
Corn on the cob (sweet), frozen, boiled and drained	94	.08
Cornflakes (cereal)	386	.08
Crab canned	101	.08
Dried pears cooked, no added sugar	126	.08
Egg noodles enriched, cooked	125	.08
Flounder baked	202	.08
French bread white, unenriched, commercial	290	.08
French fried potatoes	274	.08
French fried shrimp	225	.08
Garlic cloves raw	137	.08
Green peppers (sweet), raw	22	.08
Lettuce (cos and romaine), raw	18	.08
Lobster salad	110	.08
Macaroni enriched, cooked until tender	111	.08
Parsnips boiled and drained	66	.08
Raisins	289	.08
Spaghetti enriched, cooked until tender	111	.08
Spaghetti enriched, cooked until tender	111	.08
Summer squash boiled and drained	14	.08
Swamp cabbage boiled and drained	21	.08
Weakfish broiled	208	.08

FOOD ITEM	CALS.	UNITS
White cake homemade	375	.08
Yellow beans cut, frozen, boiled and drained	27	.08
Bamboo shoots raw	27	.07
Blue cheese & Roquefort salad dressing commercial, low calorie	76	.07
Chili con carne with beans, canned	133	.07
Chocolate chip cookies commercial	471	.07
Chocolate syrup (thin)	245	.07
Dried pears cooked, sugar added, fruit and liquid	151	.07
Dried prunes cooked, no added sugar, fruit and liquid	119	.07
Haddock fried	165	.07
Halibut (Atlantic and Pacific), broiled	171	.07
Lobster canned or cooked	95	.07
Mixed vegetables frozen, boiled and drained	64	.07
Peas and carrots frozen, boiled and drained	53	.07
Pecan pie piecrust made with unenriched flour, commercial	418	.07
Potato chips	568	.07
Potato sticks	544	.07
Red cherries (sour), frozen, unsweetened	55	.07
Rutabagas raw	46	.07
Rye bread (American), commercial	243	.07
Spaghetti with cheese in tomato sauce, homemade	104	.07
Spaghetti with meatballs in tomato sauce, canned	103	.07
Strawberries raw	37	.07
Sweet potatoes with skin, baked	141	.07
Tomato catsup bottled	106	.07
Turnips raw	30	.07
Winter squash frozen	38	.07
Zwieback	423	.07
Bananas raw	85	.06
Cane syrup	263	.06
Celeriac root, raw	40	.06
Chicken noodle dinner (baby food), commercial	49	.06
Corn sweet, frozen, boiled and drained	79	.06
Corn flour	368	.06
Dried peaches cooked, no sugar, fruit and liquid	82.	.06
Elderberries raw	72	.06
Frankfurters and beans canned	144	.06
Green beans (baby food), commercial	22	.06
Green chili peppers (hot), raw, pods without seeds	37	.06

FOOD ITEM	CALS.	UNITS
Green pea soup from mix	50	.06
Green peas (sweet), canned, regular, solids and liquid	57	.06
Green peas (sweet), canned, low sodium, solids and liquid	47	.06
Italian bread unenriched	276	.06
Jerusalem artichokes raw, freshly harvested	7	.06
Leeks bulb and lower leaf, raw	52	.06
Lentils whole, dry, cooked	106	.06
Lettuce (Boston and bibb), raw	14	.06
Lima beans dry, boiled and drained	138	.06
Pimientos canned, solids and liquid	27	.06
Purslane leaves and stems, boiled and drained	15	.06
Red beans dry, boiled and drained	90	.06
Red cabbage raw	31	.06
Red cherries (sweet), raw	70	.06
Red cherries (sour), frozen, sweetened	112	.06
Red cherries (sour), raw	58	.06
Red raspberries frozen, sweetened	98	.06
Rutabagas boiled and drained	35	.06
Salmon broiled or baked	182	.06
Strawberries sliced, frozen, sweetened	109	.06
Sweet potatoes with skin, boiled	114	.06
Assorted cookies commercial	480	.05
Barley pearled, light	349	.05
Beef and vegetable stew canned	79	.05
Beef noodle dinner (baby food), commercial	48	.05
Black currants (European), raw	54	.05
Blueberries frozen, sweetened	105	.05
Cabbage raw	24	.05
Carrots raw	42	.05
Carrots boiled and drained	31	.05
Cauliflower frozen, boiled and drained	18	.05
Chop suey with meat, canned	62	.05
Coleslaw made with salad dressing	99	.05
Corn (sweet, white and yellow), regular, solids and liquid	83	.05
Corn (sweet, white and yellow), canned, low sodium, solids and liquid	57	.05
Cowpeas (including black-eyed peas), canned, solids and liquid	70	.05
Creamed corn (sweet, white and yellow), canned, regular or low sodium, solids and liquid	82	.05

FOOD ITEM	CALS.	UNITS
Dried peaches cooked, sugar added, fruit and liquid	119	.05
Figs raw	80	.05
Finnan haddie (smoked haddock)	103	.05
Fruit pudding (baby food), commercial	96	.05
Green peas (Alaska), canned, regular, solids and liquid	66	.05
Green peas (Alaska), canned, low sodium, solids and liquid	55	.05
Hash-browned potatoes	229	.05
Lichees raw	64	.05
Lima beans frozen, boiled and drained	99	.05
Mangoes raw	66	.05
Mashed potatoes milk added	65	.05
Peaches raw	38	.05
Pumpkin canned	33	.05
Red beets raw	43	.05
Rice flakes (cereal)	390	.05
Russian salad dressing commercial, regular	494	.05
Succotash frozen, boiled and drained	93	.05
Swordfish broiled	174	.05
Tomato puree canned, regular or low sodium	39	.05
Tomatoes ripe, boiled	26	.05
Turnips boiled and drained	23	.05
Wheat flour unenriched	364	.05
Apricots raw	51	.04
Artichokes (globe or French), boiled and drained	44	.04
Blackberries raw	58	.04
Cabbage shredded, boiled and drained	20	.04
Chicken chow mein without noodles, canned	38	.04
Chinese cabbage raw	14	.04
Coconut meat dried, unsweetened	662	.04
Cornflakes sugar coated	386	.04
Cornmeal (white or yellow), degermed, enriched, cooked	50	.04
Cucumbers with skin, raw	15	.04
Eggplant boiled and drained	19	.04
Frosting (chocolate fudge), from mix, made with water and table fat	378	.04
Ginger root fresh	49	.04
Green snap beans canned, regular, solids and liquid	18	.04
Green snap beans canned, low sodium, solids and liquid	16	.04
Honey	304	.04
Kohlrabi thickened bulb-like stems, raw	29	.04

FOOD ITEM	CALS.	UNITS
Lima beans canned, regular, solids and liquid	71	.04
Lima beans canned, low sodium, solids and liquid	70	.04
Mashed potatoes dehydrated, flakes without milk	93	.04
Mashed potatoes frozen	93	.04
Mayonnaise	718	.04
Onions raw	38	.04
Oranges raw	49	.04
Papayas raw	39	.04
Peaches canned in juice, fruit and liquid	45	.04
Pears with skin, raw	61	.04
Plantains (baking bananas), raw	119	.04
Potatoes with skin, baked	93	.04
Puffed rice (cereal)	399	.04
Red bananas raw	90	.04
Red beans canned, solids and liquid	90	.04
Red beets boiled and drained	32	.04
Rhubarb frozen, cooked, sugar added	143	.04
Sauerkraut canned, solids and liquid	18	.04
Squash (yellow crookneck), frozen, boiled and drained	21	.04
Tomatoes ripe, raw	22	.04
Whole wheat crackers	403	.04
Yellow snap beans canned, regular, solids and liquid	19	.04
Apricots canned in juice, fruit and liquid	54	.03
Beer	42	.03
Blackberries canned in juice, fruit and liquid	54	.03
Brown sugar (beet or cane)	373	.03
Cantaloupe	30	.03
Carrots (baby food), commercial	29	.03
Celery (green and yellow varieties), boiled and drained	14	.03
Chayote raw	28	.03
Coconut meat shredded, dried, sweetened	548	.03
Corn grits degermed, enriched	51	.03
Dried apples cooked, sugar added	112	.03
Farina enriched, regular, cooked	42	.03
Figs canned in water, with or without artificial sweetener, fruit and liquid	48	.03
Figs canned in light syrup, fruit and liquid	65	.03
Figs canned in heavy syrup, fruit and liquid	84	.03
Figs canned in extra-heavy syrup, fruit and liquid	103	.03
Grape juice frozen concentrate, sweetened	53	.03

FOOD ITEM	CALS.	UNITS
Grapes (European), raw	67	.03
Honeydew melon	33	.03
Jams and preserves	272	.03
Kohlrabi thickened bulb-like stems, boiled and drained	24	.03
Oat cereal with toasted wheat germ and soy grits, cooked	62	.03
Onions boiled and drained	29	.03
Orange juice fresh, commercial	45	.03
Orange juice dehydrated, prepared with water	46	.03
Orange sherbert	134	.03
Pastry plain, made with unenriched flour	500	.03
Peaches canned in light syrup, fruit and liquid	58	.03
Peaches canned in water, with or without artificial sweetener, fruit and liquid	31	.03
Peaches canned in heavy syrup, fruit and liquid	78	.03
Peaches canned in extra-heavy syrup, fruit and liquid	97	.03
Pears canned in juice, fruit and liquid	46	.03
Piecrust made with unenriched flour	500	.03
Piecrust from mix	464	.03
Pineapple chunks, frozen, sweetened	85	.03
Pineapple raw	52	.03
Pineapple canned in juice, fruit and liquid	58	.03
Plums (prune type), raw	75	.03
Pomegranate pulp, raw	63	.03
Pretzels	390	.03
Prickly pears raw	42	.03
Radishes raw	17	.03
Raisins cooked, sugar sugar added, fruit and liquid	213	.03
Rose apples raw	56	.03
Shrimp raw	91	.03
Soybean milk thin	33	.03
Strawberries canned in water, with or without artificial sweetener, fruit and liquid	22	.03
Sweet potatoes canned in syrup, solids and liquid	114	.03
Sweet potatoes canned in liquid, solids and liquid, unsweetened	46	.03
Tartar sauce regular	531	.03
Tartar sauce low calorie	224	.03
Thousand Island salad dressing commercial, regular	502	.03
Thousand Island salad dressing commercial, low calorie	180	.03
Tofu (soybean curd)	72	.03

FOOD ITEM	CALS.	UNITS
Tomato juice canned or bottled, regular or low sodium	19	.03
Tomato juice canned, concentrate	20	.03
Tomatoes ripe, canned, regular, solids and liquid	21	.03
Tomatoes ripe, canned, low sodium, solids and liquid	20	.03
Watermelon raw	26	.03
Yam beans tuber, raw	55	.03
Apple juice canned or bottled	47	.02
Apples freshly harvested, with skin, raw	58	.02
Applesauce (baby food), commercial	72	.02
Apricots canned in water, with or without artificial sweetener, fruit and liquid	38	.02
Apricots canned in light syrup, fruit and liquid	66	.02
Apricots canned in heavy syrup, fruit and liquid	86	.02
Apricots canned in extra-heavy syrup, fruit and liquid	101	.02
Beef broth, bouillon, and consomme canned, condensed	26	.02
Beef noodle soup from mix	28	.02
Blackberries canned in water, with or without artificial sweetener, fruit and liquid	40	.02
Blackberries canned in extra-heavy syrup, fruit and liquid	110	.02
Blackberries canned in light syrup, fruit and liquid	72	.02
Blackberries canned in heavy syrup, fruit and liquid	91	.02
Brown rice	119	.02
Carrots canned, low sodium, solids and liquid	22	.02
Carrots canned, regular, solids and liquid	28	.02
Chicken noodle soup canned, condensed	53	.02
Chicken noodle soup from mix	22	.02
Coconut meat fresh	346	.02
French fried potatoes frozen	220	.02
Grape juice canned or bottled	66	.02
Grapefruit raw	41	.02
Grapefruit canned in water, with or without artificial sweetener, fruit and liquid	30	.02
Grapefruit juice	39	.02
Grapefruit juice frozen concentrate, unsweetened	41	.02
Hash-browned potatoes frozen, cooked	224	.02
Lemons peeled, raw	27	.02
Limes raw	28	.02
Marmalade plums	125	.02
Orange juice canned, sweetened or unsweetened	48	.02
Orange juice canned, sweetened	52	.02

FOOD ITEM	CALS.	UNITS
Peach nectar canned	48	.02
Peaches canned in heavy syrup, fruit and liquid	18	.02
Pears canned in water, with or without artificial sweetener, fruit and liquid	32	.02
Pears canned in light syrup, fruit and liquid	61	.02
Pears canned in heavy syrup, fruit and liquid	76	.02
Pears canned in extra-heavy syrup, fruit and liquid	92	.02
Pickles (dill)	11	.02
Pickles (sweet)	146	.02
Pickles (sour)	10	.02
Pineapple all styles except crushed, canned in water, with or without artificial sweetener,	39	.02
Pineapple all styles except crushed, canned in extra-heavy syrup, fruit and liquid	90	.02
Pineapple all styles except crushed, canned in light syrup, fruit and liquid	59	.02
Pineapple all styles except crushed, canned in heavy syrup, fruit and liquid	74	.02
Pineapple juice frozen concentrate, unsweetened	52	.02
Pineapple juice canned, unsweetened	50	.02
Plums (purple), canned in water, with or without artificial sweetener, fruit and liquid	46	.02
Plums (purple), canned in extra-heavy syrup, fruit and liquid	102	.02
Plums (purple), canned in heavy syrup, fruit and liquid	83	.02
Plums (purple), canned in light syrup, fruit and liquid	63	.02
Potatoes canned, solids and liquid	44	.02
Radishes (Oriental, including daikon and Chinese), raw	19	.02
Red beets canned, regular or low sodium, solids and liquid	32	.02
Red cherries sour, canned in water, fruit and liquid	43	.02
Red cherries canned in light syrup, fruit and liquid	74	.02
Red cherries canned in heavy syrup, fruit and liquid	89	.02
Red cherries canned in extra-heavy syrup, fruit and liquid	112	.02
Shallots bulbs, raw	72	.02
Strained bananas (baby food), commercial	84	.02
Tangerine juice fresh	43	.02
Tangerine juice frozen concentrate, unsweetened	46	.02
Tangerines raw	46	.02
Tomato juice cocktail canned or bottled	21	.02
Tomato soup canned, condensed	36	.02

FOOD ITEM	CALS.	UNITS
Applesauce canned, sweetened	91	.01
Applesauce canned, unsweetened or artificially sweetened	41	.01
Apricot nectar canned	57	.01
Barbecue sauce	91	.01
Blueberries canned in water, with or without artificial sweetener, fruit and liquid	39	.01
Blueberries canned in syrup, fruit and liquid	101	.01
Cranberry juice cocktail bottled	65	.01
Cranberry sauce canned, sweetened, strained	146	.01
Fruit cocktail canned in water, with or without artificial sweetener, fruit and liquid	37	.01
Fruit cocktail canned in extra-heavy syrup, fruit and liquid	90	.01
Fruit cocktail canned in heavy syrup, fruit and liquid	85	.01
Fruit cocktail canned in light syrup, fruit and liquid	59	.01
Fruit dessert with tapioca (baby food), commercial	84	.01
Grape drink canned	54	.01
Grapefruit juice frozen concentrate, sweetened	47	.01
Lemon juice canned or bottled, unsweetened	23	.01
Lemonade frozen concentrate	44	.01
Lime juice fresh, canned, or bottled, unsweetened	26	.01
Macaroni unenriched, cooked until tender	111	.01
Manhattan clam chowder canned, condensed	33	.01
Orange juice frozen concentrate, unsweetened	45	.01
Rice cereal cooked	50	.01
Tea instant	2	.01
Tomato vegetable soup with noodles from mix	27	.01
Wine	85	.01
Butterscotch candy	397	.00
Coconut milk	252	.00
Coconut water	22	.00
Italian salad dressing commercial, regular	552	.00
Italian salad dressing commercial, low calorie	50	.00
Lime ice	78	.00
Limeade frozen concentrate	41	.00

Vitamin B$_6$

FOOD ITEM	CALS.	UNITS
Torula yeast	277	3.000
Brewer's yeast debittered	283	2.500
Baker's yeast dry (active)	282	2.000
Sunflower seed kernels dried	560	1.250
Wheat germ toasted	391	1.150
Wheat bran (cereal)	240	.820
Walnuts	651	.730
Soybean flour defatted	326	.724
Smoked salmon salted	176	.700
Baker's yeast compressed	86	.600
Buckwheat flour dark	333	.578
Filberts (hazelnuts)	634	.545
Bananas raw	85	.510
Onions dried	350	.500
White rice parboiled	106	.425
Avocados raw	167	.420
Smoked mackerel (Atlantic), salted	219	.410
Peanuts roasted	582	.400
Skim milk dry, regular	363	.380
Tomato paste canned	82	.380
Ham canned	193	.360
Whole wheat flour	333	.340
Chestnuts fresh	194	.330
Peanut butter	581	.330
Cod dehydrated	375	.300
Crab cooked or canned	101	.300
Rye flour	334	.300
Wheat flakes (cereal)	354	.292
Mackerel (Atlantic), canned	183	.280
Spinach raw	26	.280
Whole milk dry	502	.270
Turnip greens raw	28	.263
Green peppers (sweet), raw	22	.260
Cornmeal (white and yellow)	355	.250
Herring kippered, canned	211	.250
Sauerkraut juice canned	10	.250
Garden cress raw	32	.247
Shredded wheat (cereal)	354	.244

FOOD ITEM	CALS.	UNITS
Prunes dried	255	.240
Elderberries raw	72	.230
Camembert cheese	299	.220
Sardines (Pacific), canned in tomato sauce, solids and liquid	197	.220
Cauliflower raw	27	.210
Popcorn popped, plain	386	.204
Corn canned	83	.200
Dried apples cooked, sugar added	112	.200
Molasses (blackstrap)	213	.200
Red cabbage raw	31	.200
Smoked herring salted	218	.200
Broccoli spears, raw	32	.195
Tomato juice canned, regular or low sodium	19	.192
Cabbage (savoy), raw	24	.190
Liverwurst	307	.190
Pecans	687	.183
Chives raw	28	.181
Potato chips	568	.180
Sardines (Atlantic), canned in oil, solids and liquid	311	.180
Whole wheat bread	243	.180
Dried figs	274	.175
Blue cheese	368	.170
Brazil nuts	654	.170
Puffed rice (cereal)	399	.170
Parsley raw	44	.164
Cabbage raw	24	.160
Herring (Atlantic), canned	208	.160
Pumpernickel bread	246	.160
Dates (domestic), natural, dry	274	.153
Tomato puree canned, regular or low sodium	39	.152
Carrots raw	42	.150
Anchovies	176	.144
American cheese food pasteurized, processed	323	.141
Cod canned	85	.140
Onions raw	38	.130
Sauerkraut canned, solids and liquid	18	.130
Watercress leaves and stem, raw	19	.129
Mushrooms raw	28	.125
Rice flakes (cereal)	390	.125
Salami dry	450	.123

FOOD ITEM	CALS.	UNITS
Roquefort cheese	368	.120
Pickled herring	223	.117
Figs raw	80	.113
Tomato catsup bottled	106	.107
Potatoes canned, solids and liquid	44	.102
Almonds dried	598	.100
Beet greens raw	24	.100
Bologna	304	.100
Dried peaches	262	.100
Fennel leaves, raw	28	.100
Rutabagas boiled and drained	35	.100
Rye bread (American), commercial	243	.100
Tomatoes ripe, raw	22	.100
Turnip greens canned	18	.100
Parmesan cheese	393	.096
Pineapple juice canned	55	.096
Almonds roasted and salted	627	.095
Cracked wheat bread	263	.092
Parsnips raw	76	.090
Rye flour light	367	.090
Tomatoes ripe, canned	21	.090
Pineapple raw	52	.088
Cantaloupe	30	.086
Limburger cheese	345	.086
Vienna sausage canned	240	.083
Cheddar cheese unprocessed	398	.080
Grapes (American), raw	69	.080
Green snap beans raw	32	.080
Lemons peeled, raw	27	.080
Rice cereal cooked	350	.080
Puffed rice (cereal)	399	.075
Radishes (Oriental, including daikon and Chinese), raw	19	.075
Swiss cheese	355	.075
Pineapple juice frozen, diluted	52	.074
Brick cheese	370	.073
Jerusalem artichokes raw, freshly harvested	7	.071
Apricots raw	51	.070
Spinach canned	19	.070
Saltine crackers	433	.068
Watermelon	26	.068

FOOD ITEM	CALS.	UNITS
Blueberries raw	62	.067
Tangerines raw	46	.067
Black currants (European)	54	.066
Sweet potatoes canned	114	.066
Cornflakes	386	.065
Red cherries (sour), raw	58	.065
Beer	42	.060
Bread flour	365	.060
Celery raw	17	.060
Condensed milk canned, sweetened	321	.060
Mushrooms canned, solids and liquid	17	.060
Oranges raw	49	.060
Red cherries sour, frozen, unsweetened	55	.060
Red raspberries raw	73	.060
Shrimp canned, wet pack, solids and liquid	80	.060
Honeydew melon	33	.056
Pumpkin canned	33	.056
Asparagus canned	18	.055
Cream cheese	374	.055
Red beets raw	43	.055
Strawberries raw	37	.055
Apricots canned in light syrup, fruit and liquid	66	.054
Apricots canned in heavy syrup, fruit and liquid	86	.054
Apricots canned in extra-heavy syrup, fruit and liquid	101	.054
French bread	290	.053
Chicken noodle soup canned, condensed	53	.052
Plums raw	66	.052
Beets canned, regular pack, solids and liquid	34	.050
Blackberries raw	58	.050
Evaporated milk canned, unsweetened	137	.050
Green peas canned, regular, solids and liquid	66	.050
Lemon juice fresh	25	.046
Yogurt	50	.046
Cake and pastry flour	364	.045
Chicory raw	15	.045
Goat's milk	67	.045
Chicken vegetable soup canned, condensed	62	.044
Coconut fresh	346	.044
Lime juice fresh	26	.043
Swiss cheese pasteurized, processed	355	.043

FOOD ITEM	CALS.	UNITS
Tomato soup canned, condensed	36	.043
Cucumbers raw	15	.042
Skim milk	36	.042
Cottage cheese	106	.040
Orange juice	45	.040
Red raspberries canned, fruit and liquid	35	.040
Whey	26	.040
White bread made with 1% - 2% nonfat dry milk	269	.040
Whole milk	502	.040
Red raspberries frozen, sweetened	98	.038
Oysters canned, solids and liquids	76	.037
Red currants	50	.037
Buttermilk	36	.036
Asparagus (white), canned	18	.035
Baking chocolate	505	.035
Orange juice canned, sweetened	52	.035
Orange juice canned, unsweetened	48	.035
Grapefruit raw	41	.034
White rice precooked	109	.034
Light cream	211	.033
Cherries (sweet), raw	70	.032
Coconut water	22	.032
Tangerine juice canned, sweetened	50	.032
Apple juice canned or bottled	47	.030
Apples freshly harvested, with skin, raw	58	.030
Rhubarb raw	16	.030
Light whipping cream	300	.029
Orange juice frozen, concentrate, unsweetened	45	.028
Plums canned	33	.027
Rhubarb frozen, cooked, sugar added	143	.025
Peaches raw	38	.024
Cranberry sauce canned	146	.022
Grape juice frozen, sweetened	53	.021
Grapefruit canned in water, with or without artificial sweetener, fruit and liquid	30	.020
Honey	304	.020
Peaches canned	31	.019
Pretzels	390	.019
Nectarines raw	64	.017
Pears raw	61	.017

FOOD ITEM	CALS.	UNITS
Marmalade (lemon or orange)	720	.016
Grapefruit juice frozen, concentrate, unsweetened	41	.014
Olives ripe	129	.014
Pears canned	32	.014
Gooseberries raw	39	.012
Grapefruit juice canned, sweetened	53	.011
Potato flour	351	.008
Butter	716	.003

Vitamin B$_{12}$

FOOD ITEM	CALS.	UNITS
Cod canned	85	.0150
Liverwurst	307	.0139
Smoked mackerel (Atlantic), salted	N.A.	.0120
Cod dehydrated, lightly salted	375	.0100
Crab cooked or canned	101	.0100
Sardines (Atlantic), canned in oil, solids and liquid	311	.0100
Herring (Atlantic), canned	208	.0080
Mackerel (Atlantic), canned	183	.0077
Smoked salmon salted	176	.0070
Skim milk dry, regular	363	.0032
Whole milk dry	502	.0023
Buttermilk powder	387	.0020
Whey dried	349	.0020
Swiss cheese	370	.0018
Herring kippered, canned	211	.0015
Blue cheese	368	.0014
Camembert cheese	299	.0013
Swiss cheese pasteurized, processed	355	.0012
Smoked haddock	103	.0011
Brick cheese	370	.0010
Cheddar cheese unprocessed	398	.0010
Limburger cheese	345	.0010
American cheese food pastuerized, processed	323	.0006
Roquefort cheese	368	.0006
Condensed milk canned, sweetened	321	.0004
Skim milk	36	.0004
Whole milk	65	.0004

FOOD ITEM	CALS.	UNITS
Buttermilk fluid	36	.0002
Cream cheese	106	.0002
Light cream	211	.0002
Light whipping cream	300	.0002
Evaporated milk canned, unsweetened	137	.0001
Heavy whipping cream	352	.0001
Goat's milk	67	.0000

Vitamin C

FOOD ITEM	CALS.	UNITS
Red chili peppers (hot), pods, raw	93	369.00
Green chili peppers (hot), pods only, canned, solids and liquid	25	359.00
Green chili peppers (hot), pods, raw	37	235.00
Lemon juice frozen concentrate, unsweetened	116	230.00
Red peppers (sweet), raw	31	204.00
Black currants (European), raw	54	200.00
Parsley	44	172.00
Collards leaves only, raw	45	152.00
Mustard spinach (tendergreen), raw	22	130.00
Green peppers (sweet), raw	22	128.00
Kale leaves and stems, raw	38	125.00
Broccoli spears, raw	32	113.00
Mustard greens raw	31	97.00
Green peppers (sweet), boiled and drained	18	96.00
Pimientos canned, solids and liquid	27	95.00
Collards leaves and stems, raw	40	92.00
Broccoli spears, boiled and drained	26	90.00
Brussels sprouts boiled and drained	36	87.00
Brussels sprouts frozen, boiled and drained	33	81.00
Horseradish raw	87	81.00
Watercress with leaves and stems, raw	19	79.00
Cauliflower raw	27	78.00
Lemons with peel, raw	20	77.00
Collards leaves, boiled and drained	33	76.00
Broccoli spears, frozen, boiled and drained	26	73.00
Oranges (California Valencias), with peel, raw	40	71.00
Garden cress raw	32	69.00
Turnip greens leaves and stems, boiled and drained	20	69.00

FOOD ITEM	CALS.	UNITS
Green chili peppers (hot), pods without seeds, canned, solids and liquid	25	68.00
Green chili peppers (hot), canned in chili sauce	20	68.00
Persimmons (native), raw	127	66.00
Mustard spinach (tendergreen), boiled and drained	16	65.00
Kale leaves and stems, boiled and drained	28	62.00
Orange juice (from California navels), fresh	48	61.00
Oranges (California navels), raw	51	61.00
Red cabbage raw	31	61.00
Strawberries raw	37	59.00
Broccoli chopped, frozen, boiled and drained	26	57.00
Lemons peeled, raw	27	53.00
Rice cereal with casein	382	53.00
Collards leaves, boiled and drained	31	51.00
Orange juice (from Florida oranges), raw	40	51.00
Spinach raw	26	51.00
Orange juice fresh, commercial	45	50.00
Orange juice (from Temple oranges), fresh	54	50.00
Oranges peeled, raw	49	50.00
Orange juice (from California Valencia oranges), fresh	47	49.00
Oranges (California Valencias), peeled, raw	51	49.00
Tomato paste canned	82	49.00
Mustard greens boiled and drained	23	48.00
Cabbage raw	24	47.00
Collards leaves and stems, boiled and drained	29	46.00
Lemon juice fresh	25	46.00
Orange juice (from Florida oranges), commercial	43	45.00
Orange juice frozen concentrate, unsweetened	45	45.00
Lemon juice frozen, unsweetened	22	44.00
Orange juice dehydrated (crystals), prepared with water	46	44.00
Kohlrabi thickened bulb-like stems, boiled and drained	24	43.00
Rutabagas raw	46	43.00
Lemon juice canned or bottled, unsweetened	23	42.00
Lichees raw	64	42.00
Cauliflower frozen, boiled and drained	18	41.00
Grapefruit juice and orange juice blend, frozen concentrate, unsweetened	44	41.00
Red currants raw	50	41.00
White currants raw	50	41.00
Green peppers stuffed with beef and bread crumbs	170	40.00

FOOD ITEM	CALS.	UNITS
Orange juice canned, unsweetened	48	40.00
Orange juice canned, sweetened	52	40.00
Grapefruit juice frozen concentrate, unsweetened	41	39.00
Grapefruit juice	38	38.00
Kale frozen, boiled and drained	31	38.00
Calf liver fried	261	37.00
Guavas (strawberry), whole, raw	65	37.00
Limes raw	28	37.00
Elderberries raw	72	36.00
Kumquats raw	65	36.00
Turnips raw	30	36.00
Dandelion greens raw	45	35.00
Mangoes raw	66	35.00
Garden cress boiled and drained	23	34.00
Grapefruit juice canned, unsweetened	41	34.00
Grapefruit juice and orange juice blend, canned, unsweetened	43	34.00
Grapefruit juice and orange juice blend, canned, sweetened	50	34.00
Cabbage shredded, boiled and drained	20	33.00
Cantaloupe	30	33.00
Collards frozen, boiled and drained	30	33.00
Gooseberries raw	39	33.00
Grapefruit juice frozen concentrate, sweetened	47	33.00
Tomato puree canned, regular or low sodium	39	33.00
Chard (Swiss), raw	25	32.00
Lime juice fresh	26	32.00
Radishes (Oriental, including daikon and Chinese), raw	19	32.00
Swamp cabbage raw	29	32.00
Fennel leaves, raw	28	31.00
Grapefruit juice canned, sweetened	53	31.00
Tangerine juice fresh	43	31.00
Tangerines raw	46	31.00
Beet greens raw	24	30.00
Grapefruit canned in water, with or without artificial sweetener, fruit and liquid	30	30.00
Grapefruit canned in syrup, fruit and liquid	70	30.00
New Zealand spinach raw	19	30.00
Red chili peppers (hot), canned in chili sauce	21	30.00
Spinach boiled and drained	23	28.00
Beef liver fried	229	27.00

FOOD ITEM	CALS.	UNITS
Tangelo juice	41	27.00
Tangerine juice frozen concentrate, unsweetened	46	27.00
Asparagus spears, cooked	26	26.00
Asparagus spears, boiled and drained	20	26.00
Radishes raw	17	26.00
Rutabagas boiled and drained	35	26.00
Chinese cabbage raw	14	25.00
Purslane leaves and stems, raw	21	25.00
Red raspberries raw	57	25.00
Loganberries raw	62	24.00
Tomatoes ripe, boiled	26	24.00
Asparagus cuts and tips, frozen, boiled and drained	22	23.00
Honeydew melon	33	23.00
Sweet potatoes firm fleshed, raw	102	23.00
Tomatoes ripe, raw	22	23.00
Chicory greens raw	20	22.00
Prickly pears raw	42	22.00
Sweet potatoes with skin, baked	141	22.00
Tangerine juice canned, unsweetened	43	22.00
Tangerine juice canned, sweetened	50	22.00
Turnips boiled and drained	23	22.00
French fried potatoes	274	21.00
French fried potatoes frozen	220	21.00
Lime juice canned or bottled, unsweetened	26	21.00
Peas edible, podded, raw	53	21.00
Red raspberries frozen, sweetened	98	21.00
Baked potatoes with skin	93	20.00
Green peas boiled and drained	71	20.00
Green tomatoes raw	24	20.00
Mustard greens frozen, boiled and drained	20	20.00
Okra boiled and drained	29	20.00
Strawberries canned in water, with or without artificial sweetener, fruit and liquid	22	20.00
Yellow snap beans raw	27	20.00
Chayote raw	28	19.00
Green snap beans raw	32	19.00
Mung bean sprouts raw	35	19.00
Potatoes fried	268	19.00
Spinach chopped frozen, boiled and drained	23	19.00
Summer squash (zucchinni and cocozelle), raw	17	19.00

FOOD ITEM	CALS.	UNITS
Turnip greens leaves and stems, canned, solids and liquid	18	19.00
Turnip greens leaves and stems, frozen, boiled and drained	23	19.00
Black raspberries raw	73	18.00
Cranberry-orange relish uncooked	178	18.00
Dandelion greens boiled and drained	33	18.00
Dried peached cooked	262	18.00
Lettuce (cos and romaine), raw	18	18.00
Lobster salad	110	18.00
Sauerkraut juice canned	10	18.00
Cowpeas (including black-eye peas), boiled and drained	108	17.00
Cowpeas (including black-eye peas), boiled and drained	34	17.00
Leeks bulb and lower leaf, raw	52	17.00
Lima beans boiled and drained	111	17.00
Lima beans frozen, boiled and drained	99	17.00
Pineapple raw	52	17.00
Sweet potatoes with skin, boiled	114	17.00
Tomatoes ripe, canned, regular, solids and liquid	21	17.00
Chard (Swiss), boiled and drained	18	16.00
Grape drink canned	54	16.00
Grape juice frozen concentrate, sweetened	53	16.00
Orange and apricot drink canned	50	16.00
Parsnips raw	76	16.00
Pineapple and grapefruit drink canned	54	16.00
Pineapple and orange drink canned	54	16.00
Potato chips	568	16.00
Potatoes with skin, boiled	76	16.00
Swamp cabbage boiled and drained	21	16.00
Tomato juice canned or bottled, regular or low sodium	19	16.00
Tomato juice dehydrated, (crystals), prepared with water	20	16.00
Tomato juice cocktail canned or bottled	21	16.00
Asparagus spears, canned, regular, solids and liquids or drained solids	16	15.00
Asparagus spears, canned, regular, solids and liquid	18	15.00
Beet greens boiled and drained	18	15.00
Garlic cloves raw	137	15.00
Spanish rice homemade	87	15.00
Tomato catsup bottled	106	15.00
Avocados raw	167	14.00
Blueberries raw	62	14.00

FOOD ITEM	CALS.	UNITS
Dried peaches cooked without sugar, fruit and liquid	340	14.00
New Zealand spinach boiled and drained	13	14.00
Peas edible podded, boiled and drained	43	14.00
Plantains (baking bananas), raw	119	14.00
Sauerkraut canned, solids and liquid	18	14.00
Spinach canned, or low sodium, solids and liquid	21	14.00
Spinach canned, regular, solids and liquid	19	14.00
Casaba melon	27	13.00
Chop suey with meat, homemade	120	13.00
Green peas frozen, boiled and drained	68	13.00
Nectarines raw	64	13.00
Potatoes canned, solids and liquid	44	13.00
Soybean sprouts raw	46	13.00
Tomato juice canned, concentrate	20	13.00
Winter squash baked	63	13.00
Yellow snap beans boiled and drained	22	13.00
Baby lima beans frozen, boiled and drained	118	12.00
Dried apricots uncooked	260	12.00
Green snap beans boiled and drained	25	12.00
Loganberries canned in juice, fruit and liquid	54	12.00
Okra cuts and pods, frozen, boiled and drained	38	12.00
Purslane leaves and stems, boiled and drained	15	12.00
Red chili peppers (hot), pods, dried	321	12.00
Cucumbers without skin, raw	14	11.00
Gooseberries canned in water, with or without artificial sweetener, fruit and liquid	26	11.00
Persimmons (Japanese or kaki), raw	77	11.00
Potatoes scalloped and au gratin without cheese	104	11.00
Summer squash (yellow crookneck and straightneck), boiled and drained	15	11.00
Apricots raw	51	10.00
Bananas raw	85	10.00
Blackberries canned in fruit and liquid	54	10.00
Dried apples cooked sulfured	275	10.00
Endive (curry endive and escarole), raw	20	10.00
Gooseberries canned in heavy syrup, fruit and liquid	90	10.00
Green peas canned, regular, drained solids	18	10.00
Green peas canned, regular, solids and liquid	22	10.00
Mashed potatoes milk added	65	10.00
Onions raw	38	10.00

FOOD ITEM	CALS.	UNITS
Parsnips boiled and drained	66	10.00
Pineapple canned in juice, fruit and liquid	58	10.00
Potatoes scalloped and au gratin with cheese	145	10.00
Red beets raw	43	10.00
Red cherries (sour), raw	58	10.00
Red cherries (sweet), raw	70	10.00
Summer squash boiled and drained	14	10.00
Sweet potatoes candied	168	10.00
Wheat germ toasted	391	10.00
Black eyed peas frozen, boiled and drained	130	9.00
Black raspberries canned in water, with or without artificial sweetener, fruit and liquid	35	9.00
Celery (green and yellow varieties), raw	17	9.00
Corn on the cob (sweet, white and yellow), boiled and drained	91	9.00
Green peas (Alaska), canned, low sodium, solids and liquid	55	9.00
Green peas (sweet), canned, low sodium, solids and liquid	47	9.00
Green peas (Alaska), canned, regular, solids and liquid	66	9.00
Green peas (sweet), canned, regular, solids and liquid	57	9.00
Hash-browned potatoes	229	9.00
Pickles fresh	73	9.00
Pineapple juice canned, unsweetened	55	9.00
Pizza with sausage, homemade	234	9.00
Spaghetti with meatballs in tomato sauce, homemade	134	9.00
Squash (zucchini and cocozelle), boiled and drained	12	9.00
Vegetable juice cocktail canned	17	9.00
Artichokes (globe or French), boiled and drained	44	8.00
Carrots raw	42	8.00
Celeriac root, raw	40	8.00
Crabapples raw	68	8.00
Hash browned potatoes frozen, cooked	224	8.00
Lettuce (Boston and bibb), raw	14	8.00
Mixed vegetables (carrots, corn, peas, green snap beans, and lima beans), frozen, boiled and drained	64	8.00
Peas and carrots frozen, boiled and drained	53	8.00
Pizza homemade	236	8.00
Shad creole, cooked	152	8.00
Shallots bulbs, raw	72	8.00
Soybeans canned, solids and liquid	75	8.00
Summer squash (yellow crookneck), frozen, boiled and drained	21	8.00

FOOD ITEM	CALS.	UNITS
Sweet potatoes canned in syrup, solids and liquid	114	8.00
Sweet potatoes canned in liquid, soilds and liquid, unsweetened	46	8.00
Winter squash boiled, mashed	38	8.00
Banana powder	340	7.00
Beef and vegetable stew with lean beef, homemade	89	7.00
Blackberries canned in water, with or without artificial sweetner, fruit and liquid	40	7.00
Blackberries canned in extra-heavy syrup, fruit and liquid	110	7.00
Blackberries canned in light syrup, fruit and liquid	72	7.00
Blackberries canned in heavy syrup, fruit and liquid	91	7.00
Blueberries canned in water, with or without artificial sweetner, fruit and liquid	39	7.00
Boysenberries canned in water, with or without artificial sweetner, fruit and liquid	36	7.00
Corn sweet, white and yellow, boiled and drained	83	7.00
Corn on the cob sweet, frozen, boiled and drained	94	7.00
Dried pears uncooked	268	7.00
Lemonade frozen concentrate	44	7.00
Lima beans canned, regular or low sodium, solids and liquid	70	7.00
Lima beans canned, regular, solids and liquid	71	7.00
Onions boiled and drained	29	7.00
Peaches raw	38	7.00
Pickles (sour)	10	7.00
Pineapple all styles except crushed, canned in water, with or without artificial	39	7.00
Pineapple all styles, canned in syrup, fruit and liquid	74	7.00
Pineapple all styles, canned in light syrup, fruit and liquid	59	7.00
Skim milk dry, regular	363	7.00
Snap beans (french style), frozen, boiled and drained	26	7.00
Watermelon raw	26	7.00
Apricots canned in juice, fruit and liquid	54	6.00
Black raspberries canned in water, with or without artificial sweetner, fruit and liquid	51	6.00
Blueberries canned in syrup, fruit and liquid	101	6.00
Carrots boiled and drained	31	6.00
Celery (green and yellow varieties), boiled and drained	14	6.00
Marmalade (lemon or orange)	720	6.00
Mung bean sprouts boiled and drained	28	6.00

FOOD ITEM	CALS.	UNITS
Pickles (dill)	11	6.00
Pickles (sweet)	146	6.00
Pineapple canned in syrup, fruit and liquid	90	6.00
Plums (Japanese and hybrid), raw	48	6.00
Red beets boiled and drained	32	6.00
Rhubarb cooked, sugar added	141	6.00
Rhubarb frozen, cooked, sugar added	143	6.00
Succotash frozen, boiled and drained	93	6.00
Tomato soup canned, condensed, prepared with milk	69	6.00
Whole milk dry	502	6.00
Yellow snap beans cut, frozen, boiled and drained	27	6.00
Barbecue sauce	91	5.00
Chicken a la king homemade	191	5.00
Chicken chow mein without noodles, canned	38	5.00
Chicken noodle soup from mix, dry	383	5.00
Corn (sweet, yellow), regular, solids and liquid	83	5.00
Corn sweet, frozen, boiled and drained	79	5.00
Creamed corn sweet, white and yellow, canned, regular pack, solids and liquid	82	5.00
Green snap beans cut, frozen, boiled and drained	25	5.00
Mashed potatoes dehydrated, flakes without milk	93	5.00
Pumpkin canned	33	5.00
Red cherries (sour), canned in water, fruit and liquid	48	5.00
Red cherries (sour), canned in light syrup, fruit and liquid	74	5.00
Red cherries (sour), canned in heavy syrup, fruit and liquid	89	5.00
Red cherries (sour), canned in extra-heavy syrup, fruit and liquid	112	5.00
Spaghetti with cheese in tomato sauce, homemade	104	5.00
Tomato soup canned, condensed	36	5.00
Yellow snap beans canned, regular, solids and liquids	19	5.00
Apples freshly harvested, with skin, raw	58	4.00
Aprcots canned in extra-heavy syrup, fruit and liquid	101	4.00
Apricots canned in water, with or without artificial sweetener, fruit and liquid	38	4.00
Apricots canned in light syrup, fruit and liquid	66	4.00
Apricots canned in heavy syrup, fruit and liquid	86	4.00
Bamboo shoots raw	27	4.00
Chicken canned, boned	198	4.00
Chicken chow mein without noodles, homemade	102	4.00
Chinese water chestnuts raw	79	4.00

FOOD ITEM	CALS.	UNITS
Dried prunes	344	4.00
Fruit dessert with tapioca (baby food), commercial	84	4.00
Ginger root fresh	49	4.00
Grapes (American), raw	69	4.00
Grapes (European), raw	67	4.00
Green pea soup canned, condensed, prepared with milk	85	4.00
Jellies	273	4.00
Mashed potatoes frozen	93	4.00
Peaches canned in juice, fruit and liquid	45	4.00
Pears with skin, raw	61	4.00
Plums prune-type, raw	75	4.00
Pomegranate pulp, raw	63	4.00
Soybean sprouts boiled and drained	38	4.00
Spaghetti with cheese in tomato sauce, canned	76	4.00
Apricot nectar canned	57	3.00
Apricots cooked, without added sugar, fruit and liquid	85	3.00
Beef and vegetable stew canned	79	3.00
Blueberry pie piecrust made with unenriched flour	242	3.00
Cherries (sweet), canned in water, with or without artificial sweetner, fruit and liquid	48	3.00
Cherries (sweet), canned in extra-heavy syrup, fruit and liquid	100	3.00
Cherries (sweet), canned in light syrup, fruit and liquid	65	3.00
Cherries (sweet), canned in heavy syrup, fruit and liquid	81	3.00
Coconut meat fresh	346	3.00
Cowpeas (including black-eyed peas), canned, solids and liquid	70	3.00
Dried apricots cooked, no sugar added	85	3.00
Eggplant boiled and drained	19	3.00
Fruit pudding (baby food), commercial	96	3.00
Fruit salad canned in water, with or without artificial sweetener, fruit and liquid	35	3.00
Green pea soup canned, condensed	53	3.00
Mashed potatoes dehydrated, flakes without milk	93	3.00
Mushrooms raw	28	3.00
Peaches canned in water, with or without artificial sweetener, fruit and liquid	31	3.00
Peaches canned in extra-heavy syrup, fruit and liquid	97	3.00
Peaches canned in light syrup, fruit and liquid	58	3.00

FOOD ITEM	CALS.	UNITS
Peaches canned in heavy syrup, fruit and liquid	78	3.00
Red beets canned, regular, solids and liquid	34	3.00
Red beets canned, low sodium, solids and liquid	32	3.00
Thousand Island salad dressing commercial, low calorie	180	3.00
Thousand Island salad dressing commercial, regular	502	3.00
Apple butter	186	2.00
Apples freshly harvested, pared, raw	54	2.00
Applesauce canned, sweetened or artificially sweetened	91	2.00
Beef with vegetables (baby food), commercial	87	2.00
Blue cheese & Roquerfort salad dressing commercial, regular	502	2.00
Blue cheese and Roquefort cheese salad commercial, low calorie	76	2.00
Carrots canned, low sodium, solids and liquid	22	2.00
Carrots canned, regular	28	2.00
Cherry pies frozen	291	2.00
Chicken with vegetables (baby food), commercial	100	2.00
Chop suey with meat, canned	62	2.00
Coconut milk	252	2.00
Coconut water	22	2.00
Corn fritters	377	2.00
Corn pudding	104	2.00
Crab steamed	93	2.00
Cranberry sauce canned, sweetened, strained	146	2.00
Cranberry sauce homemade, unstrained	178	2.00
Dried peaches cooked, no sugar added	82	2.00
Dried pears cooked, no added sugar	126	2.00
Figs raw	80	2.00
Flounder baked	202	2.00
Fruit cocktail canned in water, with or without artificial sweetener, fruit and liquid	37	2.00
Fruit cocktail canned in extra-heavy syrup, fruit and liquid	92	2.00
Fruit cocktail canned in light syrup, fruit and liquid	60	2.00
Fruit cocktail canned in heavy syrup, fruit and liquid	76	2.00
Fruit salad canned in extra-heavy syrup, fruit and liquid	90	2.00
Fruit salad canned in light syrup, fruit and liquid	59	2.00
Fruit salad canned in heavy syrup, fruit and liquid	75	2.00
Jams and preserves	272	2.00

FOOD ITEM	CALS.	UNITS
Limeade frozen concentrate	41	2.00
Mushrooms canned, solids and liquid	17	2.00
Orange sherbet	134	2.00
Pears canned in juice, fruit and liquid	46	2.00
Pecans	601	2.00
Plums (purple), canned in extra-heavy syrup, fruit and liquid	102	2.00
Plums (purple), canned in light syrup, fruit and liquid	63	2.00
Plums (purple), canned in heavy syrup, fruit and liquid	83	2.00
Prune juice canned or bottled	77	2.00
Roe canned, solids and liquid	118	2.00
Soybeans canned, drained solids	75	2.00
Spaghetti with meatballs in tomato sauce, canned	103	2.00
Tomato vegetable soup with noodles from mix	27	2.00
Walnuts	651	2.00
White beans dry or canned, solids and liquid	120	2.00
Apple juice canned or bottled	47	1.00
Applesauce canned, unsweetened	41	1.00
Beef heart lean, braised	188	1.00
Blueberry muffins homemade from enriched flour	281	1.00
Bread pudding with raisins	187	1.00
Buttermilk cultured, made from skim milk	36	1.00
Chocolate milk made with skim, commercial	76	1.00
Chocolate milk made with whole milk, commercial	88	1.00
Coconut cream	337	1.00
Condensed milk canned, sweetened	321	1.00
Cornbread (Johnnycake), homemade from whole-ground de-germed enriched cornmeal	267	1.00
Custard pudding (baby food), commercial	100	1.00
Dried prunes cooked, without added sugar, fruit and liquid	119	1.00
Dried prunes cooked, with added sugar, fruit and liquid	172	1.00
Evaporated milk canned, unsweetened	137	1.00
Figs canned in water, with or without artificial sweetener, fruit and liquid	48	1.00
Frozen custard fat content 10%	193	1.00
Goat's milk	67	1.00
Half-and-half cream	134	1.00
Heavy whipping cream	352	1.00
Honey	304	1.00
Hot chocolate homemade	95	1.00
Hot cocoa homemade	97	1.00

FOOD ITEM	CALS.	UNITS
Ice cream fat content 10%	193	1.00
Ice milk	152	1.00
Light whipping cream	300	1.00
Light cream	211	1.00
Lime ice	78	1.00
Malted milk	104	1.00
Pears canned in water, with or without artificial sweetener, fruit and liquid	32	1.00
Pears canned in extra-heavy syrup, fruit and liquid	93	1.00
Pears canned in light syrup, fruit and liquid	61	1.00
Pears canned in heavy syrup, fruit and liquid	76	1.00
Raisins	289	1.00
Skim milk	36	1.00
Split pea soup canned, condensed	118	1.00
Tapioca cream pudding	134	1.00
Tartar sauce low calorie, commercial	224	1.00
Tartar sauce regular, commercial	531	1.00
Tuna salad	170	1.00
Vanilla pudding homemade	111	1.00
Whole milk	65	1.00
Yogurt made from partially skimmed milk	50	1.00
Yogurt made from whole milk	62	1.00
Almond meal partially defatted	408	.00
Almonds dried	598	.00
Animal crackers	429	.00
Apple pie commercial	256	.00
Apple tapioca commercial	117	.00
Applesauce baby food, commercial	72	.00
Assorted cookies commercial	480	.00
Baker's yeast compressed, dry (active)	86	.00
Beef noodle soup from mix	28	.00
Biscuits made with self-rising flour, enriched	372	.00
Biscuits from mix, enriched flour, prepared with milk	325	.00
Bran sugar and malt extract added, cereal	240	.00
Brewer's yeast debittered	283	.00
Brownies with nuts, commerical	419	.00
Brownies from mix	403	.00
Caramels plain or chocolate	399	.00
Chicken and noodles homemade	153	.00
Chicken noodle soup canned, condensed	53	.00

FOOD ITEM	CALS.	UNITS
Chicken noodle soup from mix	22	.00
Chocolate chip cookies commercial	471	.00
Chocolate pudding homemade	148	.00
Chocolate syrup	330	.00
Cookies plain, from mix, made with milk	490	.00
Cornbread (spoonbread) from mix	195	.00
Cornbread from mix, made with eggs and milk	233	.00
Cracked-wheat bread toasted	313	.00
Cream puffs with custard filling	233	.00
Creamed pollack	128	.00
Custard baked	115	.00
Danish pastry commercial	422	.00
Doughnuts cake type	391	.00
Dried apples cooked, sugar added	112	.00
Eclairs with custard filling and chocolate frosting, commercial	239	.00
Filberts (hazelnuts)	634	.00
Frankfurters and beans canned	144	.00
French or Vienna bread enriched or unenriched, toasted	338	.00
Frosting (white), uncooked, homemade	376	.00
Grape juice canned or bottled	66	.00
Green pea soup from mix	50	.00
Hard rolls enriched, commercial	312	.00
Ice cream cones	377	.00
Macaroni and cheese canned	215	.00
Milk chocolate plain	520	.00
Muffins (plain), homemade from enriched flour	294	.00
Muffins from mix, made with eggs and milk	324	.00
Oyster stew prepared with milk, commercial	84	.00
Pancakes homemade from enriched or unenriched flour	231	.00
Pancakes from mix, made with milk and eggs	225	.00
Peach nectar canned	48	.00
Pear nectar canned	52	.00
Pinenuts	635	.00
Popovers homemade from enriched flour	224	.00
Pudding from mix, made with milk, cooked,	124	.00
Raisins cooked, sugar added, fruit and liquid	213	.00
Rice pudding with raisins, commercial	146	.00
Rolls from mix	299	.00
Rolls and buns homemade	339	.00
Salad dressing homemade, cooked	164	.00

FOOD ITEM	CALS.	UNITS
Soybeans	130	.00
Sweet rolls commercial	316	.00
Torula yeast	277	.00
Waffles homemade	279	.00
Whitefish (lake), stuffed, baked	215	.00

Vitamin E

FOOD ITEM	CALS.	UNITS
Rye oil	N.A.	192.11
Rice germ oil	N.A.	171.87
Barley oil	N.A.	150.29
Soybean oil crude	N.A.	111.00
Cottonseed oil crude	N.A.	105.00
Soybean oil hydrogenated	N.A.	103.00
Soybean shortening	N.A.	98.28
Soybean oil refined	N.A.	94.00
Sesame oil crude	N.A.	74.60
Margarine (from corn, soybean, and cottonseed oils), stick	N.A.	68.18
Sunflower seed oil crude	N.A.	68.00
Cottonseed oil refined	N.A.	65.00
Sunflower seed oil refined	N.A.	64.00
Grapeseed oil	N.A.	62.00
Palm oil crude	N.A.	59.00
Mayonnaise	N.A.	58.00
Sunflower seed kernels dried	560	52.18
Safflower seed oil crude	N.A.	51.63
Apricot kernel oil	N.A.	50.48
Margarine (from safflower and soybean oils)	N.A.	48.80
Corn oil partially hydrogenated, commercial	N.A.	47.45
Margarine (from corn oil), tub	N.A.	45.00
Oat oil	N.A.	40.89
Almond oil	N.A.	40.09
Palm oil nonhydrogenated	N.A.	38.40
Peanut oil crude	N.A.	38.00
Safflower seed oil refined	N.A.	38.00
Palm oil refined	N.A.	35.53
Almond meal partially defatted	408	33.40
Sesame oil refined	N.A.	29.01
Wheat germ raw, commercially milled	363	27.56

FOOD ITEM	CALS.	UNITS
Peanut oil refined	N.A.	25.00
Brazil nut oil	N.A.	24.22
Pecan oil	N.A.	23.34
Safflower seed oil hydrogenated	N.A.	23.20
Peanut oil hydrogenated	N.A.	22.89
Sesame seeds raw	563	22.70
Cod liver oil (Atlantic)	N.A.	21.96
Palm kernel oil crude	N.A.	21.06
Pecans shelled, raw	687	19.86
Walnuts (English), shelled, raw	651	19.62
Haddock liver canned	N.A.	17.50
Avocado oil	N.A.	17.23
Peanuts shelled, raw	564	16.37
Peach kernel oil	N.A.	15.00
Rice bran	N.A.	14.92
Olive oil	N.A.	13.00
Peanuts oil roasted	582	11.60
Margarine (from sunflower and palm oils), stick	N.A.	11.10
Palm oil hydrogenated	N.A.	9.70
Paprika seeds raw	N.A.	9.60
Buckwheat flour	335	7.91
Potato chips	568	7.31
Rye flour dark	327	6.68
Milk chocolate	520	6.30
Palm kernel oil refined	N.A.	6.20
Corn	N.A.	5.81
Almond roasted	627	5.65
Cashew nuts	561	4.20
Whole wheat cereal cooked	45	4.05
Rye whole grain	334	3.80
Radishes raw	17	3.76
Coconut oil refined	N.A.	3.58
Egg yolks fresh	348	3.12
Spinach raw	26	3.00
Butter oil	N.A.	2.83
Wheat crackers	403	2.81
Peas fresh	53	2.71
Peas (Alaska), canned	66	2.63
Parsley raw	44	2.53
Butter	716	2.40

FOOD ITEM	CALS.	UNITS
Oatmeal	55	2.31
Turnip greens leaves and stems, raw	28	2.30
Shredded wheat (cereal)	354	2.15
Wheat flakes (cereal)	354	2.11
Cabbage raw	24	1.67
Beef liver broiled	N.A.	1.62
Corn flour	368	1.47
Corn grits cooked	51	1.38
Haddock broiled	165	1.20
White bread made with 1% - 2% nonfat dry milk	269	1.19
Whole dry milk	502	1.08
Farina enriched, regular, cooked	42	.94
Rye flour light	357	.93
Whole wheat bread	243	.90
Brussels sprouts cooked	36	.85
Celery raw	17	.73
Tomato juice canned	19	.71
Liverwurst	307	.69
Salami	450	.68
Apples whole, raw	58	.66
Broccoli fresh	32	.64
Corn sweet	N.A.	.62
Pork chops pan fried	N.A.	.60
Bacon cured, broiled or fried, drained	611	.59
Knockwurst	278	.57
Chicken	N.A.	.55
Steak broiled	N.A.	.55
Ham fried	N.A.	.52
Carrots raw	42	.51
Bologna	304	.49
Tomatoes ripe, raw	22	.49
Carrots boiled and drained	31	.46
Cornmeal cooked	50	.42
Bananas raw	85	.32
Lamb chops broiled	359	.32
Pork sausage fried	476	.32
Cucumbers whole, raw	15	.31
Onions raw	38	.31
Mushrooms raw	28	.29
Grapefruit raw	41	.26

FOOD ITEM	CALS.	UNITS
Strawberries raw	37	.26
Green beans frozen, boiled and drained	25	.25
Oranges raw	49	.24
Orange juice fresh, commercial	45	.20
Evaporated milk canned, unsweetened	137	.18
Grapefruit juice canned, unsweetened	41	.18
Chinese cabbage raw	14	.13
Condensed milk reconstituted	321	.11
Green beans raw	32	.11
Pineapple fresh	52	.10
Cauliflower boiled and drained	22	.09
Whole milk	65	.09
Whole buttermilk	36	.07
Baked potatoes	93	.06
Boiled potatoes white	76	.06

Minerals

8

Minerals are found, in the form of inorganic compounds, in minute amounts in all our foods. They make up only 4 percent of our total body weight — and half of that is calcium, which forms the greater part of the hard tissue of our bones and teeth. Yet minerals are essential to the functioning of every single cell in our bodies.

The major minerals, such as calcium, phosphorus, magnesium, potassium, sodium, iron, and zinc, are used by our bodies in larger quantities than the trace elements. The amount of iodine, manganese, copper, fluoride, chromium, selenium, cobalt, vanadium, or molybdenum required by the body (when it is known) may often be measured in micrograms — millionths of a gram. But if these trace minerals are missing from our food, they can disrupt the functioning of our metabolism and prevent utilization of the major minerals and of other nutrients.

Why We Need Minerals

Each mineral plays a unique and often multifaceted role in the body. Taken together, minerals enable the hundreds of biochemical reactions necessary for metabolic processes to take place. In some cases, the mechanisms of these reactions have been deeply studied and are well understood. In others, we are just beginning to understand their importance.

Of course, minerals make up the hard structure of bones, teeth, nails, and hair. Calcium and phosphorus are most important in the bones and teeth; fluoride is concentrated on the surface of the teeth to make them hard and relatively impervious to infection. Zinc and sulfur, too, are present in the hair and nails.

Minerals are also important in the structure and production of the proteins of which other tissues are composed. Calcium and sulfur are present in all proteins; iron, part of the hemoglobin in each red blood cell, helps transport oxygen to the cells. Zinc is intrinsic to the structure of RNA, the chemical which encodes the arrangement of each protein produced by the cells. The glands cannot produce the hormones which regulate the body's metabolism without minerals. For example, insulin production depends upon the presence of zinc and sulfur.

Your body could not use or store energy without minerals. Phosphorus and the trace element chromium are crucial in the conversion of glucose to energy. (This is why hypoglycemics and diabetics are often helped by supplemental chromium in the form of glucose tolerance factor.) You couldn't move a muscle without minerals. The sensitivity of your nerves, and the ability of your muscles to contract, both depend upon the presence of the minerals calcium, sodium, magnesium, and potassium. (Athletes should make sure to get enough potassium after heavy exertion.)

The flow of the fluids in your body through the system and in and out of the cells is regulated by minerals. Potassium is usually found inside the cells and sodium outside them, but the permeability of the cell membranes and capillaries to these and other ionized minerals varies constantly. The acid/base balance of these fluids, too, is regulated by minerals.

Healing could not take place without minerals. The healing properties of zinc have long been known — generations of mothers have applied zinc ointment to children's cuts and babies' rashes. But few people are aware of the importance of calcium and sulfur in enabling the blood to coagulate over a wound.

Minerals are needed both for proper digestion of food, and for excretion of wastes. Minute amounts of cobalt must be present for vitamin B_{12} to be synthesized by the bacteria in the intestine, and peristalsis, the muscle action that pushes foods through the gastrointestinal tract, depends on the nerves functioning well (potassium and calcium), for two examples.

These simple functions are only the beginning of the story of the body's use of minerals. We are learning more every day about how minerals interact in the body with each other and with the enzymes that stimulate metabolic activities, and about how to balance our mineral intake.

Dietary Sources of Minerals

It is very difficult to obtain the correct amounts of all the nutrients you need, in the proper balance, if you consume the typical American meat-and-potatoes-and-junk-foods diet. For one thing, some minerals are discarded in refining, milling, and processing, while others — notoriously sodium — are added to foods in disproportionately large amounts, imbalancing the body's chemistry. For another, our soil is, in certain parts of the country, deficient in certain trace minerals. This can lead to mild, subclinical deficiencies, or to serious problems. In the goiter belt of the United States, not enough iodine is absorbed through the soil into our foods. Iodine is needed for the functioning of the thyroid gland: when not enough iodine is present for the thyroid to produce its hormones, then the gland swells up in an attempt to circumvent the lack. This swelling is called a goiter. Iodine is added to salt, a practice that has been effective in preventing goiter. (People on low-salt diets can obtain the necessary iodine from kelp.)

Much of the soil in the United States is depleted of various minerals and other nutrients because of the use of chemical fertilizers which, unlike organic fertilizer, replenish certain minerals at the expense of others. Depletion of selenium presents a more ominous threat than depletion of iodine: it has been demonstrated that those areas of the country lacking in selenium coincide with those that show increased rates of cancer, particularly breast cancer.

It is therefore important to avoid refined and processed foods, and to consume a diet high in grains, legumes, seeds, green and leafy vegetables, yellow vegetables, and fruits. (Organ meats, fish, and meat also provide certain minerals.) In addition, because of the unevenness of the distribution of the necessary minerals in our soil, it is a good idea for everyone to obtain hair and blood analyses to determine whether they have too little — or too much — of any particular minerals in their bodies.

Mineral Toxicity

Most minerals, being water-soluble, are excreted and must be replenished regularly. However, unlike the water-soluble vitamins, certain minerals are not simply excreted when the body is oversupplied. Thus, they can accumulate, with toxic effects. Lead is the best-known toxic mineral. Lead poisoning afflicts not only poor children who ingest lead-based wall paint; we all breathe lead from car exhaust and industrial sources every day. Sixty percent of Americans live in highly polluted areas. Other heavy metals that can be toxic include silver, gold, and cadmium. Copper and aluminum (while normally found in the body in traces), along with other minerals, can have toxic effects in too large quantities.

In fact, an imbalanced proportion of any mineral can be harmful, causing serious biological consequences. For example, many vegetarians take zinc supplements, since zinc is not as easily absorbable from vegetables as from meats. This helps maintain healthy hair, skin, and prostate glands (preventing the precancerous prostate condition that is almost universal among American men over the age of forty). However, without a corresponding increase in the amount of manganese, to take zinc supplements is to risk causing a relative manganese deficiency. This disruption of the body's chemistry due to the interaction of two simple nutrients can result in increased susceptibility to allergies, cerebral reactions, insomnia, or lack of energy — all of which can be alleviated when the two minerals are brought back into balance by the addition of manganese to the diet.

Another example of a common mineral imbalance is overabundance of copper. Two milligrams (mg.) of copper are frequently added to multivitamin and mineral supplements, based on studies done in the 1930s on copper deficiency in laboratory animals. However, in the 1930s most water pipes were made of galvanized lead. Today, copper is more common. As a result, many people obtain between 5 and 10 mg. of copper in their water and food. Now, excessive supplemental copper can result in imbalances in the metabolism of both chromium and molybdenum. Since chromium is involved in glucose metabolism, this can cause blood sugar problems (exacerbated by the amount of refined carbohydrates in the typical American diet). Since molybdenum helps mobilize iron from the liver, it can result in anemia (as can excess zinc or manganese).

For many years, these complex interactions were not understood, and even today, only a few clinicians are using the insights gained in the laboratory to improve their patients' mental and physical health. No one knows how many people being treated with tranquilizers, antidepressants, and other psychoactive drugs for anxiety, depression, or neurotic or psychotic behavior are the victims of environmentally caused mineral imbalances. We do know, however, that many people react to a copper/zinc, imbalance for example — too much copper causing a zinc deficiency — with depression; and that old copper pipes leech the mineral into the water. We also know that there were over three billion tablets of Valium — the most common psychoactive drug — purchased last year. How much of this might have been avoided if the recipients had instead obtained a simple and inexpensive hair mineral analysis?

The study of the interactions of the minerals in the body with each other, and with the enzyme mechanisms, is leading to new advances in the field of preventive medicine. Lead poisoning, for one example, is now known to destroy certain enzyme systems which are necessary to carry magnesium into the heart to help it beat regularly and to prevent arterial spasms. Lead is easy to detect in the hair and blood. Once detected, toxic levels of lead, as well as other minerals, may be safely eliminated through dietary changes or through a procedure for removing minerals from the blood, known as chelation, which can be done in a doctor's office.

In the future, it is to be hoped that the hair and blood tests for mineral toxicity and imbalances will be standardized, and offered by every public health facility, as tests for venereal disease and tuberculosis are today.

In the meantime, individuals must take the initiative themselves to obtain these tests, and to regulate their diets on the basis of their own biochemical individuality. A list of physicians, chiropractors, and nutritionists who approach prevention and treatment with an awareness of the importance of nutrition is available from Gary Gordon of the American Academy of Medical Preventics, Beverly Hills, California.

The unit value for the minerals listed is given in milligrams. Any food having less than .1 milligram of iron per 100-gram serving is considered to have a trace iron content and is listed as having .00 for its unit value; any food having less than 2 milligrams of potassium per 100-gram serving is considered to have a trace potassium content and is listed as having 0 for its unit value; and, any food having less than 1 milligram of calcium or phosphorous per 100-gram serving is considered to have a trace content for that mineral and as having a 0 for its unit value.

Where the symbol N. A. appears in the calorie column, the information was not available.

All figures are based on an edible portion equaling 100 grams, or approximately 3 ounces. In the case of some of the listed foods, one would not consume 100 grams in one serving. Calculations should be adjusted accordingly.

Calcium

FOOD ITEM	CALS.	UNITS
Baking powder	129	1932
Skim milk dry, regular	363	1308
Sesame seeds dry, whole	563	1160
Parmesan cheese	393	1140
Swiss cheese (domestic), unprocessed	370	925
Whole milk dry	502	909
Rice cereal (baby food), commercial	371	858
Oatmeal (baby food), commercial	375	757
Cheddar cheese	398	750
American cheese pasteurized, processed	370	697
Blackstrap molasses cane	213	684
Whey dried	349	646
Sardines (Pacific), canned in tomato sauce, solids and liquid	197	449
Almond meal partially defatted	408	424
Torula yeast	277	424

FOOD ITEM	CALS.	UNITS
Smelt (Atlantic, jack, and bay), canned, solids and liquid	200	358
Sardines (Atlantic), canned in oil, solids and liquid	311	354
Carob flour	180	352
Sunflower seed flour partially defatted	339	348
Cheese crackers	479	336
Blue cheese and Roquefort cheese unprocessed	368	315
Cottonseed flour	356	283
Milk chocolate plain	520	278
Caviar (sturgeon, granular	262	276
Soybean milk powder	429	275
Soybean flour defatted	326	265
Wheat flour self rising, enriched	352	265
Condensed milk sweetened	321	262
Salt	0	253
Evaporated milk canned, unsweetened	137	252
Turnip greens leaves and stems, raw	28	246
Almonds roasted and salted	627	235
Almonds dried	598	234
Pizza homemade	236	221
Buckwheat pancakes and waffles from mix, made with eggs, and milk	200	220
Pancakes from mix, with enriched or unenriched flour	225	215
Brewer's yeast	283	210
Filberts (hazelnuts)	634	209
Collards leaves and stems, raw	40	203
Parsley raw	44	203
Dandelion greens raw	45	187
Brazil nuts	654	186
Turnip greens leaves and stems, boiled and drained	20	184
Mustard greens raw	31	183
Kale leaves and stems, raw	38	179
Collards frozen, boiled and drained	30	176
Pickled anchovies with or without added oil, lightly salted	176	168
Ice cream cones	377	156
Ice milk	152	156
Pizza frozen	245	156
Collards leaves and stems, boiled and drained	29	152
Oysters fried	239	152
Watercress leaves and stems, raw	19	151
Caramels plain or chocolate	399	148

FOOD ITEM	CALS.	UNITS
Frozen custard fat content 10%	193	146
Ice cream fat content 10%	193	146
Maple sugar	348	143
Bran muffins homemade from enriched flour	261	142
Dandelion greens boiled and drained	33	140
Mustard greens boiled and drained	23	138
Kale leaves and stems, boiled and drained	28	134
Pistachio nuts	594	131
Goat's milk	67	129
Tofu (soybean curd)	72	128
Dried figs uncooked	274	126
Brown mustard prepared	91	124
Bread crumbs dry, grated, commercial	392	122
Baking powder biscuits homemade from enriched flour	369	121
Buttermilk cultured	36	121
Kale frozen, boiled and drained	31	121
Skim milk	36	121
Cornbread homemade from whole-ground cornmeal	207	120
Sunflower seed kernels dried	560	120
Yogurt made from partially skimmed milk	50	120
Beet greens raw	24	119
Wheat bran crude, commercially milled	213	119
Turnip greens leaves and stems, frozen, boiled and drained	65	118
Whole milk	62	118
Vanilla puddding homemade	111	117
Scallops (bay and sea), steamed	112	115
Spinach chopped, frozen, boiled and drained	23	113
Corn muffins homemade from whole-ground cornmeal	288	112
Custard baked, commercial	115	112
Yogurt made from whole milk	62	111
Sesame seeds dry, hulled	582	110
Bread pudding with raisins	187	109
Half-and-half cream	134	108
Whole wheat rolls and buns commercial	257	106
Corn muffins homemade from enriched, degermed cornmeal	314	105
Hot chocolate homemade	95	104
Maple syrup	252	104
Muffins plain, homemade from enriched or unenriched flour	294	104
Peanut flour defatted	371	104
Broccoli spears, raw	32	103

FOOD ITEM	CALS.	UNITS
Natto (fermented soybean product)	167	103
Purslane leaves and stems, raw	21	103
Pudding from mix, prepared with milk, cooked	124	102
Pancakes homemade from enriched or unenriched flour	231	101
Fennel leaves, raw	28	100
Turnip greens leaves and stems, canned, solids and liquid	18	100
Beet greens boiled and drained	18	99
Walnuts	651	99
White cake with chocolate frosting, made with eggs and water	351	99
Whole wheat bread made with 2% nonfat dry milk	243	99
Rice pudding with raisins, commercial	146	98
Chocolate pudding homemade	148	96
Popovers baked	224	96
Rhubarb raw	16	96
Cottage cheese creamed	106	94
Okra cuts and pods, frozen, boiled and drained	38	94
Spinach raw	26	94
Spinach boiled and drained	23	94
Okra boiled and drained	36	92
Cottage cheese uncreamed	86	90
Gingerbread from mix, made with water	276	90
Broccoli spears, boiled and drained	26	88
Chard (Swiss), raw	25	88
Cracked wheat bread	263	88
Chicory greens raw	20	86
Brown sugar (beet or cane)	373	85
Cornbread from mix, made with eggs and milk	233	85
Light whipping cream	300	85
Spinach canned, low sodium, solids and liquid	21	85
Spinach canned, regular, solids and liquid	19	85
Sweet rolls commercial	316	85
Blueberry muffins homemade	281	84
Pumpernickel bread	246	84
Yellow mustard prepared	75	84
Lemon candied	314	83
Soy sauce	68	82
Blue and Roquefort cheese salad dressing commercial, regular	504	81
Endive (curly endive and escarole), raw	20	81
Garden cress raw	32	81

FOOD ITEM	CALS.	UNITS
Eclairs with chocolate frosting and custard filling, commercial	239	80
Eggs scrambled	173	80
Omelets	173	80
Baking chocolate	505	78
Bitter chocolate	505	78
Rhubarb frozen, cooked, sugar added	143	78
Rice bran	276	76
Heavy whipping cream	352	75
Rye bread (American), commercial	243	75
Safflower seed meal partially defatted	355	75
Rolls and buns plain, commercial	298	74
Chard (Swiss), boiled and drained	18	73
Pecans	687	73
Soybeans dry, cooked	130	73
Swamp cabbage raw	29	73
Dark fruitcake homemade	379	72
French fried shrimp	225	72
Peanuts with skin, roasted	582	72
Wheat germ raw, commercially milled	363	72
Bran sugar and malt extract added, cereal	270	70
Chocolate cake with chocolate frosting, homemade	369	70
White bread made with 1% - 2% nonfat dry milk	269	70
Chives raw	28	69
Biscuits from mix	325	68
Gingerbread homemade from enriched flour	317	68
Lettuce (cos and romaine), raw	18	68
Light fruitcake homemade	389	68
Miso (fermented soybean product)	171	68
Dried apricots uncooked	260	67
Tomato soup canned, condensed, prepared with milk	69	67
Corn pudding commercial	104	66
Rutabagas raw	46	66
Lobster (northern), canned or cooked	95	65
Blue cheese & Roquefort salad dressing commercial, low calorie	76	64
Cake and cupcake (plain), homemade	364	64
Corn fritters commercial	377	64
Custard pudding (baby food), commercial	100	64
Kumquats raw	65	63
Peanut butter fat and salt added	581	63

FOOD ITEM	CALS.	UNITS
White cake homemade	375	63
Cream cheese natural	374	62
Peas edible-podded, raw	53	62
Raisins natural	289	62
Garden cress boiled and drained	23	61
Green olives pickled, canned or bottled	116	61
Horseradish prepared	38	61
Black currants (European), raw	54	60
Cane syrup	263	60
Eggs fried	216	60
Dates (domestic), dry	274	59
Peanuts without skins, raw	568	59
Rutabagas boiled and drained	35	59
New Zealand spinach raw	19	58
Green snap beans raw	32	56
Peas edible-podded, boiled and drained	43	56
Rolls from mix	299	56
Yellow snap beans raw	27	56
Clams canned, solids and liquid	52	55
Eggs poached	163	55
Soybeans canned, solids and liquid	75	55
Swamp cabbage boiled and drained	21	55
Eggs hard-boiled	163	54
Rye wafers whole grain	344	53
Chestnuts dried	377	52
Leeks bulb and lower leaves, raw	52	52
Artichokes (globe or French), boiled and drained	44	51
Dried prunes "softenized"	255	51
Pumpkin pie commercial	211	51
Danish pastry commercial	422	50
Parsnips raw	76	50
Spaghetti with meatballs in tomato sauce, homemade	134	50
Yellow snap beans boiled and drained	22	50
Cabbage raw	24	49
Dried peaches uncooked	262	48
Macadamia nuts	691	48
Malt extract dried	367	48
New Zealand spinach boiled and drained	13	48
Soybean sprouts raw	46	48
Hard rolls enriched, commercial	312	47

FOOD ITEM	CALS.	UNITS
Lima beans boiled and drained	111	47
Pecan pie piecrust made with unenriched flour, commercial	418	47
Rolls and buns homemade	339	47
Wheat germ toasted	391	47
Corn syrup (light and dark)	290	46
Crabs canned	101	45
Parsnips boiled and drained	66	45
Cabbage shredded, boiled and drained	20	44
Potato sticks	544	44
Celeriac root, raw	40	43
Chinese cabbage raw	14	43
Coleslaw made with salad dressing	99	43
Crab steamed	93	43
French bread enriched or unenriched	290	43
Shredded wheat (cereal)	354	43
Soybean sprouts boiled and drained	38	43
Red cabbage raw	31	42
Brownies with nuts, homemade from enriched flour	485	41
Kohlrabi thickened bulb-like stems, raw	29	41
Oranges raw	49	41
Pie crust commercial	464	41
Wheat flakes (cereal), added nutrients	354	41
Whole wheat flour	333	41
Doughnuts cake type	391	40
Gluten flour	378	40
Graham crackers plain	384	40
Green snap beans cut, frozen, boiled and drained	25	40
Haddock fried	165	40
Potato chips	568	40
Sturgeon steamed	160	40
Sweet potatoes with skin, baked	141	40
Tangerines raw	46	40
Celery (green and yellow varieties), raw	17	39
Chocolate chip cookies commercial	471	39
Turnips raw	30	39
Cashew nuts	561	38
Elderberries raw	72	38
Red beans dry, boiled and drained	118	38
Assorted cookies commercial	480	37
Carrots raw	42	37

FOOD ITEM	CALS.	UNITS
Frankfurters and beans canned	144	37
Sweet potatoes candied	168	37
Lobster salad	110	36
Sauerkraut canned, solids and liquid	18	36
Baby lima beans frozen, boiled and drained	118	35
Chop suey with meat, canned	62	35
Dried pears uncooked	268	35
Figs raw	80	35
Lettuce (Boston and bibb), raw	14	35
Loganberries raw	62	35
Marmalade (lemon or orange	720	35
Radishes (oriental, including daikon and Chinese), raw	19	35
Turnips boiled and drained	23	35
Yellow snap beans cut, frozen, boiled and drained	27	35
Chocolate chip cookies homemade from enriched flour	516	34
Green snap beans canned, regular, solids and liquid	18	34
Green snap beans canned, low sodium, solids and liquid	16	34
Yellow snap beans canned, regular, solids and liquid	19	34
Yellow snap beans canned, regular, solids and liquid	19	34
Carrots boiled and drained	31	33
Green beans (baby food), commercial	22	33
Kohlrabi thickened bulb-like stems, boiled and drained	24	33
Lichees dried	277	33
Limes raw	28	33
Ocean perch (Atlantic), fried	227	33
Potato flour	351	33
Banana powder	340	32
Blackberries raw	58	32
Brussels sprouts boiled and drained	36	32
Chili con carne with beans, canned	133	32
Potato salad homemade with cooked salad dressing and seasonings	99	32
Spaghetti with cheese in tomato sauce, homemade	104	32
Sweet potatoes with skin, boiled	114	32
Celery (green and yellow varieties), boiled and drained	14	31
Cod broiled	170	31
Mashed potatoes dehydrated, flakes without milk, prepared with water, milk, and table fat	93	31
Black raspberries raw	73	30
Radishes raw	17	30

FOOD ITEM	CALS.	UNITS
Bluefish baked or broiled	159	29
Garlic cloves raw	137	29
Lima beans dry, boiled and drained	138	29
Raisins cooked, sugar added, fruit and liquid	213	29
Red beans dry, canned, solids and liquid	90	29
Rice flakes (cereal)	390	29
Puffed wheat (cereal)	363	28
Chestnuts fresh	194	27
Chicken noodle dinner (baby food), commercial	49	27
Fruit pudding (baby food), commercial	96	27
Onions raw	38	27
Persimmons native, raw	127	27
Swordfish broiled	174	27
Tomato paste canned	82	27
Coconut meat dried, unsweetened	662	26
Lemons peeled, raw	27	26
Lima beans canned, low sodium, solids and liquid	70	26
Lima beans canned, regular, solids and liquid	71	26
Pickles (dill)	11	26
Black-eyed peas frozen, boiled and drained	130	25
Blackberries canned in juice, fruit and liquid	54	25
Carrots canned, low sodium, solids and liquid	22	25
Carrots canned, regular, solids and liquid	28	25
Cauliflower raw	27	25
Cucumbers with skin, raw	15	25
Lentils whole, dry, cooked	106	25
Mashed potatoes frozen	93	25
Peas and carrots frozen, boiled and drained	53	25
Pumpkin canned	33	25
Split pea soup canned, condensed	118	25
Summer squash boiled and drained	14	25
Chop suey with meat, homemade	120	24
Cowpeas (including black-eyed peas), boiled and drained	108	24
Dried prunes ''softenized,'' cooked, without added sugar, fruit and liquid	119	24
Mashed potatoes milk added	65	24
Onions boiled and drained	29	24
Shad baked	201	24
Carrots (baby food), commercial	29	23
Chicken chow mein without noodles, homemade	102	23

FOOD ITEM	CALS.	UNITS
Flounder baked	202	23
Ginger root fresh	49	23
Green peas boiled and drained	71	23
Guavas whole, raw	62	23
Asparagus spears, raw	26	22
Asparagus spears, frozen, boiled and drained	23	22
Blackberries canned in water, with or without artificial sweetener, fruit and liquid	40	22
Chicken with vegetables (baby food), commercial	100	22
Pretzels	390	22
Red cherries (sour)	58	22
Red cherries (sour), raw	58	22
Red raspberries raw	57	22
Smoked whitefish (lake)	155	22
Tomato catsup bottled	106	22
Asparagus spears, boiled and drained	20	21
Barbecue sauce	91	21
Blackberries canned in light syrup, fruit and liquid	72	21
Blackberries canned in heavy syrup, fruit and liquid	91	21
Brussels sprouts frozen, boiled and drained	33	21
Cauliflower boiled and drained	22	21
Jellies	273	21
Pound cake homemade	473	21
Saltine crackers	433	21
Soybean milk fluid	33	21
Spaghetti with meatballs in tomato sauce, canned	103	21
Strawberries raw	37	21
Blackberries canned in extra-heavy syrup, fruit and liquid	110	20
Butter	716	20
Coconut water	22	20
Cornmeal (white or yellow), whole ground, unbolted	355	20
Green peas (Alaska), regular, solids and liquid	66	20
Green peas (Alaska), low sodium, solids and liquid	55	20
Jams and preserves	272	20
Lettuce (iceberg), raw	13	20
Lima beans frozen, boiled and drained	99	20
Margarine	720	20
Papayas raw	39	20
Pickle relish	138	20
Prickly pears raw	42	20

FOOD ITEM	CALS.	UNITS
Puffed corn (cereal), added nutrients	399	20
Puffed rice (cereal), added nutrients, without salt	399	20
Tomato chili sauce bottled	104	20
Tuna salad	170	20
Dried prunes "softenized," cooked, sugar added, fruit and liquid	172	19
Green peas (sweet), canned, regular, solids and liquid	57	19
Green peas sweet, canned, low sodium, solids and liquid	47	19
Green peas frozen, boiled and drained	68	19
Mung bean sprouts raw	35	19
Russian salad dressing commercial, regular	494	19
Asparagus spears, canned, regular, solids and liquid	18	18
Asparagus spears, canned, low sodium, solids and liquid	16	18
Beef kidneys braised	252	18
Chicken chow mein without noodles, canned	38	18
Chicory raw	15	18
Cowpeas (including black-eyed peas), canned, solids and liquid	70	18
Gooseberries raw	39	18
Hash browned potatoes frozen, cooked	224	18
Mayonnaise commercial	718	18
Tangerine juice canned, unsweetened	42	18
Tangerine juice canned, sweetened	50	18
Tartar sauce regular	531	18
Tartar sauce low calorie	224	18
Apricots raw	51	17
Apricots canned in juice, fruit and liquid	54	17
Butterscotch candy	397	17
Cake or pastry flour	364	17
Cauliflower frozen, boiled and drained	18	17
Chocolate syrup (thin)	245	17
Cornflakes added nutrients	386	17
Cowpeas (including black-eyed peas), dry, cooked	76	17
Italian bread enriched or unenriched	276	17
Mung bean sprouts boiled and drained	28	17
Pickles (sour)	10	17
Pizza with sausage, homemade	234	17
Bread flour enriched or unenriched	365	16
Coconut meat dried, shredded, sweetened	548	16
Coconut milk	252	16

FOOD ITEM	CALS.	UNITS
Dried pears cooked, no added sugar	126	16
Frosting (chocolate fudge), made with water and table fat	378	16
Grapefruit raw	41	16
Halibut (Atlantic and Pacific), broiled	171	16
Maple syrup cane and maple blend	252	16
Orange sherbet	134	16
Pineapple canned in juice, fruit and liquid	58	16
Red beets raw	43	16
Spaghetti with cheese in tomato sauce, canned	76	16
Tuna canned in water, solids and liquid	127	16
Blueberries raw	62	15
Coconut cream	334	15
Dried peaches cooked, no sugar added	82	15
French fried potatoes	274	15
Fruit dessert with tapioca (baby food), commercial	84	15
Pineapple juice canned, unsweetened	55	15
Red cherries canned in light syrup, fruit and liquid	65	15
Red cherries (sour), canned in water, with or without artificial sweetener, fruit and liquid	48	15
Red cherries (sweet), canned in heavy syrup, fruit and liquid	81	15
Tomatoes ripe, boiled	26	15
Abalone canned	80	14
Bacon cured, boiled or fried, drained	611	14
Cantaloupe	30	14
Cherries (sweet), canned in extra-heavy syrup, fruit and liquid	100	14
Cherry pie piecrust made from unenriched flour, commercial	261	14
Cranberries raw	46	14
Figs canned in water, with or without artificial sweetener, fruit and liquid	48	14
Honeydew melon	33	14
Jerusalem artichokes raw, freshly harvested	7	14
Manhattan clam chowder canned, condensed	33	14
Pastry plain, made with enriched or unenriched flour	500	14
Piecrust made with enriched or unenriched flour, commercial	500	14
Prune juice canned or bottled	77	14
Red beets canned, regular, solids and liquid	39	14
Red beets boiled and drained	32	14
Red beets canned, low sodium, solids and liquid	32	14
Red cherries (sour), canned in light syrup, fruit and liquid	74	14
Red cherries (sour), canned in heavy syrup, fruit and liquid	89	14

FOOD ITEM	CALS.	UNITS
Red cherries (sour), canned in extra-heavy syrup, fruit and liquid	112	14
Shredded rice (cereal), added nutrients	392	14
Spanish rice homemade	87	14
Strawberries canned in water, with or without artificial sweetener, fruit and liquid	22	14
Summer squash (yellow crookneck), frozen, boiled and drained	21	14
Baker's yeast compressed	86	13
Bamboo shoots raw	27	13
Beef with vegetables (baby food), commercial	87	13
Chayote raw	28	13
Chicken all classes, dark meat, roasted, without skin	176	13
Coconut meat fresh	346	13
Corn beef hash with potatoes, canned	181	13
Figs canned in light syrup, fruit and liquid	65	13
Figs canned in heavy syrup, fruit and liquid	84	13
Figs canned in extra-heavy syrup, fruit and liquid	103	13
Grapefruit canned in water, with or without artificial sweetener, fruit and liquid	30	13
Grapefruit canned in syrup, fruit and liquid	70	13
Red cherries (sour), frozen, unsweetened	55	13
Red peppers (sweet), raw	31	13
Roe (cod and shad), baked or broiled	126	13
Succotash frozen, boiled and drained	93	13
Sweet potatoes canned in syrup, solids and liquid	114	13
Sweet potatoes canned in liquid, solids and liquid, unsweetened	46	13
Tomato puree canned, regular or low sodium	39	13
Tomatoes ripe, raw	22	13
Zwieback	23	13
Apricots canned in water, with or without artificial sweetener, fruit and liquid	38	12
Beef and vegetable stew canned	79	12
Beef noodle dinner (baby food), commercial	48	12
Cornflakes sugar coated, added nutrients	306	12
Grapes (European), raw	67	12
Hash-browned potatoes	229	12
Pickles (sweet)	146	12

FOOD ITEM	CALS.	UNITS
Pineapple all styles except crushed, canned in water, with or without artificial	39	12
Red cherries (sour), frozen, unsweetened	55	12
Veal chuck, medium fat content, braised	135	12
Vegetable juice cocktail canned	17	12
Apricots canned in light syrup, fruit and liquid	66	11
Apricots canned in heavy syrup, fruit and liquid	86	11
Apricots canned in extra-heavy syrup, fruit and liquid	101	11
Beef chuck cuts, choice grade, braised or pot roasted	327	11
Blueberry pie piecrust made from unenriched flour, commercial	242	11
Boiled ham (luncheon meat)	234	11
Chicken all classes, light meat, roasted, without skin	166	11
Chicken and noodles homemade	153	11
Eggplant boiled and drained	19	11
French salad dressing regular, commercial	410	11
French salad dressing commercial, low calorie	96	11
Grape juice canned or bottled	66	11
Hamburger regular ground, cooked	286	11
Oat and wheat cereal cooked	65	11
Orange juice fresh, commercial	45	11
Peas dry, cooked	115	11
Pineapple canned in light syrup, fruit and liquid	59	11
Pineapple canned in heavy syrup, fruit and liquid	74	11
Pineapple canned in extra-heavy syrup, fruit and liquid	90	11
Thousand Island salad dressing commercial, regular	502	11
Thousand Island salad dressing commercial, low calorie	180	11
Blueberries canned in water, with or without artificial sweetener, fruit and liquid	39	10
Egg noodles enriched, cooked	125	10
Grapefruit juice frozen concentrate, unsweetened	41	10
Green chili peppers (hot), raw, pods, without seeds	37	10
Italian salad dressing commercial, regular	552	10
Mangoes raw	66	10
Orange juice canned, unsweetened	48	10
Orange juice dehydrated	46	10
Red bananas raw	90	10
Salami cooked	311	10
Tangerine juice frozen concentrate, unsweetened	46	10
Tomato juice cocktail canned or bottled	21	10

FOOD ITEM	CALS.	UNITS
White rice fully milled or polished, enriched	109	10
Angel food cake homemade	269	9
Baked potatoes with skin	93	9
Blueberries canned in syrup, fruit and liquid	101	9
Corned beef medium fat content	372	9
French fried potatoes frozen	220	9
Fruit cocktail canned in heavy syrup, fruit and liquid	76	9
Fruit cocktail canned in light syrup, fruit and liquid	60	9
Fruit cocktail canned in extra-heavy syrup, fruit and liquid	92	9
Fruit cocktail canned in water, with or without artificial sweetener, fruit and liquid	37	9
Grapefruit juice	39	9
Green peppers (sweet), raw	22	9
Green peppers (sweet), boiled and drained	18	9
Lime juice fresh, canned, or bottled, unsweetened	26	9
Liverwurst	307	9
Orange juice frozen concentrate, unsweetened	45	9
Peaches raw	38	9
Plums (purple), canned in water, with or without artificial sweetener,fruit and liquid	46	9
Apple pie commercial	256	8
Bananas raw	85	8
Dried apples cooked, sugar added	112	8
Fruit salad canned in light syrup, fruit and liquid	59	8
Fruit salad canned in heavy syrup, fruit and liquid	75	8
Fruit salad canned in extra-heavy syrup, fruit and liquid	90	8
Fruit salad canned in water, with or without artificial sweetener, fruit and liquid	35	8
Grapefruit juice canned, sweetened	53	8
Grapefruit juice canned, unsweetened	41	8
Grapefruit juice frozen concentrate, sweetened	47	8
Green pea soup from mix	50	8
Lichees raw	64	8
Macaroni enriched or unenriched, cooked until tender	111	8
Pears with skin, raw	61	8
Pears canned in juice, solids and liquid	46	8
Plums (purple), canned in light syrup, fruit and liquid	63	8
Plums (purple), canned in heavy syrup, fruit and liquid	83	8
Spaghetti enriched, cooked until tender	111	8
Apples freshly harvested, with skin, raw	56	7

FOOD ITEM	CALS.	UNITS
Bologna	304	7
Chicken noodle soup canned, condensed	53	7
Lemon juice fresh	25	7
Lemon juice canned or bottled, unsweetened	23	7
Pimiento canned, solids and liquid	27	7
Plantains (baking bananas), raw	119	7
Tomato juice canned or bottled, regular or low sodium	19	7
Tomato juice canned, concentrate	20	7
Watermelon raw	26	7
Apple juice canned or bottled	47	6
Beef heart lean, braised	188	6
Corn flour	368	6
Cranberry sauce canned, sweetened, strained	146	6
Dried apples cooked no sugar added	93	6
Mushrooms raw	28	6
Mushrooms canned, solids and liquid	17	6
Peaches canned in juice, fruit and liquid	45	6
Tomato soup canned, condensed	36	6
Tomatoes ripe, canned, low sodium, solids and liquid	20	6
Tomatoes ripe, canned, regular, solids and liquid	21	6
Tuna canned in oil, solids and liquid	288	6
Beer	42	5
Cranberry juice cocktail bottled	65	5
Frankfurters	304	5
Green chili peppers (hot), canned in chili sauce	20	5
Honey	304	5
Pears canned in water, with or without artificial sweetener, fruit and liquid	32	5
Pears canned in extra-heavy syrup, fruit and liquid	92	5
Pears canned in light syrup, fruit and liquid	61	5
Pears canned in heavy syrup, fruit and liquid	78	5
Shredded corn (cereal), added nutrients	389	5
Applesauce canned, unsweetened or artificially sweetened	41	4
Beef noodle soup from mix	28	4
Chinese water chestnuts raw	79	4
Corn (sweet, white and yellow), canned, regular, solids and liquid	66	4
Farina enriched	42	4
Peach nectar canned	48	4
Peaches canned in extra-heavy syrup, fruit and liquid	97	4

FOOD ITEM	CALS.	UNITS
Peaches canned in water, with or without artificial sweetener, fruit and liquid	31	4
Peaches canned in light syrup, fruit and liquid	58	4
Peaches canned in heavy syrup, fruit and liquid	78	4
Chicken noodle soup from mix	22	3
Corn sweet, frozen, boiled and drained	79	3
Corn on the cob (sweet, white and yellow), boiled and drained	91	3
Corn on the cob sweet, frozen, boiled and drained	94	3
Creamed corn (white and yellow), solids and liquid	82	3
Grape drink canned	54	3
Grape juice frozen concentrate, sweetened	53	3
Pear nectar canned	52	3
Pomegranate pulp, raw	63	3
Coffee instant	1	2
Italian salad dressing commercial, low calorie	50	2
Rice cereal cooked	50	2
Corn grits degermed, enriched, cooked	51	1
Cornmeal (white or yellow), degermed, enriched, cooked	50	1
Lemonade frozen concentrate	44	1
Limeade frozen concentrate	41	1
Apples freshly harvested, pared, raw	78	0
Black walnuts	628	0
Hickory nuts	673	0
Tea instant	2	0

Iron

FOOD ITEM	CALS.	UNITS
Rice bran	276	19.40
Torula yeast	277	19.30
Brewer's yeast debittered	283	17.30
Potato flour	351	17.20
Blackstrap molasses (cane)	213	16.10
Rice polish	265	16.10
Wheat bran crude, commercially milled	213	14.90
Sunflower seed flour partially defatted	339	13.20
Beef kidneys braised	252	13.10
Caviar (sturgeon), granular	262	11.80
Pumpkin and squash seed kernels dried	553	11.20
Soybean flour defatted	326	11.10

FOOD ITEM	CALS.	UNITS
Cocoa powder high fat	299	10.70
Sesame seeds dry, whole	563	10.50
Wheat germ raw, commercially milled	363	9.40
Irish moss (seaweed), raw	N.A.	8.90
Wheat germ toasted	391	8.90
Beef liver fried	229	8.80
Malt extract dried	367	8.70
Almond meal partially defatted	408	8.50
Oysters fried	239	8.10
Pistachio nuts	594	7.30
Sunflower seed kernels dried	560	7.10
Butternuts	629	6.80
Proso millet whole grain	327	6.80
Baking chocolate	505	6.70
Bitter chocolate	505	6.70
Agar (seaweed), raw	N.A.	6.30
Parsley	44	6.20
Black walnuts	628	6.00
Dried peaches uncooked	262	6.00
Puffed corn (cereal)	399	5.80
Coffee instant, powder	129	5.60
Dried apricots uncooked	260	5.50
Liverwurst	307	5.40
Baker's yeast compressed	86	4.90
Soy sauce	68	4.80
Almonds roasted and salted	627	4.70
Almonds dried	598	4.70
Wheat flakes (cereal)	354	4.40
Puffed wheat (cereal)	363	4.20
Clams canned, solids and liquid	52	4.10
Corn syrups (light and dark)	290	4.10
Prune juice canned or bottled	77	4.10
Sardines (Pacific), canned in tomato sauce, solids and liquid	197	4.10
Dried prunes uncooked	255	3.90
Rye wafers whole grain	344	3.90
Cashew nuts	561	3.80
Bran muffins homemade from enriched flour	261	3.70
Natto (fermented soybean product)	167	3.70
Rye whole grain	334	3.70
Breadcrumbs dry, grated	392	3.60

FOOD ITEM	CALS.	UNITS
Cane syrup	263	3.60
Peanut flour defatted	371	3.50
Purslane leaves and stems, raw	21	3.50
Raisins	289	3.50
Sardines (Atlantic), canned in oil, solids and liquid	311	3.50
Shredded wheat (cereal)	354	3.50
Tomato paste canned	82	3.50
Veal chuck, medium fat content, braised	235	3.50
Wheat whole grain, soft red winter	326	3.50
Brazil nuts	654	3.40
Brown sugar (beet or cane)	373	3.40
Filberts (hazelnuts)	634	3.40
Wheat whole grain, hard red winter	330	3.40
Bacon cured, broiled or fried, drained	611	3.30
Beet greens raw	24	3.30
Chestnuts dried	377	3.30
Coconut meat dried, unsweetened	662	3.30
Whole wheat flour	333	3.30
Chard, Swiss raw	25	3.20
Hamburger regular ground, cooked	286	3.20
Pickles (sour)	10	3.20
Buckwheat whole grain	335	3.10
Chicken gizzard all classes, simmered	148	3.10
Dandelion greens raw	45	3.10
Lima beans dry, cooked	138	3.10
Spinach raw	26	3.10
Walnuts	651	3.10
Wheat whole grain, hard red spring	330	3.10
Dates (domestic), dry	274	3.00
Dried figs	274	3.00
Mustard greens raw	31	3.00
Scallops (bay and sea), steamed	112	3.00
Wheat whole grain, white	335	3.00
Bread flour enriched, self rising	352	2.90
Corned beef medium fat content	216	2.90
Soybeans canned, solids and liquid	75	2.90
Bananas dried	340	2.80
Black-eyed peas frozen, boiled and drained	130	2.80
Boiled ham (luncheon meat)	234	2.80
Cowpeas boiled and drained	130	2.80

FOOD ITEM	CALS.	UNITS
Pecan pie commercial	418	2.80
Soybeans dry, cooked	130	2.70
Baby lima beans frozen, boiled and drained	118	2.60
Dark fruitcake homemade	379	2.60
New Zealand spinach raw	19	2.60
Rye flour medium	350	2.60
Salami cooked	311	2.60
Lima beans boiled and drained	111	2.50
Persimmons (native), raw	127	2.50
Swamp cabbage raw	29	2.50
Bread (pumpernickel, rye, and white), enriched	246	2.40
Cornmeal (white or yellow), whole ground, unbolted	355	2.40
Eggs fried	216	2.40
Hickory nuts	673	2.40
Lima beans canned, regular, solids and liquid	71	2.40
Pecans	687	2.40
Pork sausage links or bulk	476	2.40
Red beans dry, boiled and drained	118	2.40
Sesame seeds dry, hulled	582	2.40
Shredded corn (cereal)	389	2.40
Whole wheat rolls and buns commercial	257	2.40
Biscuits from mix	325	2.30
Eggs hard-boiled	163	2.30
Gingerbread homemade from enriched flour	317	2.30
Hard rolls enriched, commercial	312	2.30
Roe (cod and shad), baked or broiled	126	2.30
Whole wheat bread commercial	243	2.30
Beef tongue medium fat content, braised	244	2.20
Breads (French, Vienna, and Italian), enriched	290	2.20
Peanuts with skins, roasted	582	2.20
Poached eggs	163	2.20
Spinach boiled and drained	23	2.20
Chocolate chip cookies homemade from enriched flour	516	2.10
Cowpeas (including black-eyed peas), immature seeds, boiled and drained	108	2.10
Ginger-root fresh	49	2.10
Lentils whole, dry, cooked	106	2.10
Rolls and buns homemade	339	2.10
Spinach canned, regular, solids and liquid	19	2.10
Spinach chopped, frozen, boiled and drained	23	2.10

FOOD ITEM	CALS.	UNITS
Spinach canned, low sodium, solids and liquid	21	2.10
Barley pearled, light	349	2.00
Coconut meat dried, shredded, sweetened	548	2.00
Corned beef hash with potatoes, canned	181	2.00
French fried shrimp	225	2.00
Lettuce (Boston and Bibb), raw	14	2.00
Macadamia nuts	691	2.00
Peanut butter fat and salt added	581	2.00
Peanuts without skin, raw	568	2.00
Sturgeon steamed	160	2.00
Yellow mustard prepared	75	2.00
Beet greens boiled and drained	18	1.90
Brownies with nuts, homemade from enriched flour	485	1.90
Chop suey with meat homemade	120	1.90
Chop suey with meat, canned	62	1.90
Dried peaches cooked, no sugar added	82	1.90
Frankfurters and beans canned	144	1.90
Green peas frozen, boiled and drained	68	1.90
Rolls and buns plain, commercial	298	1.90
Tofu (soybean curd)	72	1.90
Bologna	304	1.80
Brown mustard prepared	91	1.80
Chard, Swiss boiled and drained	18	1.80
Chocolate chip cookies commercial	471	1.80
Coconut cream	334	1.80
Corn flour	368	1.80
Dandelion greens boiled and drained	33	1.80
Dried prunes cooked, no added sugar	119	1.80
French fried potatoes frozen	220	1.80
Green peas boiled and drained	71	1.80
Mustard greens boiled and drained	23	1.80
Potato chips	568	1.80
Potato sticks	544	1.80
Puffed rice (cereal), added nutrients without salt	399	1.80
Red beans canned, solids and liquid	90	1.80
Shredded rice (cereal), added nutrients	392	1.80
Turnip greens leaves and stems, raw	28	1.80
Asparagus spears, canned, regular, solids and liquid	18	1.70
Asparagus spears, canned, low sodium, solids and liquid	16	1.70

FOOD ITEM	CALS.	UNITS
Carrots canned, low sodium, solids and liquid	22	1.70
Chestnuts fresh	194	1.70
Chicken all classes, dark meat, roasted, without skin	176	1.70
Chili con carne with beans, canned	133	1.70
Chives raw	28	1.70
Coconut meat fresh	346	1.70
Corn muffins homemade from enriched degermed cornmeal	314	1.70
Eggs scrambled	173	1.70
Endive (curly endive and escarole), raw	20	1.70
Green peas (Alaska), canned, regular, solids and liquid	66	1.70
Green peas (Alaska), canned, low sodium, solids and liquid	55	1.70
Lichees dried	277	1.70
Lima beans frozen, boiled and drained	99	1.70
Miso (fermented soybean product)	171	1.70
Omelets	173	1.70
Smelt (Atlantic, jack, and bay), canned, solids and liquid	200	1.70
Split peas cooked	115	1.70
Tomato puree canned, regular	39	1.70
Waffles homemade	279	1.70
Watercress leaves and stems, raw	19	1.70
Baking powder biscuits homemade from enriched flour	369	1.60
Blueberry muffins homemade from enriched flour	281	1.60
Chocolate syrup (thin)	245	1.60
Coconut milk	252	1.60
Dried peaches sulfured, cooked, sugar added, fruit and liquid	N.A.	1.60
Elderberries raw	72	1.60
Green olives pickled, canned or bottled	116	1.60
Light fruitcake homemade	389	1.60
Raisins cooked, sugar added, fruit and liquid	213	1.60
Rice flakes (cereal)	390	1.60
Rye bread (American), commercial	243	1.60
Tuna canned in water, solids and liquid	127	1.60
Turnip greens leaves and stems, canned, solids and liquid	18	1.60
Turnip greens frozen, boiled and drained	23	1.60
Corn muffins from mix, made with eggs and milk	324	1.50
Cowpeas (including black-eyed peas), canned, solids and liquid	70	1.50
Frankfurters cooked	304	1.50
Garlic cloves raw	137	1.50
Graham crackers plain	384	1.50

FOOD ITEM	CALS.	UNITS
Green peas (sweet), canned, regular, solids and liquid	57	1.50
Green peas (sweet), canned, low sodium, solids and liquid	47	1.50
Jellies	273	1.50
Mustard greens frozen, boiled and drained	20	1.50
New Zealand spinach boiled and drained	13	1.50
Pimientos canned, solids and liquid	27	1.50
Popovers baked, homemade	224	1.50
Pretzels	390	1.50
Spaghetti with meatballs in tomato sauce, homemade	134	1.50
Swamp cabbage boiled and drained	21	1.50
Butterscotch	397	1.40
Caramels plain or chocolate	399	1.40
Corn muffins homemade from whole-ground cornmeal	288	1.40
Cornflakes added nutrients	386	1.40
Doughnuts cake type	391	1.40
Flounder baked	202	1.40
Lettuce (cos and romaine), raw	18	1.40
Maple sugar	348	1.40
Smoked herring kippered	211	1.40
Whey dried	349	1.40
Buckwheat pancakes and waffles from mix, made with eggs and milk	200	1.30
Chicken all classes, light meat, roasted, without skin	166	1.30
Cowpeas (including black-eyed peas), dry, cooked, mature seeds	76	1.30
Dried pears	268	1.30
French fried potatoes	274	1.30
Garden cress raw	32	1.30
Mixed vegetables (carrots, corn, peas, green snap beans, and lima beans), frozen, boiled and drained	64	1.30
Mung bean sprouts	35	1.30
Ocean perch (Atlantic), fried	227	1.30
Pancakes homemade from enriched flour	231	1.30
Spaghetti with meatballs in tomato sauce, canned	103	1.30
Swordfish broiled	174	1.30
Tuna salad	170	1.30
Asparagus cuts and tips, frozen, boiled and drained	22	1.20
Beef with vegetables (baby food), commercial	87	1.20
Cornbread from mix, made with eggs and milk	233	1.20
Green snap beans canned, regular, solids and liquid	18	1.20

FOOD ITEM	CALS.	UNITS
Green snap beans canned, low sodium, solids and liquid	16	1.20
Haddock fried	165	1.20
Hash-browned potatoes frozen, cooked	224	1.20
Kale leaves and stems, boiled and drained	28	1.20
Loganberries raw	62	1.20
Maple syrup	252	1.20
Pancakes from mix, made with eggs and milk	225	1.20
Pickles (sweet)	146	1.20
Pizza with sausage, homemade	234	1.20
Purslane leaves and stems, boiled and drained	15	1.20
Roe (cod, haddock, and herring), canned, solids and liquid	118	1.20
Saltine crackers	433	1.20
Shallots bulbs, raw	72	1.20
Yellow snap beans canned, regular, solids and liquid	19	1.20
Yellow snap beans canned, low sodium, solids and liquid	15	1.20
Artichokes (globe or French), boiled and drained	44	1.10
Asparagus spears, frozen, boiled and drained	23	1.10
Black currants (European), raw	54	1.10
Bread pudding with raisins, commercial	187	1.10
Broccoli spears, raw	32	1.10
Brussels sprouts boiled and drained	36	1.10
Cauliflower raw	27	1.10
Corn muffins from mix, made with eggs and water	297	1.10
Cornbread homemade from whole-ground cormeal	207	1.10
Cracked wheat bread	263	1.10
Cucumbers with skin, raw	15	1.10
Green beans (baby food), commercial	22	1.10
Leeks bulb and lower-leaf portion, raw	52	1.10
Oat cereal with toasted wheat germ and soy grits, cooked	62	1.10
Peas and carrots frozen, boiled and drained	53	1.10
Spaghetti with cheese in tomato sauce, canned	76	1.10
Split pea soup canned, condensed	118	1.10
Tuna canned in oil, solids and liquid	288	1.10
Turnip greens leaves and stems, boiled and drained	20	1.10
Asparagus spears, raw	26	1.00
Blueberries raw	62	1.00
Cheddar cheese unprocessed	398	1.00
Chicken chow mein without noodles, homemade	102	1.00
Chocolate cake with chocolate frosting, homemade	369	1.00
Cod broiled	170	1.00

FOOD ITEM	CALS.	UNITS
Collards leaves and stems, raw	40	1.00
Collards frozen, boiled and drained	30	1.00
Cornflakes sugar coated, added nutrients	386	1.00
Jams and preserves	272	1.00
Kale frozen, boiled and drained	31	1.00
Pickles (dill)	11	1.00
Pizza with cheese, homemade	236	1.00
Plums (purple), canned in water, with or without artificial sweetener,fruit and liquid	46	1.00
Radishes raw	17	1.00
Soybean sprouts raw	46	1.00
Strawberries raw	37	1.00
Succotash frozen, boiled and drained	93	1.00
American cheese pasteurized, processed	370	.90
Beef and vegetable stew canned	79	.90
Blackberries raw	58	.90
Blackberries canned in juice, fruit and liquid	54	.90
Bread flour unenriched, wheat	365	.90
Cheese crackers	479	.90
Chicken and noodles homemade	153	.90
Chicory greens raw	20	.90
Clam chowder (Manhattan), canned, condensed	66	.90
Danish pastry commercial	422	.90
Egg noodles enriched, cooked	125	.90
Guavas whole, raw	62	.90
Hash-browned potatoes	229	.90
Horseradish prepared	38	.90
Lobster salad	110	.90
Macaroni enriched, cooked until tender	111	.90
Mung bean sprouts boiled and drained	28	.90
Plums (purple), canned in light syrup, fruit and liquid	63	.90
Plums (purple), canned in heavy syrup, fruit and liquid	83	.90
Plums (purple), canned in extra-heavy syrup, fruit and liquid	102	.90
Raspberries raw	73	.90
Spaghetti enriched, cooked until tender	111	.90
Spaghetti with cheese in tomato sauce, homemade	104	.90
Sweet potatoes candied	168	.90
Swiss cheese (domestic), unprocessed	370	.90
Tartar sauce regular	531	.90
Tartar sauce low calorie	224	.90

FOOD ITEM	CALS.	UNITS
Tomato juice canned or bottled, regular or low sodium	19	.90
Tomato juice canned, concentrate	20	.90
Tomato juice cocktail canned or bottled	21	.90
White rice enriched, cooked	109	.90
Barbecue sauce	91	.80
Broccoli spears, boiled and drained	26	.80
Brussels sprouts frozen, boiled and drained	33	.80
Corn frozen, boiled and drained, off the cob	79	.80
Corn on the cob frozen, boiled and drained	94	.80
Crab steamed	93	.80
Crab canned	101	.80
Garden cress boiled and drained	23	.80
Green snap beans raw	32	.80
Halibut (Atlantic and Pacific), broiled	171	.80
Lemon candied	314	.80
Lemon peel raw	N.A.	.80
Lobster (northern), canned or cooked	95	.80
Mushrooms raw	28	.80
Orange peel raw		.80
Pickle relish (sweet)	138	.80
Pound cake homemade	473	.80
Red bananas raw	90	.80
Red cabbage raw	31	.80
Rhubarb raw	16	.80
Soybean milk fluid	33	.80
Sweet rolls commercial	316	.80
Tomato catsup bottled	106	.80
Yellow snap beans raw	27	.80
Apple butter	186	.70
Assorted cookies commercial	480	.70
Baked potatoes with skin	93	.70
Bananas raw	85	.70
Blueberries canned in water, with or without artificial sweetener, fruit and liquid	39	.70
Bread French, unenriched	290	.70
Broccoli chopped, frozen, boiled and drained	26	.70
Carrots raw	42	.70
Carrots canned, regular, solids and liquid	28	.70
Cauliflower boiled and drained	22	.70
Eclairs with custard filling and chocolate frosting	239	.70

FOOD ITEM	CALS.	UNITS
Green peppers (hot), pods without seeds, raw	37	.70
Green peppers (sweet), raw	22	.70
Green snap beans frozen, cut, boiled and drained	25	.70
Oat and wheat cereal cooked	65	.70
Peas edible podded, raw	53	.70
Plantains (baking bananas), raw	119	.70
Red beets raw	43	.70
Rhubarb frozen, cooked, sugar added	143	.70
Rice cereal added nutrients, cooked	50	.70
Shad canned, solids and liquid	152	.70
Soybean sprouts boiled and drained	38	.70
Strawberries canned in water, with or without artificial sweetener, fruit and liquid	22	.70
Summer squash (yellow crookneck), frozen, boiled and drained	21	.70
Sweet potatoes canned in syrup, solids and liquid	114	.70
Sweet potatoes canned in liquid, solids and liquid, unsweetened	46	.70
Yellow snap beans cut, frozen, boiled and drained	27	.70
Apple juice canned or bottled	47	.60
Asparagus spears, boiled and drained	20	.60
Avocados raw	167	.60
Blackberries canned in water, with or without artificial sweetener, fruit and liquid	40	.60
Blackberries canned in light syrup, fruit and liquid	72	.60
Blackberries canned in heavy syrup, fruit and liquid	91	.60
Blackberries canned in extra-heavy syrup, fruit and liquid	110	.60
Blueberries canned in syrup, fruit and liquid	101	.60
Blueberry pie baked piecrust made from unenriched flour	242	.60
Carrots boiled and drained	31	.60
Celeriac root, raw	40	.60
Chinese cabbage raw	14	.60
Collards leaves and stems, boiled and drained	29	.60
Corn on the cob sweet, white and yellow, boiled and drained	91	.60
Creamed corn white and yellow, solids and liquid	82	.60
Dried pears cooked, no added sugar	126	.60
Eggplant boiled and drained	19	.60
Figs raw	80	.60
Green snap beans boiled and drained	25	.60

FOOD ITEM	CALS.	UNITS
Lemons peeled, raw	27	.60
Limes raw	28	.60
Marmalade citrus	257	.60
Mashed potatoes frozen	93	.60
Muffins homemade from unenriched flour	294	.60
Okra raw	36	.60
Pancakes homemade from unenriched flour	231	.60
Parsnips boiled and drained	66	.60
Potato salad homemade with cooked salad dressing and seasonings	99	.60
Potatoes raw, boiled in skin	76	.60
Radishes (Oriental, including daikon and Chinese), raw	19	.60
Red beets canned, regular, solids and liquid	34	.60
Red beets canned, low sodium, solids and liquid	32	.60
Red peppers (sweet), raw	31	.60
Red raspberries frozen, sweetened	98	.60
Rhubarb cooked, sugar added	141	.60
Rolls from mix	299	.60
Russian salad dressing commercial	494	.60
Shad baked	201	.60
Skim milk dry, regular	363	.60
Spanish rice homemade	87	.60
Thousand Island salad dressing commercial, regular	502	.60
Thousand Island salad dressing commercial, low calorie	180	.60
Tomatoes ripe, boiled	26	.60
Water chestnuts raw	79	.60
Yellow snap beans boiled and drained	22	.60
Zwieback	423	.60
Applesauce canned, sweetened	91	.50
Applesauce canned, artificially sweetened or unsweetened	41	.50
Apricots raw	51	.50
Apricots canned in juice, fruit and liquid	54	.50
Bamboo shoots raw	27	.50
Beef noodle dinner (baby food), commercial	48	.50
Brown rice cooked	119	.50
Cake or pastry flour	364	.50
Carrots (baby food), commercial	29	.50
Cauliflower frozen, boiled and drained	18	.50
Chayote raw	28	.50
Chicory raw	15	.50

FOOD ITEM	CALS.	UNITS
Chocolate pudding homemade	148	.50
Corn sweet, yellow, whole kernel, canned, vacuum pack, solids and liquid	83	.50
Corn pudding	104	.50
Cranberries raw	46	.50
Dried apples cooked, no sugar added	78	.50
Gooseberries raw	39	.50
Honey	304	.50
Kohlrabi thickened bulb-like stems, raw	29	.50
Lettuce (iceberg), raw	13	.50
Mayonnaise	718	.50
Mushrooms canned, solids and liquid	17	.50
Nectarines raw	64	.50
Okra cuts and pods, frozen, boiled and drained	38	.50
Onions raw	38	.50
Pastry plain, made with unenriched flour	500	.50
Peaches raw	38	.50
Peaches canned in juice, solids and liquid	45	.50
Peas edible podded, boiled and drained	43	.50
Peppers sweet, boiled and drained	18	.50
Piecrust made with unenriched flour	500	.50
Pineapple raw	52	.50
Plums (prune type), raw	75	.50
Pumpkin pie commercial	211	.50
Red beets boiled and drained	32	.50
Red cherries (sour), frozen, sweetened	112	.50
Sauerkraut canned, solids and liquid	18	.50
Tomatoes ripe, raw	22	.50
Tomatoes ripe, canned, regular, solids and liquid	21	.50
Tomatoes ripe, canned, low sodium, solids and liquid	20	.50
Turnips raw	31	.50
Watermelon raw	26	.50
White cake with chocolate frosting, from mix, made with egg whites and water	351	.50
Whitefish (lake), stuffed, baked	215	.50
Whole milk dry	502	.50
Applesauce (baby food), commercial	72	.40
Beef broth, bouillon, and consomme canned, condensed	26	.40
Cabbage raw	24	.40
Cantaloupe	30	.40

FOOD ITEM	CALS.	UNITS
Chicken noodle soup canned, condensed	53	.40
Corn (sweet, white and yellow), canned, regular, solids and liquid	66	.40
Corn (sweet, white and yellow), canned, low sodium, solids and liquid	57	.40
Cornmeal (white or yellow), degermed, enriched, cooked	50	.40
Cottage cheese uncreamed	86	.40
Custard baked, commercial	115	.40
Figs canned in water, with or without artificial sweetener, fruit and liquid	48	.40
Figs canned in light syrup, fruit and liquid	65	.40
Figs canned in heavy syrup, fruit and liquid	84	.40
Figs canned in extra-heavy syrup, fruit and liquid	103	.40
French salad dressing commercial, regular	410	.40
French salad dressing commercial, low calorie	96	.40
Fruit cocktail canned in water, with or without artificial sweetener, fruit and liquid	37	.40
Fruit cocktail canned in heavy syrup, fruit and liquid	76	.40
Fruit cocktail canned in extra-heavy syrup, fruit and liquid	92	.40
Fruit cocktail canned in light syrup, fruit and liquid	60	.40
Fruit dessert with tapioca (baby food), commercial	84	.40
Grapefruit raw	41	.40
Grapefruit juice canned, sweetened	53	.40
Grapefruit juice canned, unsweetened	41	.40
Grapes (American), raw	69	.40
Green chili peppers (hot), canned in chili sauce	20	.40
Green pea soup canned, condensed	53	.40
Honeydew melon	33	.40
Hot cocoa homemade	97	.40
Ice cream cones	377	.40
Kumquats raw	65	.40
Lichees raw	64	.40
Macaroni unenriched, cooked until tender	111	.40
Mangoes raw	66	.40
Manhattan clam chowder canned, condensed	33	.40
Mashed potatoes milk added	65	.40
Onions boiled and drained	29	.40
Orange juice canned, sweetened	52	.40
Orange juice canned, unsweetened	48	.40

FOOD ITEM	CALS.	UNITS
Oranges peeled, raw	49	.40
Parmesan cheese	393	.40
Piecrust from mix, prepared with water	464	.40
Pineapple canned in juice, fruit and liquid	58	.40
Pumpkin canned	33	.40
Red cherries (sweet), raw	70	.40
Red cherries (sour), raw	58	.40
Rice pudding with raisins, commercial	146	.40
Rutabagas raw	46	.40
Summer squash boiled and drained	14	.40
Tangerines raw	46	.40
Tapioca cream pudding	134	.40
Turnips boiled and drained	23	.40
Wine	85	.40
Apples freshly harvested, with skin, raw	58	.30
Apples freshly harvested, without skin, raw	54	.30
Apricots canned in water, with or without artificial sweetener, fruit and liquid	38	.30
Apricots canned in light syrup, fruit and liquid	66	.30
Apricots canned in heavy syrup, fruit and liquid	86	.30
Apricots canned in extra-heavy syrup, fruit and liquid	101	.30
Cabbage shredded, boiled and drained	20	.30
Celery (green and yellow varieties), raw	17	.30
Cherries (sweet), canned in water, with or without artificial sweetener, fruit and liquid	48	.30
Cherries (sweet), canned in extra-heavy syrup, fruit and liquid	100	.30
Cherries (sweet), canned in light syrup, fruit and liquid	65	.30
Cherries (sweet), canned in heavy syrup, fruit and liquid	81	.30
Cherries (sweet), canned in extra-heavy syrup, fruit and liquid	100	.30
Chicken noodle dinner (baby food), commercial	49	.30
Chocolate pudding from mix	124	.30
Coconut water	22	.30
Corn grits degermed, enriched, cooked	51	.30
Cottage cheese creamed	106	.30
Cranberry juice cocktail bottled	65	.30
Custard pudding all flavors, (baby food), commercial	96	.30
Farina enriched, regular, cooked	42	.30
Fruit pudding (baby food), commercial	96	.30
Fruit salad canned in water, with or without artificial sweetener, fruit and liquid	35	.30

FOOD ITEM	CALS.	UNITS
Fruit salad canned in light syrup, fruit and liquid	59	.30
Fruit salad canned in heavy syrup, fruit and liquid	75	.30
Fruit salad canned in extra-heavy syrup, fruit and liquid	90	.30
Grape juice canned or bottled	66	.30
Grapefruit canned in water, with or without artificial sweetener, fruit and liquid	30	.30
Grapefruit canned in syrup, fruit and liquid	70	.30
Kohlrabi thickened bulb-like stems, boiled and drained	24	.30
Mashed potatoes dehydrated, flakes without milk, prepared with water, milk, and fat	93	.30
Papayas raw	39	.30
Peaches canned in water, with or without artificial sweetener, fruit and liquid	31	.30
Peaches canned in light syrup, fruit and liquid	58	.30
Peaches canned in heavy syrup, fruit and liquid	78	.30
Peaches canned in extra-heavy syrup, fruit and liquid	97	.30
Pears with skin, raw	61	.30
Pears canned in juice, fruit and liquid	46	.30
Pies apple, piecrust made with unenriched flour, frozen, baked	254	.30
Pies cherry, piecrust made with unenriched flour, frozen, baked	291	.30
Pineapple all styles except crushed, canned in water, with or without artificial sweetener	39	.30
Pineapple canned in light syrup, fruit and liquid	59	.30
Pineapple canned in heavy syrup, fruit and liquid	74	.30
Pineapple canned in extra-heavy syrup, fruit and liquid	90	.30
Pineapple juice canned, unsweetened	55	.30
Pomegranate pulp, raw	63	.30
Prickly pears raw	42	.30
Red cherries (sour), canned in water or syrup, fruit and liquid	43	.30
Rutabagas boiled and drained	35	.30
Tomato soup canned, condensed	36	.30
Tomato soup canned, condensed, prepared with milk	69	.30
Whole wheat crackers	403	.30
Angel food cake homemade	269	.20
Apricot nectar canned	57	.20
Beef noodle soup from mix, prepared with water	28	.20
Celery (green and yellow varieties), boiled and drained	14	.20
Cranberry sauce canned, sweetened, strained	146	.20
Cream cheese	374	.20

FOOD ITEM	CALS.	UNITS
Grapefruit juice	39	.20
Hot chocolate homemade	95	.20
Italian salad dressing commercial, low calorie	50	.20
Italian salad dressing commercial, regular	552	.20
Lemon juice canned or bottled, unsweetened	23	.20
Lemon juice fresh, unsweetened	25	.20
Lime juice fresh, canned or bottled, unsweetened	26	.20
Milk (chocolate)	85	.20
Orange juice fresh, commercial	45	.20
Peach nectar canned	48	.20
Pears canned in heavy syrup, fruit and liquid	76	.20
Pears canned in extra-heavy syrup, fruit and liquid	92	.20
Pears canned in water, with or without artificial sweetener, fruit and liquid	32	.20
Pears canned in light syrup, fruit and liquid	61	.20
Salad dressing (blue cheese and Roquefort cheese), commercial, regular	504	.20
Tangerine juice canned, unsweetened	43	.20
Tangerine juice fresh	41	.20
Tangerine juice frozen concentrate, unsweetened	46	.20
Tangerine juice canned, sweetened	50	.20
Chicken noodle soup from mix, prepared with water	22	.10
Coffee instant	1	.10
Evaporated milk canned, condensed	137	.10
Frozen custard fat content 10%	193	.10
Grape drink canned	54	.10
Grape juice frozen concentrate, sweetened	53	.10
Ice cream fat content 10%	193	.10
Ice cream fat content 12%	207	.10
Ice milk	152	.10
Pear nectar canned	48	.10
Salt	0	.10
Sugar (beet or cane), powdered	385	.10
Sugar (beet or cane), granulated	385	.10
Tomato vegetable soup with noodles from mix	27	.10
Beer	42	.00
Buttermilk cultured, fluid	36	.00
Cream (half and half)	134	.00
Cream light whipping	300	.00

FOOD ITEM	CALS.	UNITS
Cream heavy whipping	352	.00
Crystallized sugar	335	.00
Lemonade frozen concentrate, diluted with water	44	.00
Limeade frozen concentrate	41	.00
Orange sherbet	134	.00
Tea instant	2	.00
Vanilla pudding with starch base, homemade	111	.00
Whole milk	65	.00
Yogurt made from partially skimmed milk	50	.00
Yogurt made from whole milk	62	.00

Phosphorus

FOOD ITEM	CALS.	UNITS
Baking powder	129	2904
Brewer's yeast debittered	283	1753
Torula yeast	277	1713
Rice bran	276	1386
Wheat bran crude, commercially milled	213	1276
Bran (cereal), sugar and malt extract added	240	1176
Pumpkin and squash seed kernels dried	553	1144
Wheat germ raw, commercially milled	363	1118
Wheat germ toasted	391	1084
Condensed milk	321	1016
Skim milk dry, regular	363	1016
Almond meal partially defatted	408	914
Sunflower seed kernels dried	560	837
Parmesan cheese	393	781
American cheese pasteurized, processed	370	771
Oatmeal (baby food), commercial	375	734
Peanut flour defatted	371	720
Whole milk dry	502	708
Brazil nuts	654	693
Soybean flour defatted	326	655
Rice cereal (baby food), commercial	371	646
Safflower seed meal partially defatted	355	620
Sesame seeds dry, whole	563	616
Sesame seeds dry, hulled	582	592

FOOD ITEM	CALS.	UNITS
Whey dried	349	589
Black walnuts	628	570
Swiss cheese (domestic), unprocessed	370	563
Almonds roasted and salted	627	504
Almonds dried	598	504
Pistachio nuts	594	500
Bran flakes (cereal)	303	495
Cheddar cheese unprocessed	398	478
Sardines (Pacific), canned in tomato sauce, solids and liquid	197	478
Wheat flour self-rising, enriched	352	466
Sardines (Atlantic), canned in oil, solids and liquid	311	434
Salmon broiled or baked	182	414
Peanuts without skins, raw	568	409
Peanut butter fat and salt added	581	407
Peanuts with skins, roasted	582	407
Bran muffins homemade	261	405
Roe (cod and shad), baked or broiled	126	402
Baker's yeast compressed	86	394
Rye wafers whole grain	344	388
Shredded wheat (cereal)	354	388
Bitter chocolate	505	384
Baking chocolate	505	383
Corn muffins from mix, made with eggs and milk	324	380
Walnuts	651	380
Rye whole grain	334	376
Cashew nuts	561	373
Whole wheat flour	333	372
Smelt (Atlantic), canned, solids and liquid	200	370
Hickory nuts	673	360
Caviar (sturgeon)	262	355
Roe (cod, haddock and herring), canned, solids and liquid	118	346
Flounder baked	202	344
Blue cheese and Roquefort cheese unprocessed	368	339
Scallops (bay and sea), steamed	112	338
Buckwheat pancakes and waffles from mix	200	337
Puffed wheat (cereal)	363	322
Shad baked	201	313
Cheese crackers	479	309
Miso (fermented soybean product)	171	309

FOOD ITEM	CALS.	UNITS
Wheat flakes (cereal)	354	309
Malt extract dried	367	294
Tuna canned in oil, solids and liquid	288	294
Pecans	687	289
Bluefish baked or broiled	159	287
Whole wheat rolls and buns commercial	257	281
Swordfish broiled	174	275
Cod broiled	170	274
Smoked whitefish (lake)	155	274
Cornbread from mix, made with eggs, and milk	233	268
Chicken all classes, light meat, roasted, without skin	166	265
Sturgeon steamed	160	263
Rye flour medium	350	262
Pancakes from mix, made with eggs and milk	225	260
Cornmeal (white or yellow), whole ground	355	256
Smoked herring kippered	211	254
Halibut (Atlantic and Pacific), broiled	171	248
Haddock fried	165	247
Whitefish (lake), stuffed, baked	215	246
Smoked salmon	176	245
Oysters fried	239	241
Liverwurst	307	238
Biscuits from mix, with enriched flour, made with milk	325	232
Milk chocolate plain	520	231
Chicken all classes, dark meat, roasted, without skin	176	229
Pumpernickel bread	246	229
Whole wheat bread made with 2% nonfat dry milk	243	228
Bacon cured, broiled or fried, drained	611	224
Corn muffins homemade from whole-ground cornmeal	288	216
Cornbread homemade from whole-ground cornmeal	207	211
Anchovies pickled	176	210
Condensed milk canned, sweetened	321	206
Eggs hard-boiled	163	205
Evaporated milk canned, unsweetened	137	205
Eggs poached	163	203
Garlic cloves raw	137	202
Salami cooked	311	200
Ice cream cones	377	198
Pizza with cheese, homemade	236	195
Hamburger regular ground, cooked	286	194

FOOD ITEM	CALS.	UNITS
Lobster (northern), canned or cooked	95	192
French fried shrimp	225	191
Doughnuts cake type	391	190
Tuna canned in water, solids and liquid	127	190
Whole wheat crackers commercial	403	190
Eggs scrambled	173	189
Omelets	173	189
Dried coconut unsweetened	662	187
Welsh rarebit	179	186
Crab canned	101	182
Natto (fermented soybean product)	167	182
Beef heart lean, braised	188	181
Lichees dried	277	181
Soybeans dry, cooked	130	179
White cake with chocolate frosting, from mix	351	179
Potato flour	351	178
Baking powder biscuits homemade from enriched flour	369	175
Cottage cheese uncreamed	86	175
Crab steamed	93	175
Corn muffins homemade from enriched, degermed cornmeal	314	169
Black-eyed peas frozen, boiled and drained	130	168
Boiled ham (luncheon meat)	234	166
Assorted cookies commercial	480	163
Chestnuts dried	377	162
Pork sausage links or bulk	476	162
Macadamia nuts	691	161
Corn fritters commercial	377	155
Lima beans dry, boiled and drained	138	154
Cottage cheese creamed	106	152
Muffins (plain), homemade from enriched or unenriched flour	294	151
Veal chuck, medium fat content, braised	235	151
Graham crackers plain	384	149
Brownies with nuts, homemade from enriched flour	485	148
Rye bread (American), commercial	243	147
Cowpeas (including black-eyed peas), boiled and drained	108	146
Tuna salad	170	142
Breadcrumbs dry, grated, commercial	392	141
Beef chuck cuts, choice grade, braised or pot roasted	327	140
Gluten flour	378	140

FOOD ITEM	CALS.	UNITS
Popovers homemade	224	140
Red beans dry, boiled and drained	118	140
Potato chips	568	139
Potato sticks	544	139
Clams canned, solids and liquid	52	137
Brown mustard prepared	91	134
Blueberry muffins homemade from enriched flour	281	132
Rice flakes (cereal)	390	132
Chocolate cake with chocolate frosting, homemade	369	131
Pretzels	390	131
Abalone canned	80	128
Bologna	304	128
Cracked wheat bread	263	128
Baby lima beans frozen, boiled and drained	118	126
Chili con carne with beans, canned	133	126
Coconut cream	334	126
Tofu (soybean curd)	72	126
Ice milk	152	124
Caramels plain or chocolate	399	122
Split pea soup canned, condensed	118	122
Lima beans boiled and drained	111	121
Frankfurters and beans canned	144	119
Lentils whole, dry, cooked	106	119
Beef tongue medium fat content, braised	244	117
Chicken chow mein without noodles, homemade	102	117
Custard commercial	115	117
Dried peaches uncooked	262	117
Chop suey with meat, canned	62	116
Mushrooms raw	28	116
Celeriac root, raw	40	115
Frozen custard fat content 10%	193	115
Ice cream fat content 10%	193	115
Light fruitcake homemade	389	115
Bread pudding with raisins	187	114
Chocolate chip cookies commercial	471	114
Dark fruitcake homemade	379	113
Hot cocoa homemade	97	113
Coconut meat dried, shredded, sweetened	548	112
Cowpeas (including black-eyed peas), canned, solids and liquid	70	112

FOOD ITEM	CALS.	UNITS
Eclairs with custard filling and chocolate frosting, commercial	239	112
French fried potatoes	274	111
Danish pastry commercial	422	109
Red beans canned, solids and liquid	90	109
Dried apricots uncooked	260	108
Sweet rolls commercial	316	107
Goat's milk	67	106
Banana powder	340	104
Soy sauce	68	104
Chicken and noodles homemade	153	103
Pecan pie piecrust made with unenriched flour, commercial	418	103
Cake (plain), homemade	364	102
Frankfurters	304	102
Rolls and buns homemade	339	102
Raisins natural	289	101
Coconut milk	252	100
Gingerbread from mix, made with water	276	100
Soybeans canned, solids and liquid	75	100
Chocolate chip cookies homemade from enriched flour	516	99
Chop suey with meat, homemade	120	99
Green peas boiled and drained	71	99
Chocolate pudding homemade	148	98
Rolls from mix	299	97
Corn on the cob (sweet), frozen, boiled and drained	94	96
Oat cereal with toasted wheat germ and soy grits, cooked	62	96
Bread flour enriched or unenriched	365	95
Buttermilk cultured	36	95
Chocolate pudding from mix	124	95
Coconut meat fresh	346	95
Cowpeas (including black-eyed peas), dry, cooked	76	95
Cream cheese	374	95
Lobster salad	110	95
Shredded rice (cereal)	392	95
Skim milk	36	95
Spaghetti with meatballs in tomato sauce, homemade	134	95
Hot chocolate homemade	95	94
Rice pudding with raisins, commercial	146	94
Yogurt made from partially skimmed milk	50	94
Corned beef medium fat content, cooked	372	93
Whole milk (3.5% fat)	65	93

FOOD ITEM	CALS.	UNITS
Chocolate syrup (thin)	245	92
Hard rolls enriched, commercial	312	92
Pizza with sausage, homemade	234	92
Vanilla pudding homemade	111	91
White cake homemade, without icing	375	91
Lima beans frozen, boiled and drained	99	90
Peas edible podded, raw	53	90
Puffed corn (cereal)	399	90
Corn on the cob (sweet, white and yellow), boiled and drained	91	89
Split peas cooked	115	89
Chestnuts fresh	194	88
White bread made with 1% - 2% nonfat dry milk	269	87
Yogurt made from whole milk	62	87
French fried potatoes frozen	220	86
Green peas frozen, boiled and drained	68	86
Chicken with vegetables (baby food), commercial	100	85
French bread enriched or unenriched	290	85
Half-and-half cream	134	85
Pie crust from mix	464	85
Rolls and buns plain, commercial	298	85
Succotash frozen, boiled and drained	93	85
Beef with vegetables (baby food), commercial	87	84
Blackstrap molasses (cane)	213	84
Corn pudding commercial	104	84
Carob flour	180	81
Dried prunes "softenized", uncooked	255	79
Hash browned potatoes	229	79
Pound cake homemade	473	79
Jerusalem artichokes raw, freshly harvested	7	78
Dried figs uncooked	274	77
Italian bread enriched or unenriched	276	77
Parsnips raw	76	77
Garden cress raw	32	76
Peas edible podded, boiled and drained	43	76
Oat and wheat cereal cooked	65	75
Blue cheese & Roquefort salad dressing commercial, regular	504	74
Brown rice cooked	119	73

FOOD ITEM	CALS.	UNITS
Cake or pastry flour	364	73
Corn (sweet, yellow), canned, solids and liquid	83	73
Corn (sweet), frozen, boiled and drained	79	73
Kale leaves and stems, raw	38	73
Brussels sprouts boiled and drained	36	72
Tomato paste canned	82	70
Artichokes (globe or French), boiled and drained	44	69
Pumpkin pie piecrust made with unenriched flour	211	69
Zwieback	423	69
Mushrooms canned, solids and liquid	17	68
Asparagus spears, frozen, boiled and drained	23	67
Corned beef hash with potatoes, canned	181	67
Light whipping cream	300	67
Lima beans canned, regular, solids and liquid	71	67
Lima beans canned, low sodium, solids and liquid	70	67
Soybean sprouts raw	46	67
Dandelion greens raw	45	66
Frosting chocolate fudge, from mix, made with water and table fat	378	66
Green peas (Alaska), canned, regular, solids and liquid	66	66
Green peas (Alaska), canned, low sodium, solids and liquid	55	66
Baked potatoes with skin	93	65
Chinese water chestnuts raw	79	65
Gingerbread homemade from enriched flour	317	65
Asparagus cuts and tips, frozen, boiled and drained	22	64
Mung bean sprouts raw	35	64
Potato salad homemade with cooked salad dressing and seasonings	99	64
Collards leaves and stems, raw	40	63
Dates (domestic), dry	274	63
Mixed vegetables (carrots, corn, peas, green snap beans, and lima beans), frozen, boiled and drained	64	63
Parsley raw	44	63
Asparagus spears, raw	26	62
Broccoli spears, boiled and drained	26	62
Custard pudding (baby food), commercial	100	62
Parsnips boiled and drained	66	62
Tomato soup canned, condensed, prepared with milk	69	62
Brussels sprouts frozen, boiled and drained	33	61
Shallots bulbs, raw	72	60

FOOD ITEM	CALS.	UNITS
Bamboo shoots raw	27	59
Egg noodles enriched, cooked	125	59
Heavy whipping cream	352	59
Green peas (sweet), canned, regular, solids and liquid	57	58
Green peas (sweet), canned, low sodium, solids and liquid	47	58
Sweet potatoes with skin, baked	141	58
Turnip greens leaves and stems, raw	28	58
Peas and carrots frozen, boiled and drained	53	57
Broccoli chopped, frozen, boiled and drained	26	56
Cauliflower raw	27	56
Endive (curly endive and escarole), raw	20	54
Spaghetti with cheese in tomato sauce, homemade	104	54
Watercress leaves and stems, raw	19	54
Potatoes with skin, boiled	76	53
Tomato chili sauce bottled	104	52
Collards frozen, boiled and drained	30	51
Fennel leaves, raw	28	51
Kohlrabi thickened bulb-like stems, raw	29	51
Spinach raw	26	51
Swamp cabbage raw	29	51
Asparagus spears, boiled and drained	20	50
Hash-browned potatoes frozen, cooked	224	50
Leeks bulb and lower-leaf portion, raw	52	50
Macaroni enriched or unenriched, cooked until tender	111	50
Mustard greens raw	31	50
Pastry (plain), made with enriched or unenriched flour	500	50
Piecrust commercial	500	50
Soybean sprouts boiled and drained	38	50
Spaghetti enriched, cooked until tender	111	50
Tomato catsup bottled	106	50
Mashed potatoes milk added	65	49
Corn (sweet, white and yellow), canned, regular, solids and liquid	66	48
Corn (sweet, white and yellow), canned, low sodium, solids and liquid	57	48
Garden cress boiled and drained	23	48
Kale frozen, boiled and drained	31	48
Mung bean sprouts boiled and drained	28	48
Soybean milk fluid	33	48
Winter squash baked	63	48

FOOD ITEM	CALS.	UNITS
Blue cheese & Roquefort salad dressing commercial, low calorie	76	47
Mashed potatoes dehydrated, flakes without milk, prepared with water, milk, and table fat	93	47
Raisins cooked, sugar added, fruit and liquid	213	47
Sweet potatoes with skin, boiled	114	47
Kale leaves and stems, boiled and drained	28	46
New Zealand spinach raw	19	46
Beef and vegetable stew canned	79	45
Cornflakes commercial	386	45
Spaghetti with meatballs in tomato sauce, canned	103	45
Chives raw	28	44
Green snap beans raw	32	44
Spinach chopped, frozen, boiled and drained	23	44
Asparagus spears, regular, solids and liquid	16	43
Asparagus spears, canned, low sodium, solids and liquid	16	43
Mustard greens frozen, boiled and drained	20	43
Okra cuts and pods, frozen, boiled and drained	38	43
Sweet potatoes candied	168	43
Yellow snap beans raw	27	43
Avocados raw	167	42
Cauliflower boiled and drained	22	42
Dandelion greens boiled and drained	33	42
Guavas whole, raw	62	42
Lichees raw	64	42
Mashed potatoes frozen	93	42
Kohlrabi thickened bulb-like stems, boiled and drained	24	41
Okra boiled and drained	29	41
Beet greens raw	24	40
Black currants (European), raw	54	40
Chicory greens raw	20	40
Chinese cabbage raw	14	40
Chard (Swiss), raw	25	39
Collards leaves and stems, boiled and drained	29	39
Purslane leaves and stems, raw	21	39
Rutabagas raw	46	39
Spanish rice homemade	87	39
Turnip greens leaves and stems, frozen, boiled and drained	23	39
Cauliflower frozen, boiled and drained	18	38
Spinach boiled and drained	23	38

FOOD ITEM	CALS.	UNITS
Dried peaches cooked without added sugar, fruit and liquid	82	37
Dried peaches cooked, no sugar added	82	37
Dried prunes "softenized," cooked without added sugar, fruit and liquid	119	37
Green snap beans boiled and drained	25	37
Russian salad dressing commercial, regular	494	37
Turnip greens leaves and stems, boiled and drained	20	37
Yellow snap beans boiled and drained	22	37
Apple butter	186	36
Carrots raw	42	36
Ginger root fresh	49	36
Onions raw	38	36
Red cabbage raw	31	35
Spaghetti with cheese in tomato sauce, canned	76	35
Chicken chow mein without noodles, canned	38	34
Fruit pudding (baby food), commercial	96	34
Tomato puree canned, regular or low sodium	39	34
Red beets raw	43	33
Green snap beans cut, frozen, boiled and drained	25	32
Horseradish prepared	38	32
Mustard greens boiled and drained	23	32
Summer squash (yellow crookneck), frozen, boiled and drained	21	32
Swamp cabbage boiled and drained	21	32
Tartar sauce regular	531	32
Tartar sauce low calorie	224	32
Tomatoes ripe, boiled	26	32
Winter squash boiled, mashed	38	32
Carrots boiled and drained	31	31
Radishes raw	17	31
Rutabagas boiled and drained	35	31
Yellow snap beans cut, frozen, boiled and drained	27	31
Beer	42	30
Chicken noodle dinner (baby food), commercial	49	30
Chicken noodle soup canned, condensed	53	30
Dried prunes "softenized," cooked, sugar added, fruit and liquid	172	30
Plantains (baking bananas), raw	119	30
Red peppers (sweet), raw	31	30
Turnip greens leaves and stems, canned, solids and liquid	18	30

FOOD ITEM	CALS.	UNITS
Turnips raw	30	30
Beef noodle dinner (baby food), commercial	48	29
Cabbage raw	24	29
Cane syrup	263	29
Greek olives	338	29
Onions boiled and drained	29	29
Sweet potatoes canned in liquid, solids and liquid, unsweetened	46	29
Sweet potatoes canned in syrup, solids and liquid	114	29
Celery (green and yellow varieties), raw	17	28
Coleslaw made with salad dressing	99	28
Elderberries raw	72	28
Mayonnaise	718	28
New Zealand spinach boiled and drained	13	28
Prickly pears raw	42	28
White rice fully milled or polished, enriched, cooked	109	28
Cucumbers with skin, raw	15	27
Tomatoes ripe, raw	22	27
Bananas raw	85	26
Beef broth, bouillon and consomme canned, condensed	26	26
Chayote raw	28	26
Lettuce (Boston and bibb), raw	14	26
Persimmons (native), raw	127	26
Pumpkin canned	33	26
Radishes (Oriental, including daikon and Chinese), raw	19	26
Spinach canned, regular, solids and liquid	19	26
Spincah canned, low sodium, solids and liquid	21	26
Beet greens boiled and drained	18	25
Cherry pie commercial	261	25
Green beans (baby food), commercial	22	25
Green chili peppers (hot), raw, pods without seeds	37	25
Lettuce (cos and romaine), raw	18	25
Squash (zucchini and cocozelle), boiled and drained	12	25
Chard (Swiss), boiled and drained	18	24
Cornflakes sugar coated, added nutrients	386	24
Lemon candied	314	24
Nectarines raw	64	24
Purslane leaves and stems, boiled and drained	15	24
Turnips boiled and drained	23	24
Apricots raw	51	23

FOOD ITEM	CALS.	UNITS
Blueberry pie commercial	242	23
Dried pears cooked, no added sugar	126	23
Kumquats raw	65	23
Red beets boiled and drained	32	23
Angel food cake homemade	269	22
Apple pie commercial	256	22
Black raspberries raw	73	22
Celery (green and yellow varieties), boiled and drained	14	22
Figs raw	80	22
Green peppers (sweet), raw	22	22
Lettuce (iceberg), raw	13	22
Red cherries (sour), frozen, unsweetened	55	22
Red raspberries raw	57	22
Vegetable juice cocktail canned	17	22
Carrots (baby food), commercial	29	21
Chicory raw	15	21
Eggplant boiled and drained	19	21
Green snap beans canned, regular, solids and liquid	18	21
Green snap beans canned, low sodium, solids and liquid	16	21
Pickles (dill)	11	21
Strawberries raw	37	21
Yellow snap beans canned, regular, solids and liquid	19	21
Yellow snap beans canned, low sodium, solids and liquid	15	21
Barbecue sauce	91	20
Cabbage shredded, boiled and drained	20	20
Carrots canned, regular, solids and liquid	28	20
Carrots canned, low sodium, solids and liquid	22	20
Dried pears cooked, with added sugar, fruit and liquid	151	20
Grapes (European), raw	67	20
Oranges raw	49	20
Prune juice canned or bottled	77	20
Blackberries raw	58	19
Brown sugar (beet or cane)	373	19
Manhattan clam chowder canned, condensed	33	19
Peaches raw	38	19
Peaches canned in juice, fruit and liquid	45	19
Red cherries (sweet), raw	70	19
Red cherries (sour), raw	58	19
Tomato juice canned, concentrate	20	19
Tomatoes ripe, canned, regular, solids and liquid	21	19

FOOD ITEM	CALS.	UNITS
Tomatoes ripe, canned, low sodium, solids and liquid	20	19
Limes raw	28	18
Orange juice canned, unsweetened	48	18
Orange juice canned, sweetened	52	18
Red bananas raw	90	18
Rhubarb raw	16	18
Sauerkraut canned, solids and liquid	18	18
Tangerines raw	46	18
Tomato juice canned or bottled, regular or low sodium	19	18
Blackberries canned in juice, fruit and liquid	54	17
Grapefruit juice frozen concentrate, unsweetened	41	17
Green olives pickled, canned or bottled	116	17
Loganberries raw	62	17
Orange juice fresh, commercial	45	17
Pimientos canned, solids and liquid	27	17
Red beets canned, regular, solids and liquid	34	17
Red beets canned, low sodium, solids and liquid	32	17
Red raspberries frozen, sweetened	98	17
Thousand Island salad dressing commercial, regular	502	17
Thousand Island salad dressing commercial, low calorie	180	17
Apricots canned in water, with or without artificial sweetener, fruit and liquid	38	16
Butter	716	16
Cantaloupe	30	16
Corn syrup (light and dark)	90	16
Grapefruit raw	41	16
Green peppers (sweet), boiled and drained	18	16
Honeydew melon	33	16
Lemons peeled, raw	27	16
Margarine	720	16
Orange juice frozen concentrate, unsweetened	45	16
Orange juice dehydrated	46	16
Pickles (sweet)	146	16
Apricots canned in light syrup, fruit and liquid	66	15
Apricots canned in heavy syrup, fruit and liquid	86	15
Apricots canned in extra-heavy syrup, fruit and liquid	101	15
Gooseberries raw	39	15
Pickles (sour)	10	15
Rhubarb cooked, sugar added	141	15
Cornmeal (white or yellow), degermed, enriched, cooked	50	14

FOOD ITEM	CALS.	UNITS
Figs canned in water, with or without artificial sweetener, fruit and liquid	48	14
French salad dressing commercial, regular	410	14
French salad dressing commercial, low calorie	96	14
Grapefruit canned in water, with or without artificial sweetener, fruit and liquid	30	14
Grapefruit canned in syrup, fruit and liquid	70	14
Grapefruit juice frozen concentrate, sweetened	47	14
Green chili peppers (hot), canned in chili sauce	20	14
Pickle relish (sweet), finely cut or chopped	138	14
Strawberries canned in water, with or without artificial sweetener, fruit and liquid	22	14
Tangerine juice canned, unsweetened	43	14
Tangerine juice frozen concentrate, unsweetened	46	14
Tangerine juice fresh	43	14
Tangerine juice canned, sweetened	50	14
Tomato soup canned, condensed	36	14
Blackberries canned in water, with or without artificial sweetener, fruit and liquid	40	13
Cherries (sweet), canned in water, with or without artificial sweetener, fruit and liquid	48	13
Dried apples cooked, sugar added	112	13
Red cherries (sour), canned in water with or without artificial sweetener, fruit and liquid	43	13
Red cherries (sour), canned in light syrup, fruit and liquid	65	13
Red cherries (sweet), canned in syrup, fruit and liquid	81	13
Red cherries canned in light syrup, fruit and liquid	65	13
Farina enriched, regular, cooked	42	12
Fruit cocktail canned in extra-heavy syrup, fruit and liquid	92	12
Fruit cocktail canned in light syrup, fruit and liquid	60	12
Fruit cocktail canned in heavy syrup, fruit and liquid	76	12
Grape juice canned or bottled	66	12
Grapes (American), raw	69	12
Peaches canned in extra-heavy syrup, fruit and liquid	97	12
Peaches canned in heavy syrup, fruit and liquid	78	12
Rhubarb frozen, cooked, sugar added	143	12
Beef noodle soup from mix, prepared with water	28	11
Fruit salad canned in water, with or without artificial sweetener, fruit and liquid	35	11

FOOD ITEM	CALS.	UNITS
Lime juice fresh, canned or bottled, unsweetened	26	11
Maple sugar	348	11
Pears with skin, raw	61	11
Apples freshly harvested, without skin, raw	54	10
Apples freshly harvested, with skin, raw	58	10
Corn grits degermed, enriched	51	10
Lemon juice canned or bottled, unsweetened	23	10
Lemon juice fresh	25	10
Plums (purple), canned in water, with or without artificial sweetener	46	10
Plums (purple), canned in heavy syrup, fruit and liquid	83	10
Plums (purple), canned in light syrup, fruit and liquid	63	10
Strained bananas (baby food), commercial	84	10
Watermelon raw	26	10
Wine	85	10
Apple juice canned or bottled	47	9
Blueberries canned in water, with or without artificial sweetener, fruit and liquid	39	9
Fruit dessert with tapioca (baby food), commercial	84	9
Jams and preserves	272	9
Pineapple juice canned, unsweetened	55	9
Plums (purple), canned in extra-heavy syrup, fruit and liquid	102	9
Chicken noodle soup from mix	22	8
Maple syrup	252	8
Pineapple raw	52	8
Pineapple canned in juice	58	8
Pineapple juice frozen concentrate, unsweetened	52	8
Pomegranate pulp, raw	63	8
Applesauce (baby food), commercial	72	7
Jellies	273	7
Pears canned in water, with or without artificial sweetener, fruit and liquid	32	7
Pears canned in extra-heavy syrup, fruit and liquid	92	7
Pears canned in light syrup, fruit and liquid	61	7
Pears canned in heavy syrup, fruit and liquid	76	7
Butterscotch candy	397	6
Honey	304	6
Applesauce canned, unsweetened or artificially sweetened	41	5
Italian salad dressing commercial, low calorie	50	5
Pear nectar canned	52	5

FOOD ITEM	CALS.	UNITS
Pineapple canned in extra-heavy syrup, fruit and liquid	90	5
Pineapple all styles except crushed, canned in water, with or without artificial sweetener	39	5
Pineapple canned in light syrup, fruit and liquid	59	5
Pineapple canned in heavy syrup, fruit and liquid	74	5
Coffee instant	1	4
Cranberry sauce canned, sweetened, strained	146	4
Grape drink canned	54	4
Grape juice frozen concentrate, sweetened	53	4
Italian salad dressing commercial, regular	552	4
Cranberry juice cocktail bottled	65	3
Lemonade frozen concentrate	44	1
Limeade frozen concentrate	41	1
Syrup cane and maple blend	252	1

Potassium

FOOD ITEM	CALS.	UNITS
Kelp raw	N.A.	5273
Blackstrap molasses (cane)	213	2927
Irish moss (seaweed), raw	N.A.	2844
Torula yeast	277	2046
Brewer's yeast debittered	283	1894
Soybean flour defatted	326	1820
Skim milk dry, regular	363	1745
Potato flour	351	1588
Rice bran	276	1495
Banana powder	340	1477
Almond meal partially defatted	408	1400
Whole milk dry	502	1330
Peanut flour defatted	371	1186
Potato chips	568	1130
Potato sticks	544	1130
Wheat bran crude, commercially milled	213	1121
Lichees dried	277	1100
Sunflower seed flour partially defatted	339	1080
Dried apricots uncoooked	260	979
Pistachio nuts	594	972
Dried peaches uncooked	262	950
Wheat germ toasted	391	947

FOOD ITEM	CALS.	UNITS
Tomato paste canned	82	888
Chestnuts dried	377	875
French fried potatoes	274	853
Baking chocolate	505	830
Bitter chocolate	505	830
Wheat germ commercially milled	363	827
New Zealand spinach raw	19	795
Almonds dried	598	773
Almonds roasted and salted	627	773
Raisins	289	763
Parsley raw	44	727
Sesame seeds dry, whole	563	725
Brazil nuts	654	715
Rice polish	265	714
Filberts (hazelnuts)	634	704
Peanuts with skins, roasted	582	701
Dried prunes uncooked	255	694
Peanuts without skins, raw	568	674
Peanut butter	581	670
French fried potatoes frozen	220	652
Dates (domestic), dried, unsulfured	274	648
Dried figs	274	640
Lima beans dry, boiled and drained	138	612
Baker's yeast compressed	86	610
Garden cress raw	32	606
Avocados raw	167	604
Pecans	687	603
Rye wafers whole grain	344	600
Coconut meat dried, unsweetened	662	588
Flounder baked	202	587
Dried pears uncoooked	268	573
Beet greens raw	24	570
Dried apples uncooked	275	569
Sardines (Atlantic), canned in oil, solids and liquid	311	560
Chard (Swiss), raw	25	550
Parsnips raw	76	541
Soybeans dry, cooked	130	540
Bamboo shoots raw	27	533
Garlic cloves raw	137	529
Halibut (Atlantic and Pacific), broiled	171	525

FOOD ITEM	CALS.	UNITS
Baked potatoes with skin	93	503
Chinese water chestnuts raw	79	500
Dark fruitcake homemade	379	496
Scallops (bay and sea), steamed	112	476
Hash-browned potatoes	229	475
Spinach raw	26	470
Rye whole grain	334	467
Cashew nuts	561	464
New Zealand spinach boiled and drained	13	463
Black walnuts	628	460
Chestnuts fresh	194	454
Gingerbread homemade from enriched flour	317	454
Pumpernickel bread	246	454
Hamburger regular ground, cooked	286	450
Walnuts	651	450
Rockfish oven steamed	107	446
Salmon broiled or baked	182	443
Bran muffins homemade from enriched flour	261	431
Lima beans frozen, boiled and drained	99	426
Tomato puree canned, regular or low sodium	39	426
Cane syrup	263	425
Lima beans boiled and drained	111	422
Chicory greens raw	20	420
Mushrooms raw	28	414
Chicken all classes, light meat, roasted, without skin	166	411
Cod broiled	170	407
Potatoes with skin, boiled	76	407
Collards leaves and stems, raw	40	401
Dandelion greens raw	45	397
Fennel leaves, raw	28	397
Baby lima beans frozen, boiled and drained	118	394
Plantains (baking bananas), raw	119	385
Graham crackers plain	384	384
Broccoli spears, raw	32	382
Cowpeas (including black-eyed peas), boiled and drained	108	379
Parsnips boiled and drained	66	379
Kale leaves and stems, raw	38	378
Mustard greens raw	31	377
Shad baked	201	377
Oatmeal (baby food), commercial	375	374

FOOD ITEM	CALS.	UNITS
Black currants (European), raw	54	372
Kohlrabi thickened bulb-like stems, raw	29	372
Red bananas raw	90	370
Whole wheat flour	333	370
Soy sauce	68	366
Tomato catsup bottled	106	363
Apricots canned in juice, solids and liquid	54	362
Raisins cooked, sugar added, fruit and liquid	213	355
Coconut meat shredded, dried, sweetened	548	353
Garden cress boiled and drained	23	353
Cowpeas (including black-eyed peas), canned, solids and liquid	70	352
Haddock fried	165	348
Shredded wheat (cereal)	354	348
Leeks bulb and lower leaf, raw	52	347
Brown sugar beet or cane	373	344
Carrots raw	42	341
Celery (green and yellow varieties), raw	17	341
Puffed wheat (cereal)	363	340
Red beans dry, boiled and drained	118	340
Black-eyed peas frozen, boiled and drained	130	337
Red beets raw	43	335
Miso (fermented soybean product)	171	334
Spinach chopped, frozen, boiled and drained	23	333
Beet greens boiled and drained	18	332
Dried prunes cooked, without added sugar, fruit and liquid	119	327
Dried prunes cooked, no added sugar	119	327
Beef kidneys braised	252	324
Coconut cream (from grated coconut)	334	324
Spinach boiled and drained	23	324
Radishes raw	17	322
Chard Swiss, boiled and drained	18	321
Chicken all classes, dark meat, roasted, without skin	176	321
Sardines (Pacific), canned in tomato sauce, solids and liquid	197	320
Potato salad homemade with cooked salad dressing and seasonings	99	319
Condensed milk canned, sweetened	321	314
Persimmons (native), raw	127	310
Evaporated milk canned, unsweetened	137	303
Artichokes (globe or French), boiled and drained	44	301

FOOD ITEM	CALS.	UNITS
Tuna canned in oil, solids and liquid	288	301
Celeriac root, raw	40	300
Elderberries raw	72	300
Sweet potatoes with skin, baked	141	300
Dried peaches cooked, no sugar added	82	297
Split peas cooked	115	296
Brussels sprouts frozen, boiled and drained	33	295
Cauliflower raw	27	295
Endive (curly endive and escarole), raw	20	294
Nectarines raw	64	294
Whole wheat rolls and buns commercial	257	292
Whitefish (lake), stuffed, baked	215	291
Horseradish prepared	38	290
Guavas whole, raw	62	289
Tomatoes ripe, boiled	26	287
Mashed potatoes from flakes	93	286
Ocean perch (Atlantic), fried	227	284
Hash-browned potatoes frozen, cooked	224	283
Chocolate syrup (thin)	245	282
Watercress leaves and stems, raw	19	282
Apricots raw	51	281
Tuna canned in water, solids and liquid	127	279
Asparagus spears, raw	26	278
Gingerbread from mix	276	274
Whole wheat bread made with 2% nonfat dry milk	243	273
Pork sausage links, bulk, cooked	476	269
Red cabbage raw	31	268
Spaghetti with meatballs in tomato sauce, homemade	134	268
Turnips raw	28	268
Broccoli spears, boiled and drained	26	267
Ginger root fresh	49	264
Lettuce (Boston and bibb), raw	14	264
Lobster salad	110	264
Macadamia nuts	691	264
Red beans canned, solids and liquid	90	264
Frankfurters and beans canned	144	262
Mashed potatoes milk added	65	261
Kohlrabi thickened bulb-like stems, boiled and drained	24	260
Pomegranate pulp, raw	63	259
Coconut meat fresh	346	256

FOOD ITEM	CALS.	UNITS
Chinese cabbage raw	14	253
Apple butter	186	252
Cantaloupe	30	251
Honeydew melon	33	251
Rhubarb raw	16	251
Chives raw	28	250
Potatoes canned, solids and liquid	44	250
Spinach canned, low sodium, solids and liquid	19	250
Lentils whole, dry, cooked	106	249
Natto (fermented soybean product)	167	249
Apricots canned in water, with or without artificial sweetener, fruit and liquid	38	246
Succotash frozen, boiled and drained	93	246
Buckwheat pancakes and waffles from mix, made with eggs and milk	200	245
Dried pears sugar added, fruit and liquid	151	244
Ice cream cones	377	244
Tomatoes ripe, raw	22	244
Green snap beans raw	32	243
Sweet potatoes with skin, boiled	114	243
Turnip greens leaves and stems, canned, solids and liquid	18	243
Yellow snap beans raw	27	243
Maple sugar	348	242
Pumpkin canned	33	240
Apricots canned in light syrup, fruit and liquid	66	239
Celery (green and yellow varieties), boiled and drained	14	239
Rutabagas raw	46	239
Asparagus spears, frozen, boiled and drained	23	238
Creamed pollack	128	238
Bacon cured, boiled or fried, drained	611	236
Collards frozen, boiled and drained	30	236
Kumquats raw	65	236
Prune juice canned or bottled	77	235
Sturgeon steamed	160	235
Tomato juice canned concentrate	20	235
Apricots canned in heavy syrup, fruit and liquid	86	234
Collards leaves and stems, boiled and drained	29	234
Papayas raw	39	234
Cabbage raw	24	233

FOOD ITEM	CALS.	UNITS
Chile con carne with beans, canned	133	233
Light fruitcake homemade	389	233
Beef heart lean, braised	188	232
Dandelion greens boiled and drained	33	232
Corn on the cob frozen, boiled and drained	94	231
Spanish rice homemade	87	231
Apricots canned in extra-heavy syrup, fruit and liquid	101	230
Bologna	304	230
Malt extract dried	367	230
Cowpeas (including black-eyed peas), dry, cooked	76	229
French fried shrimp	225	229
Tomato juice canned or bottled, regular or low sodium	19	227
Mung bean sprouts raw	35	223
Carrots boiled and drained	31	222
Lima beans canned, regular, solids and liquid	71	222
Lima beans canned, low sodium, solids and liquid	70	222
Tomato juice cocktail canned or bottled	21	221
Asparagus cuts and tips, frozen, boiled and drained	22	220
Mustard greens boiled and drained	23	220
Split pea soup canned, condensed	118	220
Tomatoes canned, regular, solids and liquid	21	217
Tomatoes canned, low sodium, solids and liquid	20	217
Bread pudding with raisins, commercial	187	215
Mashed potatoes frozen, heated	93	215
Green peppers (sweet), raw	22	213
Broccoli chopped, frozen, boiled and drained	26	212
Red beets boiled and drained	32	208
Rice cereal (baby food), commercial	371	208
Cauliflower frozen, boiled and drained	18	207
Cauliflower boiled and drained	22	206
Peaches canned in juice, fruit and liquid	45	205
Oysters fried	239	203
Rhubarb cooked, sugar added	141	203
Rye flour medium	350	203
Peaches raw	38	202
Corned beef hash with potatoes, canned	181	200
Orange juice fresh, commercial	45	200
Oranges raw	49	200
Pickles (dill)	11	200
Black raspberries raw	73	199

FOOD ITEM	CALS.	UNITS
Orange juice canned, unsweetened	48	199
Mushrooms canned, soilds and liquid	17	197
Corn on the cob (white and yellow), boiled and drained	91	196
Ice milk	152	195
Figs raw	80	194
Kale frozen, boiled and drained	31	193
Caramels plain or chocolate	299	192
Coleslaw made with salad dressing	99	192
Mixed vegetables (carrots, corn, peas, green snap beans, and lima beans), frozen, boiled and drained	64	191
Red cherries (sour) raw	58	191
Red cherries (sweet), raw	70	191
Brownies with nuts, homemade from enriched flour	485	190
Sweet potatoes candied	168	190
Chicken chow mein without noodles, homemade	102	189
Mangoes raw	66	189
Red cherries (sour), frozen, unsweetened	55	188
Tomato soup canned, condensed	72	188
Turnips boiled and drained	23	188
Orange juice frozen concentrate, unsweetened	45	186
Corn sweet, frozen, boiled and drained	79	184
Asparagus spears, boiled and drained	20	183
Chicory raw	15	182
Carrots (baby food), commercial	29	181
Frozen custard medium fat content 10%	193	181
Ice cream medium fat content 10%	193	181
Caviar (sturgeon)	262	180
Goat's milk	67	180
Lobster (northern), canned or cooked	95	180
Radishes (Oriental, including daikon and Chinese), raw	19	180
Rice flakes (cereal)	390	180
Tangerine juice fresh	43	178
Tangerine juice canned, sweetened	50	178
Tangerine juice canned, unsweetened	43	178
Rice pudding with raisins, commercial	146	177
Maple syrup	252	176
Rhubarb frozen, cooked, sugar added	143	176
Lettuce (iceberg), raw	13	175
Barbecue sauce	91	174
Beef and vegetable stew canned	79	174

FOOD ITEM	CALS.	UNITS
Okra boiled and drained	29	174
Tangerine juice frozen concentrate, unsweetened	46	174
Grapes (European), raw	67	173
Chocolate pudding homemade	148	171
Blackberries raw	58	170
Blackberries canned in juice, fruit and liquid	54	170
Chop suey with meat, homemade	120	170
Grapefruit juice frozen concentrate, unsweetened	41	170
Lichees raw	64	170
Loganberries raw	62	170
Peas edible, podded, raw	53	170
Plums (prune type), raw	75	170
Corn pudding	104	169
Fruit cocktail canned in water, with or without artificial sweetener, fruit and liquid	37	168
Pizza with sausage	234	168
Red raspberries raw	57	168
Chicken chow mein without noodles, canned	38	167
Red beets canned, regular, solids and liquid	34	167
Red beets canned, low sodium, solids and liquid	32	167
Rutabagas boiled and drained	35	167
Summer squash (yellow crookneck), frozen, boiled and drained	21	167
Tomato soup canned, condensed, prepared with milk	69	167
Asparagus spears, canned, regular, solids and liquid	18	166
Asparagus spears, canned, low sodium, solids and liquid	16	166
Prickly pears raw	42	166
Beef tongue meduim fat content, braised	244	164
Fruit cocktail canned in light syrup, fruit and liquid	60	164
Okra cuts and pods, frozen, boiled and drained	38	164
Strawberries raw	37	164
Yellow snap beans cut, frozen, boiled and drained	27	164
Cabbage shredded, boiled and drained	20	163
Spaghetti with cheese in tomato sauce, homemade	104	163
Grapefruit juice fresh	39	162
Grapefruit juice canned, sweetened	53	162
Grapefruit juice canned, unsweetened	41	162
Fruit cocktail canned in heavy syrup, fruit and liquid	76	161
Cucumbers with skin, raw	15	160
Pumpkin pie homemade from unenriched flour	211	160

FOOD ITEM	CALS.	UNITS
Beef noodle dinner (baby food), commercial	48	159
Fruit cocktail canned in extra-heavy syrup, fruit and liquid	92	159
Grapes (American), raw	69	158
Cornbread (southern style), homemade from whole-ground cornmeal	207	157
Mustard greens frozen, boiled and drained	20	157
Onions raw	38	157
Peas and carrots frozen, boiled and drained	53	157
Russian salad dressing regular, commercial	494	157
Mung bean sprouts boiled and drained	28	156
Figs canned in water, with or without artificial sweetener, fruit and liquid	48	155
Gooseberries raw	39	155
Chocolate cake with chocolate frosting, homemade	369	154
Pancakes from mix, made with eggs and milk	225	154
Breadcrumbs dry, grated	392	152
Figs canned in light syrup, fruit and liquid	65	152
Green snap beans cut, frozen, boiled and drained	25	152
Apricot nectar canned	57	151
Green snap beans boiled and drained	25	151
Yellow snap beans boiled and drained	22	151
Baking powder	129	150
Corned beef medium fat content, cooked	372	150
Eggplant boiled and drained	19	150
Popovers homemade with enriched flour	224	150
Swamp cabbage raw	29	150
Zwieback	423	150
Figs canned in heavy syrup, fruit and liquid	84	149
Parmesan cheese	393	149
Peppers sweet, boiled and drained	18	149
Pineapple juice canned, unsweetened	55	149
Turnip greens leaves and stems, frozen, boiled and drained	23	149
Hot chocolate homemade	95	148
Plums (purple), canned in water, with or without artificial sweetener,fruit and liquid	46	148
Coconut water	22	147
Pineapple canned in juice, fruit and liquid	58	147
Chocolate milk	85	146
Custard baked, commercial	115	146
Eggs scrambled	173	146

FOOD ITEM	CALS.	UNITS
Figs canned in extra-heavy syrup, fruit and liquid	103	146
Omelets	173	146
Pineapple raw	52	146
Hot cocoa homemade	97	145
Plums canned in light syrup, fruit and liquid	63	145
Rye bread (American), commercial	243	145
Skim milk	36	145
Dried apples cooked, with sugar added	112	144
Grapefruit canned in water, with or without artificial sweetener, fruit and liquid	30	144
Grapefruit juice frozen concentrate, sweetened	47	144
Whole milk 3.5% fat	65	144
Yogurt made from partially skimmed milk	50	143
Plums canned in heavy syrup, fruit and liquid	83	142
Lemon juice fresh	25	141
Lemon juice canned or bottled, unsweetened	23	141
Summer squash boiled and drained	14	141
Buttermilk cultured	36	140
Clams canned, solids and liquid	52	140
Eggs fried	216	140
Sauerkraut juice canned	10	140
Fruit salad canned in water, with or without artificial sweetener, fruit and liquid	35	139
Plums canned in extra-heavy syrup, fruit and liquid	102	139
Chop suey with meat, canned	62	138
Lemons peeled, raw	27	138
Vanilla pudding homemade	111	138
Welsh rarebit	179	138
Peaches canned in water, with or without artificial sweetener, fruit and liquid	31	137
Fruit salad canned in light syrup, fruit and liquid	59	136
Pineapple juice frozen concentrate, unsweetened	52	136
Pudding chocolate, from mix, made with milk, cooked	124	136
Corn muffins homemade from enriched degermed cornmeal	314	135
Grapefruit raw	41	135
Grapefruit canned in syrup, fruit and liquid	70	135
Green peas frozen, boiled and drained	68	135
Cracked wheat bread commercial	263	134
Fruit salad canned in heavy syrup, fruit and liquid	75	134
Corn fritters commercial	377	133

FOOD ITEM	CALS.	UNITS
Peaches canned in light syrup, fruit and liquid	58	133
Corn muffins homemade from whole-ground cornmeal	288	132
Roe (cod and shad), baked or broiled	126	132
Yogurt made from whole milk	62	132
Fruit salad canned in extra-heavy syrup, fruit and liquid	90	131
Brown mustard prepared	91	130
Cherries (sweet), canned in water, with or without artificial sweetener, fruit and liquid	48	130
Peaches canned in heavy syrup, fruit and liquid	78	130
Pears with skin, raw	61	130
Pears canned in juice, solids and liquid	46	130
Pizza with cheese, homemade	236	130
Pretzels	390	130
Red cherries (sour), canned in water, fruit and liquid	43	130
Yellow mustard prepared	75	130
Eggs hard-boiled	163	129
Half-and-half cream	134	129
Cherries (sweet), canned in light syrup, fruit and liquid	65	128
Eggs poached	163	128
Peaches canned in extra-heavy syrup, fruit and liquid	97	128
Cornbread from mix, made with eggs, and milk	233	127
Red cherries (sour), canned in light syrup, fruit and liquid	74	126
Tangerines raw	46	126
Muffins plain, homemade from enriched or unenriched flour	294	125
Red cherries (sour), canned in heavy syrup, fruit and liquid	89	124
Sweet rolls commercial	316	124
Cherries (sweet) canned in extra-heavy syrup, fruit and liquid	100	123
Pancakes homemade from enriched or unenriched flour	231	123
Pecan pie piecrust made with unenriched flour	418	123
Rolls from mix	299	123
Eclairs with custard filling and chocolate frosting, commercial	239	122
Red cherries (sour), canned in extra-heavy syrup, fruit and liquid	112	121
Spaghetti with cheese in tomato sauce, canned	76	121
Carrots canned, regular, solids and liquid	28	120
Carrots canned, low sodium, solids and liquid	22	120
Cornflakes (cereal)	386	120
Lemon candied	314	120
Pea soup canned, condensed	53	120
Sweet potatoes canned in liquid, solids and liquid	46	120

FOOD ITEM	CALS.	UNITS
Peas edible podded, boiled and drained	43	119
Strained bananas (baby food), commercial	84	118
Baking powder biscuits homemade from enriched flour	369	117
Chocolate chip cookies homemade from enriched flour	516	117
Rolls and buns homemade	339	117
Biscuits from mix, with enriched flour, prepared with milk	325	116
Grape juice canned or bottled	66	116
White cake with chocolate frosting, from mix, made with egg whites and water	351	116
Blackberries canned in water, with or without artificial sweetener, fruit and liquid	40	115
Blueberry muffins homemade	281	115
Beef with vegetables (baby food), commercial	87	113
Thousand Island salad dressing regular	502	113
Thousand Island salad dressing low calorie	180	113
Danish pastry commercial	422	112
Blackberries canned in light syrup, fruit and liquid	72	111
Strawberries canned in water, with or without artificial sweetener, fruit and liquid	22	111
Apples freshly harvested, with skin, raw	58	110
Apples freshly harvested, without skin, raw	54	110
Corn muffins from mix, made with eggs and milk	324	110
Crab canned	101	110
Onions boiled and drained	29	110
Blackberries canned in heavy syrup, fruit and liquid	91	109
Cheese crackers commmercial	479	109
Beef broth, bouillon, and consomme canned, condensed	26	108
Blackberries canned in extra-heavy syrup, fruit and liquid	110	107
Pie (cherry), piecrust made with unenriched flour	261	105
Corn muffins from mix, made with eggs and water	294	104
Lime juice canned or bottled, unsweetened	26	104
Swiss cheese (domestic), unprocessed	370	104
Light whipping cream	300	102
Apple juice canned or bottled	47	101
Cider vinegar	14	100
Puffed rice (cereal)	399	100
Watermelon raw	26	100
Pineapple all styles except crushed, canned in water, with or without artificial	39	99

FOOD ITEM	CALS.	UNITS
Spaghetti with meatballs in tomato sauce, canned	103	98
Corn (sweet, white and yellow), canned, regular, solids	66	97
Corn (sweet, white and yellow), canned, low sodium, solids and liquid	57	97
Hard rolls enriched, commercial	312	97
Pineapple canned in light syrup, fruit and liquid	74	97
Green peas (sweet), low sodium, solids and liquid	47	96
Green peas (sweet), canned, regular, solids and liquid	57	96
Green peas (Alaska), canned, regular, solids and liquid	65	96
Green peas (Alaska), canned, low sodium, solids and liquid	55	96
Pineapple canned in heavy syrup, fruit and liquid	74	96
Bread flour enriched or unenriched	365	95
Green snap beans canned, regular, solids and liquid	18	95
Green snap beans canned, low sodium, solids and liquid	16	95
Rolls and buns plain, commercial, enriched	312	95
Yellow snap beans canned, regular, solids and liquid	19	95
Yellow snap beans canned, low sodium, solids and liquid	15	95
Cake or pastry flour	364	94
Custard pudding (baby food), commercial	100	94
Pineapple canned in extra-heavy syrup, fruit and liquid	90	94
Green beans (baby food), commercial	22	93
Wine	85	92
Doughnuts cake type	391	90
French bread enriched or unenriched	290	90
Heavy whipping cream	352	89
Angel food cake homemade	269	88
Jams and preserves	272	88
Pears canned in water, with or without artificial sweetener, fruit and liquid	32	88
Swamp cabbage boiled and drained	21	88
Boysenberries canned in water, with or without artificial sweetener, fruit and liquid	36	85
Cottage cheese creamed	106	85
Pears canned in light syrup, fruit and liquid	61	85
White bread made with 1% - 2% nonfat dry milk	269	85
Pears canned in heavy syrup, fruit and liquid	76	84
Pears canned in extra-heavy syrup, fruit and liquid	92	83
Cheddar cheese unprocessed	398	82
Cranberries raw	46	82
American cheese pasteurized, processed	370	80

FOOD ITEM	CALS.	UNITS
French salad dressing commercial, regular	410	79
French salad dressing commercial, low calorie	96	79
Plain cake or cupcakes homemade, without icing	364	79
Applesauce canned, unsweetened or artificially sweetened	41	78
Peach nectar canned	48	78
Tartar sauce regular	531	78
Tartar sauce low calorie	224	78
White cake homemade, without icing	375	76
Fruit pudding (baby food), commercial	96	75
Jellies	273	75
Manhattan clam chowder canned, condensed	33	75
Cream cheese natural	374	74
Italian bread enriched or unenriched	276	74
Fruit dessert with tapioca (baby food), commercial	84	73
Cottage cheese uncreamed	86	72
Chicken with vegetables (baby food), commercial	100	71
Brown rice cooked	119	70
Assorted cookies commercial	480	67
Applesauce canned, sweetened	91	65
Blueberry pie piecrust made with unenriched flour	242	65
Frosting (chocolate fudge), from mix, made with water and table fat	378	63
Chicken and noodles homemade	153	62
Macaroni enriched or unenriched, cooked until tender	111	61
Spaghetti enriched, cooked until tender	111	61
Blueberries canned in water, with or without artificial sweetener, fruit and liquid	39	60
Gluten flour	378	60
Pound cake homemade	473	60
Piecrust from mix	464	56
Blueberries canned in extra-heavy syrup, fruit and liquid	101	55
Green olives pickled, canned or bottled	116	55
Honey	304	51
Piecrust made with enriched or unenriched flour	500	50
Chicken noodle soup canned, condensed	53	46
Pastry plain, made with enriched or unenriched flour	500	46
Egg noodles enriched, cooked	125	44
Chicken noodle dinner (baby food), commercial	49	42
Tofu (soybean curd)	72	42
Pear nectar canned	52	39

FOOD ITEM	CALS.	UNITS
Blue cheese & Roquefort salad dressing commercial, regular	504	37
Coffee instant	1	36
Grape drink canned	54	35
Blue cheese and Roquefort cheese special dietary, commercial	76	34
Grape juice frozen concentrate, sweetened	53	34
Mayonnaise	718	34
Marmalade citrus	257	33
Cranberry sauce canned, sweetened, strained	146	30
White rice fully milled or polished, enriched	109	28
Maple syrup (cane and maple)	252	26
Beer 4.5% alcohol by volume	42	25
Tea instant	2	25
Butter	716	23
Margarine	720	23
Orange sherbet	134	22
Beef noodle soup from mix	28	17
Cornmeal (white or yellow), degermed, enriched, cooked	50	16
Lemonade frozen concentrate	44	16
Limeade frozen concentrate	41	13
Tomato vegetable soup with noodles from mix	27	12
Corn grits degermed, enriched, cooked	51	11
Cranberry juice cocktail bottled	65	10
Farina enriched, regular, cooked	42	9
Chicken noodle soup from mix	22	8
Corn syrup (light and dark)	290	4
Salt	0	4
Sugar (beet or cane), granulated	385	3
Sugar (beet or cane), powdered	385	3
Alcoholic beverages gin, rum, vodka, and whisky	231	2
Butterscotch candy	397	2
Cornstarch	362	0
Oat cereal with toasted wheat germ and soy grits, cooked	62	0
Rice cereal cooked	50	0

Index

P=Protein, C=Carbohydrates, F=Fat, Ch=Cholesterol, Fi=Fiber, S=Sodium, V=Vitamins, M=Minerals

---

P=Protein, **C**=Carbohydrates, **F**=Fat, **Ch**=Cholesterol, **Fi**=Fiber, **S**=Sodium, **V**=Vitamins, **M**=Minerals

---

P=Protein, C=Carbohydrates, F=Fat, Ch=Cholesterol, Fi=Fiber, S=Sodium, V=Vitamins, M=Minerals

Cocoa powder, high fat content, processed with alkali C48
Cocoa powder, high fat, with alkali V184
Cocoa powder, high to medium fat content P14
Cocoa powder, low fat P13, F73, Fi104, S139, V166, 184
Cocoa powder, low to medium fat content P14, V184
Cocoa powder, medium fat V185
Cocoa powder, medium fat content F68
Cocoa powder, medium fat, processed with alkali V184
Cocoa powder, with nonfat dry milk C46, V184
Coconut bar P21
Coconut bar cookies F67
Coconut (chocolate-coated) P26, F68
Coconut cream P23, F65, V180, 217, M241, 250, 267, 282
Coconut custard pie P21, C50, F70
Coconut custard pie, from mix F73
Coconut custard pie, frozen F71
Coconut, dried, unsweetened C50
Coconut, fresh V203
Coconut frosting P28, F73
Coconut meat, dried, shredded, sweetened M240, 250, 267
Coconut meat, dried, sweetened P20, 24, V175, 194
Coconut meat, dried, unsweetened F63, Fi105, M238, 248, 280
Coconut meat, fresh P25, F65, Fi105, S137, V176, 197, 215, M242, 251, 268, 283
Coconut meat, shredded, dried, sweetened Fi104, V177, 195, M282
Coconut meat, shredded, sweetened F65
Coconut milk P25, F67, V178, 199, 216, M240, 251, 268
Coconut oil V221
Coconut water F81, V183, 199, 204, 216, M239, 260, 288
Cod, boiled P11, C55, F74, S135, V161, 173, 189, M237, 253, 265, 281
Cod, canned V191, 201, 205
Cod, dehydrated V200
Cod, dehydrated, lightly salted P10, V205
Cod, dried, lightly salted V185
Cod, dried, salted P11, V221
Coffee, instant P31, C55, S142, M246, 262, 279, 294
Coffee, instant, powder P21, S135, M247
Coho salmon, canned F73
Colas C52
Coleslaw, made with French dressing P30
Coleslaw, made with mayonnaise P29
Coleslaw, made with salad dressing Fi110, M236, 274, 286

Coleslaw, made with salas dressing V161, 176, 193
Coleslaw, with French dressing F69, 71
Collard greens, boiled P24
Collards, boiled F81
Collards, frozen, boiled Fi108, S137, V153, 175, 188, 208, M231, 254, 271, 284
Collards, leaves and stems, boiled Fi109, S137, V171, 187, 207, M231, 256, 272, 284
Collards, leaves and stems, cooked V153
Collards, leaves and stems, raw Fi109, S136, V153, 170, 206, M231, 254, 270, 281
Collards, leaves, boiled V153, 206, 207
Collards, leaves only, raw V206
Collards, leaves, raw V152
Collards, raw C53
Condensed milk M263
Condensed milk, canned, sweetened P19, S135, V159, 173, 185, 203, 205, 217, M265, 282
Condensed milk, reconstituted V223
Condensed milk, sweetened C47, F73, M231
Condiments See specific type
Consomme See specific type
Cookies See also specific type
Cookies (chocolate) P20, F69
Cookies, plain F67
Cookies, plain, from mix V219
Cookies (sandwich) P23, F67
Cookies (shortbread) F67
Corn F81, V221
Corn beef hash, with potatoes, canned S131, M242
Corn bread (Johnny cake) P18
Corn bread, made with degermed meal F74
Corn, canned P27, V201
Corn flakes C45
Corn flakes and puffed corn (cereal), sugar coated Fi113
Corn flakes (cereal) Fi113
Corn flour P19, C45, F77, Fi110, V159, 170, 192, 222, M245, 250
Corn fritters P19, C48, F67, Fi112, S131, V159, 171, 187, 216, M234, 266, 289
Corn, frozen, boiled M255
Corn grits, cooked P30, C52, V222
Corn grits, degermed P18, F81
Corn grits, degermed, cooked S134
Corn grits, degermed, enriched V195, M278
Corn grits, degermed, enriched, cooked Fi117, V163, 177, M246, 260, 294
Corn muffins, from mix S132
Corn muffins, from mix, made with eggs and milk Fi116, S131, V160, 170, 187, M251, 264, 291

P=Protein, C=Carbohydrates, F=Fat, Ch=Cholesterol, Fi=Fiber, S=Sodium, V=Vitamins, M=Minerals

P=Protein, C=Carbohydrates, F=Fat, Ch=Cholesterol, Fi=Fiber, S=Sodium, V=Vitamins, M=Minerals

Fruit pie   *See specific type*
Fruit pudding (baby food)   **P**30, **F**82,
  Fi115, **S**134, **V**162, 178, 194, 215, **M**238,
  260, 273, 293
Fruit salad   **P**31
Fruit salad, canned in extra-heavy syrup
  Fi114, **S**143, **V**158, 216, **M**244, 261, 290
Fruit salad, canned in heavy syrup   **Fi**114,
  S143, **V**158, 216, **M**244, 261, 289
Fruit salad, canned in light syrup   **Fi**114,
  S142, **V**158, 216, **M**244, 261, 289
Fruit salad, canned in water   **Fi**113, **S**142,
  V158, 182, 215, **M**244, 260, 277, 289
Fruits   *See specific type*
Fudge (chocolate-coated), with caramel and
  peanuts   **P**19, **F**67, 68

G

Garden cress   **V**152
Garden cress, boiled   **Fi**109, **V**153, 175,
  188, 208, **M**235, 255, 271, 282
Garden cress, raw   **Fi**108, **S**137, **V**174,
  185, 200, 206, **M**233, 252, 269, 280
Garlic cloves, raw   **P**21, **C**49, **F**82, **Fi**107,
  S137, **V**166, 170, 191, 210, **M**238, 251,
  265, 280
Gelatin dessert   **P**29
Gelatin dessert powder   **P**18, **S**132
Gelatin, dry   **P**10, **F**82
Giblets, simmered   **P**13
Ginger root   **C**53
Ginger root (candied)   **F**82
Ginger root, fresh   **P**29, **F**80, **Fi**108, **S**139,
  V166, 180, 194, 215, **M**239, 249, 273, 283
Ginger snaps   **P**22, **F**72
Gingerbread   **C**47
Gingerbread cake, from mix   **P**25
Gingerbread, from mix   **S**132, **V**178, 191,
  M233, 268, 283
Gingerbread, homemade   **P**24, **F**72, **Fi**117,
  S133, **V**163, 172, 189, **M**234, 249, 270, 281
Gingerroot (candied)   **Fi**110
Gingersnaps   **C**45
Gizzards   *See specific type*
Gluten flour   **F**78, **Fi**114, **M**236, 266, 293
Goat's milk   **P**25, **C**54, **F**76, **S**136, **V**177,
  189, 203, 206, 217, **M**232, 268, 286
Gooseberries, canned in extra-heavy syrup
  V161
Gooseberries, canned in heavy syrup
  V161, 211
Gooseberries, canned in water   **V**161, 211
Gooseberries, raw   **P**31, **F**82, **Fi**106, **S**143,
  V160, 205, 208, **M**240, 258, 276, 288
Graham crackers (chocolate-coated)   **F**67
Graham crackers (chocolate-covered)
  P22
Graham crackers, honey-coated   **P**20, **F**71

Graham crackers, plain   **P**19, **Fi**108, **S**130,
  V177, 186, **M**236, 251, 266, 281
Grains   *See specific type*
Grape drink, canned   **Fi**118, **S**143, **V**182,
  199, 210, **M**246, 262, 279, 294
Grape juice, canned or bottled   **P**31,
  Fi118, **S**141, **V**177, 197, 219, **M**243, 261,
  277, 291
Grape juice, frozen concentrate, sweetened
  C52, **Fi**118, **S**143, **V**180, 195, 210, **M**246,
  262, 279, 294
Grape juice, frozen, sweetened   **V**204
Grapefruit, canned in juice   **S**143, **V**166
Grapefruit, canned in syrup   **S**143, **V**166,
  208, **M**242, 261, 277, 289
Grapefruit, canned in water   **S**139, **V**166,
  178, 197, 204, 208, **M**242, 261, 277, 289
Grapefruit, canned, sweetened   **V**166
Grapefruit juice   **P**55, **Fi**118, **S**143, **V**163,
  177, 197, 208, **M**244, 262
Grapefruit juice and orange juice, blend,
  canned, sweetened   **V**208
Grapefruit juice and orange juice, blend,
  canned, unsweetened   **V**208
Grapefruit juice and orange juice, blend,
  frozen concentrate, un sweeten   **V**207
Grapefruit juice and orange juice, blend,
  frozen, unsweetened   **C**52
Grapefruit juice, canned, sweetened
  Fi118, **V**205, 208, **M**244, 259, 287
Grapefruit juice, canned, unsweetened
  Fi118, **V**208, 223, **M**244, 259, 287
Grapefruit juice, fresh   **M**287
Grapefruit juice, frozen   **C**49
Grapefruit juice, frozen concentrate, sweet-
  ened   **Fi**118, **S**143, **V**166, 179, 199, 208,
  M244, 277, 289
Grapefruit juice, frozen concentrate, un-
  sweetened   **Fi**118, **S**143, **V**166, 177, 197,
  205, 208, **M**243, 276, 287
Grapefruit pulp, raw   **V**177
Grapefruit, raw   **P**31, **C**52, **F**82, **Fi**116,
  S143, **V**163, 180, 204, 222, **M**241, 259,
  276, 289
Grapefruit segments, canned in light syrup
  Fi116
Grapefruit segments, canned in water
  Fi116
Grapes (American), raw   **P**29, **F**80, **Fi**111,
  S140, **V**162, 202, 215, **M**259, 277, 288
Grapes, canned   **P**31
Grapes (European), raw   **P**31, **C**51, **Fi**113,
  S140, **V**176, 196, 215, **M**242, 275, 287
Grapeseed oil   **V**220
Greek olives   **P**27, **C**53, **F**65, **Fi**105, **M**274
Green beans (baby food)   **F**82, **Fi**110,
  S134, **V**159, 192, **M**237, 253, 274, 292
Green beans, boiled   **P**29, **C**53

P=Protein, **C**=Carbohydrates, **F**=Fat, **Ch**=Cholesterol, **Fi**=Fiber, **S**=Sodium, **V**=Vitamins, **M**=Minerals

P=Protein, C=Carbohydrates, F=Fat, Ch=Cholesterol, Fi=Fiber, S=Sodium, V=Vitamins, M=Minerals

Luncheon meat   *See specific type*
Lychees, raw   S140

M

Macadamia nuts   P19, C51, F63, Fi105, V169, 190, M235, 250, 266, 283
Macaroni and cheese, baked, homemade C51, F71, Ch98
Macaroni and cheese, canned   P24, F76, V219
Macaroni, cooked until firm   P22, C50, F83
Macaroni, cooked until tender   P25, Fi117, S143, M244, 271, 293
Macaroni, enriched, cooked until tender V171, 191, M254
Macaroni, tomatoes, meat, and cereal (baby food)   P26, F78, V158
Macaroni, unenriched, cooked until tender V182, 199, M259
Macaroons   P22, F67
Mackerel (Atlantic), broiled   P13, F69, Ch96, V157
Mackerel (Atlantic), canned   P13, V158, 171, 175, 200, 205
Mackerel, broiled   C55
Mackerel, canned   F71
Mackerel (Pacific), canned   P13, F72, V165, 179
Mackerel, salted   P14, F66
Malt, dry   C45, F78
Malt extract, dried   P21, Fi119, S135, V169, 185, M235, 247, 265, 285
Malted milk   P15, 23, F75, V218
Malted milk powder   C46, F73, V184
Mangoes, raw   P32, C51, F83, Fi109, S138, V153, 176, 194, 208, M243, 259, 286
Manhattan clam chowder, canned, condensed   F80, Fi115, S130, 132, V156, 182, 199, M241, 259, 275, 293
Manzanilla olives, ripe   F70
Maple sugar   C45, S137, M232, 252, 278, 284
Maple syrup   C46, S138, M232, 253, 278, 286
Maple syrup (cane and maple)   M241, 294
Maraschino cherries, bottled   C50, F83, Fi115
Marble cake, with white frosting   P23
Margarine   P32, F63, S130, M239, 276, 294
Margarine (from corn oil), tub   V220
Margarine (from corn, soybean, and cotton-seed oils), stick   V220
Margarine (from safflower and soybean oils) V220
Margarine (from sunflower and palm oils), stick   V221
Margarine, salted   V154

Margarine, two thirds animal fat, one third vegetable fat   Ch97
Marmalade, citrus   F83, Fi114, M257, 294
Marmalade (lemon or orange)   S137, V181, 205, 213, M237
Marmalade plums   V197
Marshmallow cookies   P24, F70
Marshmallows   P28, F83
Mashed potatoes, dehydrated, flakes without milk   Fi115, S134, V162, 177, 195, 214, 215, M237, 261, 272
Mashed potatoes, from flakes   M283
Mashed potatoes, frozen   F77, S132, V195, 215, M238, 257, 272
Mashed potatoes, frozen, heated   Fi114, M285
Mashed potatoes, made from flakes   F76
Mashed potatoes, made from granules F76
Mashed potatoes, made from granules, pre-pared with milk   F77
Mashed potatoes, made with milk and table fat   P27, F75
Mashed potatoes, milk added   P27, Fi114, S132, V165, 174, 194, 211, M238, 259, 271, 283
Mayonnaise   P30, F63, Fi119, S131, V160, 181, 195, 220, M240, 258, 274, 294
Mayonnaise salad dressing   Ch97
Mayonnaise salad dressing, low calorie F70
Meal (powder)   *See specific type*
Meat   *See specific type*
Meatloaf   P15, F70
Meatloaf TV dinner   P19
Melon   *See specific type*
Menhaden (Atlantic), canned   P14, F72
Milk *See also specific type*
Milk chocolate   V221, M262
Milk chocolate candy   Fi114
Milk (chocolate), made with skim   P25
Milk chocolate, plain   P20, C47, F65, S135, V160, 175, 185, 219, M231, 265
Milk chocolate, with almonds   P18, C47, V185
Milk chocolate, with peanuts   P16
Milk, human   P30
Milk, part skim   P23, F78
Millet, whole grain   C46, F77, Fi105
Mince pie   P26, F71
Minced ham   P16
Minestrone soup   P28, F79
Minestrone soup, canned, condensed V156
Miso (fermented soybean product)   P17, F75, Fi105, S129, V164, 175, 190, M234, 251, 264, 282
Mission olives, large   F68

P=Protein, **C**=Carbohydrates, **F**=Fat, **Ch**=Cholesterol, **Fi**=Fiber, **S**=Sodium, **V**=Vitamins, **M**=Minerals

Mixed cereal (baby food), precooked or dry **V**184

Mixed fruits *See specific type*

Mixed vegetables (baby food)   **P**29, **F**83

Mixed vegetables (carrots, corn, peas, green snap beans, and lima   **P**25, **F**83, **Fi**108, **S**136, **V**153, 172, 212, **M**252, 270, 286

Mixed vegetables, frozen, boiled   **C**52, **V**192

Molasses (blackstrap)   **V**201

Molasses cookies   **P**21, **F**72

Molasses, medium   **C**47

Mortadella   **F**67

Muffins *See also specific type*

Muffins, from mix   **P**20, **V**219

Muffins, homemade from unenriched flour **M**257

Muffins (plain), homemade   **P**19, **C**48, **Ch**97, **Fi**117, **S**131, **V**162, **M**232, 266, 290

Muffins (plain), homemade from enriched flour   **V**171, 186, 219

Muffins (plain), homemade from unenriched flour   **V**177, 188

Mung bean sprouts   **M**252

Mung bean sprouts, boiled   **P**25, **Fi**111, **S**139, **V**165, 173, 190, 213, **M**240, 254, 271, 288

Mung bean sprouts, raw   **P**24, **Fi**111, **S**139, **V**165, 172, 189, 209, **M**240, 270, 285

Mushrooms, canned   **P**28, **F**83, **Fi**112, **S**132, **V**167, 181, 186, 203, 217, **M**245, 258, 270, 286

Mushrooms, raw   **P**26, **C**54, **Fi**110, **S**137, **V**167, 172, 184, 201, 215, 222, **M**245, 255, 267, 281

Mussels (pacific), canned   **P**14, **F**76

Mustard *See specific type*

Mustard greens, boiled   **P**27, **F**83, **Fi**109, **S**137, **V**153, 174, 188, 207, **M**232, 250, 273, 285

Mustard greens, frozen, boiled   **Fi**109, **S**138, **V**153, 179, 190, 209, **M**252, 272, 288

Mustard greens, raw   **Fi**108, **S**137, **V**153, 172, 186, 206, **M**231, 248, 271, 281

Mustard spinach (tendergreen), boiled **P**28, **V**152, 207

Mustard spinach (tendergreen), raw   **F**83, **V**152, 206

N

Natto (fermented soybean product)   **F**73, **V**174, 184, **M**233, 247, 266, 284

Nectar *See specific type*

Nectarines, raw   **P**32, **Fi**114, **S**139, **V**155, 204, 211, **M**258, 274, 283

New England clam chowder, frozen, made with milk   **P**24, **F**75

New England clam chowder, frozen, made with water   **P**28, **F**76

New Zealand spinach, boiled   **P**28, **F**83, **S**135, **V**179, 190, 211, **M**235, 252, 274, 281

New Zealand spinach, raw   **Fi**111, **S**134, **V**177, 187, 208, **M**235, 249, 272, 280

Nonfat dry milk, instant   **Ch**98

Noodles *See also specific type*

Noodles, cooked   **F**78

Nougats and caramels (chocolate-coated) **P**24

Nougats (chocolate-coated)   **F**70

Nuts *See specific type*

O

Oat and wheat cereal, cooked   **P**26, **F**83, **Fi**113, **V**173, **M**243, 256, 269

Oat and wheat cereals   **S**134

Oat cereal, sugar coated   **F**76

Oat cereal, with toasted wheat germ and soy   **S**132

Oat cereal, with toasted wheat germ and soy grits, cooked   **F**78, **V**175, 196, **M**253, 268, 294

Oat flakes (cereal), maple flavored   **F**83

Oat flakes (cereal), maple flavored, cooked **P**26

Oat granules (cereal), maple flavored   **F**83

Oat oil   **V**220

Oatmeal   **V**220

Oatmeal (baby food)   **P**15, **C**46, **F**74, **Fi**107, **S**131, **M**230, 263, 281

Oatmeal (baby food), precooked or dry **V**184

Oatmeal (cereal) with wheat germ and soy grits   **P**25

Oatmeal cookies, with raisins   **P**21, **F**69

Oatmeal or rolled oats   **F**80

Oats and wheat (cereal)   **P**15

Oats (cereal), maple flavored   **P**15

Oats with toasted wheat germ and soy (cereal), cooked   **Fi**112

Ocean perch (Atlantic)   **P**14

Ocean perch (Atlantic), breaded, frozen fried **P**14

Ocean perch (Atlantic), fried   **S**134, **V**172, 190, **M**237, 252, 283

Ocean perch, breaded, frozen, fried, reheated   **F**68

Ocean perch, fried   **F**70

Oils   **P**32, *See also specific type*

Oils, salad or cooking   **C**55

Okra, boiled   **P**28, **F**83, **Fi**109, **S**141, **V**158, 209, **M**233, 272, 287

Okra, cuts and pods, frozen, boiled   **Fi**109, **S**141, **V**158, 171, 187, 211, **M**233, 258, 272, 287

Okra, raw   **C**53, **M**257

Olive oil   **V**221

Olives *See also specific type*

Olives, ripe   **V**205

Olives, ripe, extra large   **F**70

Omelets   **F**70, **S**133, **V**155, **M**234, 251, 266, 289

Omelets, with milk and fat   **Ch**96

P=Protein, C=Carbohydrates, F=Fat, Ch=Cholesterol, Fi=Fiber, S=Sodium, V=Vitamins, M=Minerals

---

P=Protein, **C**=Carbohydrates, **F**=Fat, **Ch**=Cholesterol, **Fi**=Fiber, **S**=Sodium, **V**=Vitamins, **M**=Minerals

P=Protein, C=Carbohydrates, F=Fat, Ch=Cholesterol, Fi=Fiber, S=Sodium, V=Vitamins, M=Minerals

Rice cereal, added nutrients, cooked   S134, M256

Rice cereal (baby food)   P21, Fi113, S131, V168, 184, M230, 263, 285

Rice cereal, cooked   Fi119, V175, 199, 202, M246, 294

Rice cereal, with casein   P10, V168, 207

Rice cereal, with wheat gluten   P13, V183

Rice flakes (cereal)   P22, F85, S130, V169, 194, 201, M238, 251, 267, 286

Rice germ oil   V220

Rice polish   V168, M246, 280

Rice pudding, with raisins   P24, C50, F76, Ch98, Fi118, S135, V162, 179, 188, 219, M233, 260, 268, 286

Rice, with casein   C47, F85

Rockfish, oven steamed   F77, V176, 189, M281

Roe, canned   V217

Roe (cod and shad), baked or broiled   P13, F77, S135, M242, 249, 264, 290

Roe (cod, haddock and herring), canned   M253, 264

Rolls and buns   *See also specific type*

Rolls and buns, homemade   Fi116, S133, V163, 170, 185, 219, M236, 249, 268, 291

Rolls and buns, plain, commercial   Fi116, S131, V169, 187, M234, 250, 269, 292

Rolls, from mix   P18, C47, F75, Fi116, S132, V167, 176, 189, 219, M235, 257, 268, 290

Rolls, homemade   P19, C47, F73

Romaine lettuce   C54

Root beer soda   C52

Roots   *See specific type*

Roquefort cheese   V202, 205

Rose apples, raw   P32, V181, 196

Russian salad dressing   M257

Russian salad dressing, regular   P29, C52, F64, Fi115, S130, V157, 176, 194, M240, 273, 288

Rutabagas, boiled   P32, F85, S139, V157, 175, 190, 202, 209, M235, 261, 273, 287

Rutabagas, raw   Fi108, S139, V157, 175, 192, 207, M234, 260, 272, 284

Rutabagas, raw, boiled   Fi108

Rye bread (American)   P17, 18, C47, F79, 80, Fi114, S131, V170, 192, 202, M234, 251, 266, 289

Rye bread, salt-rising   P19

Rye flour   V200

Rye flour, dark   P15, C46, V221

Rye flour, light   P18, C45, V173, 222

Rye flour, medium   P17, C46, Fi109, V169, 189, M249, 265, 285

Rye oil   V220

Rye wafers, whole grain   P16, C45, F79, Fi106, S130, V169, M235, 247, 264, 280

Rye, whole grain   P17, C46, F78, V169, 186, 221, M247, 264, 281

S

Safflower seed kernels   F64

Safflower seed meal, partially defatted   P10, C49, F73, Fi104, V168, 185, M234, 263

Safflower seed oil, crude   V220

Safflower seed oil, hydrogenated   V221

Safflower seed oil, refined   V220

Salad   *See specific type*

Salad dressing   *See also specific type*

Salad dressing (blue cheese and Roquefort cheese), low calorie   Fi118

Salad dressing (blue cheese and Roquefort cheese), regular   V182, M262

Salad dressing, cooked   V158, 219

Salad greens   *See specific type*

Salami   V222

Salami, cooked   P14, C54, F66, V170, 186, M243, 249, 265

Salami, dry   P12, F65, V201

Salmon (Atlantic), canned   C55, F71

Salmon, broiled or baked   V161, 171, 193, M264, 281

Salmon (Chinook), canned   P13, F69

Salmon (chum), canned   F75

Salmon (Coho), canned   P13

Salmon, cooked, broiled, or baked   P11, F73, S135

Salmon rice loaf   F75

Salmon (sockeye), canned   P13, V160

Salt   C55, S129, M231, 262, 294

Salt rising bread, toasted   F77

Salt sticks (Vienna bread)   C45, F76

Saltine crackers   P18, C46, F71, Fi114, V202, M239, 253

Sapotes (marmalade plums)   F85

Sapotes (marmalade plums), raw   V159

Sardines (Atlantic), canned in oil   P13, S131, V161, 181, 188, 201, 205, M231, 248, 264, 280

Sardines (Atlantic), canned in oil, drained solids   F71

Sardines (Atlantic), canned in oil, solids and liquid   F67

Sardines, canned in oil   Ch96

Sardines (Pacific), canned in brine   F71

Sardines (Pacific), canned in brine or mustard   P14

Sardines (Pacific), canned in tomato sauce   P14, F71, S132, V165, 182, 185, 201, M230, 247, 264, 282

Sauces   *See specific type*

Sauerkraut, canned   P30, F85, Fi111, S130, V164, 179, 195, 201, 211, M237, 258, 276

P=Protein, C=Carbohydrates, F=Fat, Ch=Cholesterol, Fi=Fiber, S=Sodium, V=Vitamins, M=Minerals

P=Protein, C=Carbohydrates, F=Fat, Ch=Cholesterol, Fi=Fiber, S=Sodium, V=Vitamins, M=Minerals

P=Protein, C=Carbohydrates, F=Fat, Ch=Cholesterol, Fi=Fiber, S=Sodium, V=Vitamins, M=Minerals

Vegetable beef soup, canned, condensed **F**85

Vegetable juice cocktail, canned **P**33, **F**86, **Fi**116, **V**156, 212, **M**243, 275

Vegetable soup (baby food) **F**86

Vegetable soup, with beef broth, canned **F**86

Vegetable with beef soup, canned, condensed **V**155

Vegetable with beef soup, frozen **F**79

Vegetables *See also specific type*

Vegetables and bacon with cereal (baby food) **P**29, **F**77

Vegetables and beef and cereal (baby food) **F**78

Vegetables and beef with cereal **P**26

Vegetables and chicken with cereal (baby food) **P**28, **F**79, **V**156

Vegetables and ham, with cereal **F**78

Vegetables and ham with cereal (baby food) **P**26, **V**156

Vegetables and lamb with cereal (baby food) **P**27, **V**154

Vegetables and liver with cereal (baby food) **P**25, **F**86

Vegetables and turkey with cereal (baby food) **P**28, **F**86

Vegetables, liver and bacon with cereal (baby food) **P**27, **F**78

Vegetables with beef broth **P**30

Vegetables, with peanuts and soya, canned **P**17

Vegetables, with wheat and soy protein **F**74

Vegetables, with wheat and soy protein, canned **P**15

Vegetables, with wheat protein and nuts, canned **P**13

Vegetables, with wheat protein, canned **F**86

Vegetarian vegetable soup, canned, condensed **F**86, **V**154, 155

Vienna sausage, canned **P**16, **C**56, **F**68, **V**202

Vinegar, cider **P**33

W

Waffles *See also specific type*

Waffles, from mix **Fi**118

Waffles, from mix, made with eggs and milk **C**49, **Ch**97

Waffles, from mix, made with water **P**23, **C**48

Waffles, frozen **P**20, **C**48, **S**130

Waffles, homemade **P**18, **C**49, **Fi**118, **S**131, **V**159, 171, 186, 220, **M**251

Walnuts **P**15, **F**63, **Fi**106, **S**141, **V**165, 169, 189, 200, 217, **M**233, 248, 264, 281

Walnuts (English), shelled, raw **V**221

Water chestnuts, raw **P**29, **C**51, **Fi**110, **M**257

Watercress, leaves and stems, raw **P**27, **Fi**111, **S**136, **V**153, 174, 188, 201, 206, **M**231, 251, 271, 283

Watermelon **V**202

Watermelon, raw **P**33, **C**53, **Fi**116, **S**144, **V**157, 179, 197, 213, **M**245, 258, 278, 291

Weakfish, broiled **P**12, **C**56, **S**131, **V**173, 191

Welsh onions **P**28, **F**86

Welsh rarebit **Ch**98, **S**132, **V**178, 186, **M**266, 289

Wheat and malted barley flakes (cereal) **P**18, **F**79

Wheat and malted barley (hot cereal) **P**28

Wheat bran (cereal) **V**200

Wheat bran, crude **P**15, **C**46, **F**75, **Fi**104, **S**138, **V**168, 185, **M**232, 246, 263, 279

Wheat cereal, cooked **F**86

Wheat crackers **V**221

Wheat flakes (cereal) **P**17, **C**45, **F**78, **Fi**107, **S**129, **V**169, 200, 222, **M**247, 265

Wheat flakes (cereal), added nutrients **V**188, **M**236

Wheat flour **F**79

Wheat flour, all purpose **P**17

Wheat flour, enriched **Fi**116, **V**185

Wheat flour, from straight, hard wheat **C**46

Wheat flour, self rising, enriched **S**129, **M**231, 264

Wheat flour, soft, all purpose **F**80

Wheat flour, unenriched **V**194

Wheat flour, 45% gluten, 55% patent **P**10

Wheat germ **M**280

Wheat germ, raw **P**12, **C**48, **F**71, **Fi**105, **S**140, **V**168, 220, **M**234, 247, 263

Wheat germ, toasted **P**11, **F**71, **Fi**106, **V**162, 168, 200, 212, **M**236, 247, 263, 279

Wheat, whole grain, hard red spring **M**248

Wheat, whole grain, hard red spring or winter **V**189

Wheat, whole grain, hard red winter **M**248

Wheat, whole grain, soft red winter **V**190, **M**248

Wheat, whole grain, white **V**189, **M**248

Whey **V**204

Whey, dried **F**80, **V**164, 169, 183, 205, **M**230, 252, 264

Whey, fluid **F**86

White beans, boiled **F**86

White beans, dry or canned **V**217

White beans, with pork and sweet sauce **F**75

White beans, with pork and tomato sauce **F**77

White bread, enriched, made with 1% - 2% nonfat dry milk **V**170, 187

White bread, made with 1% - 2% nonfat dry milk **C**47, **Fi**117, **S**131, **V**173, 204, 222, **M**234, 269, 292

P=Protein, **C**=Carbohydrates, **F**=Fat, **Ch**=Cholesterol, **Fi**=Fiber, **S**=Sodium, **V**=Vitamins, **M**=Minerals